Handbook of Headache

Handbook of Headache

2nd Edition

Randolph W. Evans, M.D.

Chief of Neurology
Park Plaza Hospital

Clinical Associate Professor
Department of Neurology
University of Texas Medical School at Houston

Clinical Associate Professor
Department of Family and Community Medicine
Baylor College of Medicine
Houston, Texas

Ninan T. Mathew, M.D., F.R.C.P. (C).

Director
Houston Headache Clinic

Clinical Professor
Department of Neurology
University of Texas Medical School
Houston, Texas

Former President
American Headache Society

Past President
International Headache Society

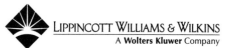

LIPPINCOTT WILLIAMS & WILKINS
A **Wolters Kluwer** Company

Philadelphia • Baltimore • New York • London
Buenos Aires • Hong Kong • Sydney • Tokyo

Acquisitions Editor: Anne M. Sydor
Developmental Editor: Sarah M. Granlund
Production Manager: Bridgett Dougherty
Senior Manufacturing Manager: Ben Rivera
Marketing Manager: Adam Glazer
Production Services: Nesbitt Graphics, Inc.
Printer: R.R. Donnelley

Library of Congress Cataloging-in-Publication Data

Evans, Randolph W.
Handbook of headache / Randolph W. Evans, Ninan T. Mathew.-- 2nd ed.
    p. ; cm.
  Includes bibliographical references and index.
  ISBN 0-7817-5223-X
  1. Headache--Handbooks, manuals, etc. I. Mathew, Ninan T. II. Title.
  [DNLM: 1. Headache--diagnosis--Handbooks. 2. Headache--therapy--Handbooks. 3. Headache Disorders--Handbooks. WL 39 H2355 2005]
RB128.H346 2005
616.8'491--dc22   2004023514

Care has been taken to confirm the accuracy of the information presented and to describe generally accepted practices. However, the authors, editors, and publisher are not responsible for errors or omissions or for any consequences from application of the information in this book and make no warranty, expressed or implied, with respect to the currency, completeness, or accuracy of the contents of the publication. Application of this information in a particular situation remains the professional responsibility of the practitioner.

The authors, editors, and publisher have exerted every effort to ensure that drug selection and dosage set forth in this text are in accordance with current recommendations and practice at the time of publication. However, in view of ongoing research, changes in government regulations, and the constant flow of information relating to drug therapy and drug reactions, the reader is urged to check the package insert for each drug for any change in indications and dosage and for added warnings and precautions. This is particularly important when the recommended agent is a new or infrequently employed drug.

Some drugs and medical devices presented in this publication have Food and Drug Administration (FDA) clearance for limited use in restricted research settings. It is the responsibility of the health care provider to ascertain the FDA status of each drug or device planned for use in their clinical practice.

10 9 8 7 6 5 4 3 2 1

Contents

Preface to the First Edition

Ninety percent of men and 95% of women have unprovoked headaches annually. Twenty-three million people in the United States have severe migraine headaches. The incidence of post-traumatic headaches is over 1 million persons per year. Furthermore, 9% of adults see physicians annually for headaches, making headaches one of the most common complaints of patients seeing primary care physicians.

Unfortunately, headache education during medical school and residency is frequently inadequate, and many physicians are less than enthusiastic about this topic. After reading this succinct volume, however, the primary care physician will be able to successfully diagnose and manage the great majority of headache patients. This book may also be of interest to neurologists since many uncommon topics are also examined.

The book begins with a general diagnostic approach to headaches. Then migraine, tension-type, chronic daily, cluster, first or worst, and posttraumatic headaches are reviewed. Chapters follow on headaches affecting various demographic groups including children and adolescents, women, and persons over the age of 50. Subsequent chapters cover short lasting head pains, vascular disorders, neoplasms, high and low pressure, HEENT disorders, other secondary headaches, and associated disorders. The final chapters feature interactive cases in "What's my Headache," and question and answer reviews in "The Headache Quiz." The book concludes with patient resources, educational materials, and a summary of alternative treatments.

With new diagnostic approaches and treatments becoming available, this is an exciting time for physicians and headache sufferers. We hope that, after you complete this book, you will be more confident and even enthusiastic in the evaluation and management of your patients with headaches.

We thank our editor at Lippincott Williams & Wilkins, Anne M. Sydor, Ph.D., for her encouragement and advice and the production team for their excellent work. Dr. Evans is indebted to his mentors in headache and neurology, K.M.A. Welch and Stanley H. Appel. He also appreciates the love and support of his wife, Marilyn, and children, Elliott, Rochelle, and Jonathan. Dr. Mathew appreciates the loving understanding of his wife, Sushila, whose support and encouragement have sustained him throughout his professional career. Dr. Mathew also appreciates the hard work of his transcriptionist, Ofelia F. Phillips, his office manager, Debbie Kennedy, and his study coordinator, Paula Gentry.

Randolph W. Evans, M.D.
Ninan T. Mathew, M.D.
October, 1999

Preface to the Second Edition

We have been delighted with the enthusiastic reception for the first edition. Underscoring the growing worldwide interest in headaches, translations are available in Chinese (Science Press, 2002) and French (Edisem, 2003). This second edition updates advances made in the last 5 years. We hope that we provide a succinct review of the specialty of headache with material that will be of interest to primary care physicians, neurologists, headache specialists, and any other physician or health professional who treats patients with headaches.

In the first chapter on diagnosis of headaches, there is a new section on medicolegal aspects. Although facets of migraine are covered in numerous chapters throughout the book, the principle migraine chapter is now expanded into three chapters, "Migraine," "Treatment of Acute Attacks of Migraine," and "Preventive Treatment of Migraine." New treatments covered include topirimate, almotriptan, frovatriptan, eletriptan, and botulinum toxin. All the chapters have been updated and revised. The new *International Classification of Headache Disorders,* 2nd edition (2004) of the International Headache Society is used.

We again thank our editor at Lippincott Williams & Wilkins, Anne M. Sydor, PhD, for her encouragement and advice. We also thank our developmental editor, Sarah Granlund, our production manager, Bridgett Dougherty, and our project manager, Maria McColligan, for their excellent work.

Randolph W. Evans, MD
Ninan T. Mathew, MD
Houston, Texas
October, 2004

About the Authors

Randolph W. Evans, M.D., is chief of Neurology at Park Plaza Hospital, and Clinical Associate Professor in both the Department of Neurology, University of Texas Medical School at Houston and the Department of Family and Community Medicine, Baylor College of Medicine. After receiving his B.A. from Rice University in 1974 and M.D. from Baylor College in 1978, Dr. Evans completed his internship and residency in Neurology at Baylor College of Medicine in 1982. He is board certified in Neurology and a fellow of the American Academy of Neurology and the American Headache Society. Dr. Evans is the senior editor of *Prognosis of Neurological Disorders* (2nd edition 2000); editor of *Neurology and Trauma* (2nd edition 2005); *Diagnostic Testing in Neurology* (1999); and Saunders Manual of Neurological Practice (2003). He is the expert opinion section editor for *Headache*. Dr. Evans is also an associate editor for *Medlink Neurology;* the editor of six issues of *Neurologic Clinics;* and an issue each of *Seminars in Neurology, Medical Clinics of North America,* and *Primary Care.* He is also the author of over 130 journal publications and 68 book chapters.

Ninan T. Mathew, M.D., is Director of the Houston Headache Clinic and Clinical Professor in the Department of Neurology, University of Texas Medical School at Houston. He is a past president of the International Headache Society, and past-chairman of the Headache and Pain Section of the American Academy of Neurology. He is also the former president of the American Headache Society. He is a reviewer for *Neurology, Archives of Neurology, Cephalalgia, Headache,* and *Lancet.* Dr. Mathew has published more than 180 peer-reviewed articles and edited two volumes of *Neurologic Clinics* and one issue of *Medical Clinics of North America* on headache and a monograph on cluster headaches.

Handbook of Headache

Diagnosis of Headaches and Medicolegal Aspects

Randolph W. Evans

Headaches are a nearly universal experience, with a 1-year period prevalence of 90% and a lifetime prevalence of 99%. Twenty-eighty million Americans have migraines per year. Worldwide, an estimated 600 million persons suffer migraines yearly. Five percent of women and 2.8% of men have headaches 180 days or more per year. It is not surprising that headaches are one of the most common complaints seen by primary care physicians. Headache is the chief complaint of 20% of the patients seen by the general neurologist. During a 1-year period in the United States, 9% of adults see physicians for headaches and 83% self-medicate. Television advertisements touting headache treatment with triptans, Tylenol, Motrin, and Excedrin Migraine are common.

The differential diagnosis of headaches is one of the longest in medicine, with more than 300 different types and causes (Table 1-1). The physician must diagnose headaches as precisely as possible. Although most headaches are of benign and still poorly understood origin, some secondary headaches can have serious and sometimes life-threatening causes. As more specific medications become available, such as selective serotonin ($5\text{-}HT_1$) receptor agonists for migraine and cluster headaches or topiramate for prophylaxis of migraine, accurate diagnosis is needed to choose the proper pharmacological treatment.

For many of the headaches described in this book, the criteria of the 2004 International Headache Society, 2nd edition (ICHD-II), are presented (1). Since their introduction in 1988, the criteria have become the worldwide standard for classification. Primary headaches, where there is no other underlying cause, include migraine, tension type, cluster, and miscellaneous headaches (such as primary exertional headaches). There are a large number of secondary headaches (Table 1-1), and the headaches are classified based on their causes. A careful history, examination, and, in some cases, diagnostic testing usually permits headaches to be diagnosed correctly. However, sometimes a precise diagnosis may be impossible. For example, some benign headaches have both migraine- and tension-type features. Patients with chronic daily headaches may be difficult to classify.

PAIN-SENSITIVE STRUCTURES

Similar headaches can have different causes because there are a limited number of pain-sensitive structures (Table 1-2). Paradoxically, although all pain is felt in the brain, the brain parenchyma itself is not pain sensitive. The arachnoid, ependyma, and dura (except portions near vessels) are also not sensitive to pain. However, cranial nerves V, VII, IX, and X; the circle of Willis and proximal continuations; meningeal arteries; large veins in the

Migraine

Tension-type headache

Cluster headache and other trigeminal autonomic cephalalgias

Other primary headaches

Primary stabbing, cough, exertional, thunderclap, and associated with sexual activity; hypnic; hemicrania continua; new daily persistent

Headache attributed to head and/or neck trauma

Headache attributed to cranial or cervical vascular disorder
Ischemic stroke or transient ischemic attack, non-traumatic intracranial

Hemorrhage, unruptured vascular malformation, arteritis, carotid or carotid artery pain, cerebral venous thrombosis, other vascular disorders

Headache attributed to non-vascular intracranial disorder
High and low cerebrospinal fluid pressure, non-infectious inflammatory disease, intracranial neoplasm, intrathecal injection, epileptic seizure, Chiari malformation type I, HaNDL

Headache attributed to a substance or its withdrawal
Acute substance use or exposure, medication-overuse headache, chronic medication, substance withdrawal

Headache attributed to infection
Intracranial, systemic, HIV/AIDS, chronic post-infection

Headache attributed to disorder of homeostasis
Hypoxia and/or hypercapnia, dialysis, arterial hypertension, hypothyroidism, fasting, cardiac cephalalgia

Headache or facial pain attributed to disorder of cranium, neck, eyes, ears, nose, sinuses, teeth, mouth, or other facial or cranial structures

Headache attributed to psychiatric disorder
Somatisation disorder, psychotic disorder

Cranial neuralgias and central causes of facial pain
Neuralgias: trigeminal, glossopharyngeal, nervus intermedius, superior laryngeal, nasociliary, supraorbital, other terminal branch, and occipital; neck-tongue syndrome; external compression and cold-stimulus headache; caused by compression, irritation or distortion of cranial nerves or upper cervical roots by structural lesions; optic neuritis; ocular diabetic neuropathy; herpes zoster; Tolosa-Hunt; ophthalmoplegic "migraine;" central causes of facial pain

Source: Excerpted from Headache Classification Subcommittee of the International Headache Society. *The international classification of headache disorders,* 2nd ed. *Cephalalgia* 2004;24[Suppl 1]:1–232.

brain and dura; and structures external to the skull (including scalp and neck muscles, cutaneous nerves and skin, the mucosa of paranasal sinuses, teeth, cervical nerves and roots, and the external carotid arteries and branches) are sensitive to pain.

Table 1-2. Pain-sensitive structures that can cause headaches

Not the brain parenchyma

Transmitted through the trigeminal nerve and upper cervical segments

Intracranial structures

Dura near vessels

Cranial nerves V, VII, IX, X

Circle of Willis and proximal continuations

Meningeal arteries

Large veins in the brain and dura external to the skull

Scalp and neck muscles

Cervical nerves and roots

Cutaneous nerves and skin

Mucosa of the paranasal sinuses

Teeth

External carotid arteries and branches

In some cases, the location and source of the pain may be the same (e.g., cheek or forehead pain from maxillary or frontal sinusitis). However, because of referral patterns, the location of the pain may not be the same as the source. For example, supratentorial structures are innervated by the ophthalmical division of the trigeminal nerve, and the infratentorial or posterior fossa structures are supplied by C_2 and C_3. Thus a cerebellar hemisphere lesion generally refers pain posteriorly and an occipital lobe lesion refers pain anteriorly.

In addition, the caudal nucleus of the trigeminal nerve, which is located from the midpons to the third cervical segment, also receives painful messages from the upper cervical roots as well as the trigeminal nerve. Thus pain from the upper cervical spine or posterior fossa can also be referred to the front of the head.

THE HEADACHE HISTORY

Most of the time, the headache history is essential to establishing the diagnosis (2–5). In the absence of an adequate headache history, unnecessary scans of the brain may be obtained or, alternatively, a necessary scan may not be obtained. The key elements of the headache history are the following: temporal profile, headache features, associated symptoms and signs, aggravating or precipitating factors, relieving factors, evaluation and treatment history, psychosocial history, family history, and a complete medical and surgical history (Table 1-3). Table 1-4 gives examples of questions to ask to gather the key elements.

Unfortunately for the busy clinician, some patients have more than one type of headache. The presence of more than one type may not be apparent at first. Both open-ended ("What are your headaches like?") and close-ended ("Do you have nausea with the headache?") approaches are necessary. Without specific prodding, some patients will not remember to tell you about

Table 1-3. Elements of the headache history

Temporal profile
    Age of onset
    Time to maximum intensity
    Frequency
    Time of day
    Duration
    Recurrence

Headache features
    Location
    Quality of pain
    Severity of pain

Associated symptoms and signs
    Before headache
    During headache
    After headache

Aggravating or precipitating factors
    Trauma
    Medical conditions
    Triggers
    Trigger zones
    Activity
    Pharmacological

Relieving factors
    Nonpharmacological
    Pharmacological

Evaluation and treatment history
    Physicians and other health care providers

Psychosocial history
    Substance use
    Occupational and personal life

Psychological history
    Sleep history
    Impact of headache

Patient's own diagnosis

Family history

Complete medical and surgical history

their "sinus" or perimenstrual headaches or those they had when they were younger that required bed rest. Other patients will need to be told the term *headache* includes any type and quality of head and facial pain. A detailed account of each type is important. In some cases, it is helpful to ask about a history of mild headaches and bad headaches. Some patients cannot clearly remember or articulate features of the headache and say something like, "It's just a headache, Doc."

Some migraineurs will say no when asked whether light or noise bothers them during a headache. But if you then inquire about their behavior during a headache, you may get different information. You may discover that, if possible, they prefer to lie

Table 1-4.   Helpful questions to ask for the headache history

Do you have different types of headaches or just one?

Where does the headache hurt?

When did you first start having these headaches?

What were you doing when the headache started?

How long before the headache is of maximal intensity?

How long does the headache last?

Does the headache recur?

How often do they occur?

What is the pain like? Is it a pressure, throbbing, pounding, aching, or stabbing?

Is the pain mild, moderate, or severe?

On a scale of 1 to 10, with 10 the worst and 1 the least, how would you rate the headache?

Do you have trouble with your vision before or during the headache?

Do you have other symptoms (e.g., nausea, vomiting, light sensitivity, noise sensitivity, discomfort with eye movement) with the headache?

During a headache, do you prefer that loud music not be playing or that you not be in bright light?

Are signs (e.g., fever, ptosis, miosis) present?

Do you have triggers (e.g., menses, stress, foods, beverages, lack of sleep, oversleeping, strong odors, trigger zones) of your headaches?

Do activities (e.g., coughing, bending over, physical activity) make the headaches worse?

What (e.g., sleep, lying down in a quiet room) makes the headache better?

Do your headaches have any impact on your life?

Do you take over-the-counter medications, vitamins, or herbs for your headaches? If so, how much and how often? Do you drink caffeinated beverages and, if so, what types and how many?

What prescription drugs have you tried and with what effect?

What doctors have you seen in the past for your headaches?

What other treatments (e.g., acupuncture, chiropractic, biofeedback, stress management, massage) have you tried and with what success?

Have you been under much stress lately?

Have you been depressed?

Do you have any parents or siblings with a history of migraines or bad headaches?

---

down during a migraine attack and prefer a dark and quiet room. ("Would loud music bother you during a headache? Would bright light or sunlight bother you more than if you did not have a headache?") Patients may sometimes also deny nausea with migraine attacks but agree they feel like they want to vomit, or "barf," with a headache. When the patient has chronic headaches, sometimes it is necessary to provide a headache diary or have them record features of the headache(s) and then return for a later appointment. Examples follow of how the elements help you diagnose the headache.

Temporal Profile

Age of Onset

Migraines usually begin before the age of 40; it is uncommon for them to start after the age of 50. In contrast, temporal arteritis typically begins after age 50 and is rare earlier.

Time to Maximum Intensity

Thunderclap headaches, a severe headache with maximum intensity within 1 minute, can be caused by subarachnoid hemorrhage, carotid artery dissection, and migraine. Severe headaches can also have a gradual onset, such as migraine or viral meningitis.

Frequency

Primary headaches have widely variable frequency, ranging from a few migraines in a lifetime to cluster headaches that occur up to eight times each day.

Time of Day

Cluster headaches often occur during certain times of the day and may awaken the sufferer from sleep about the same time nightly. Although headaches that awaken people from sleep are usually benign (such as migraine, cluster, and hypnic), headaches can also result from brain tumors, meningitis, and subarachnoid hemorrhage. Tension-type headaches often occur in the afternoon.

Duration

Typical attack durations without treatment for primary headaches are as follows: migraine, 4 to 72 hours in adults; cluster headaches, 15 to 180 minutes; and tension-type headaches, 30 minutes to days. Trigeminal neuralgia is characterized by volleys of pain lasting a few seconds to less than 2 minutes.

Recurrence

Headache recurrence is an initial response to medication followed by recurrence within 24 hours. Recurrence includes a mild, moderate, or severe headache that completely goes away and then recurs or a moderate-severe headache that becomes mild and then becomes moderate-severe again. Recurrence can occur with any medication taken for migraine. For triptans, the recurrence rate varies from about 15% to 40% depending on the drug.

Headache Features

Location

Cluster headaches are always unilateral, whereas about 60% of migraines are unilateral. Trigeminal neuralgia typically occurs unilaterally and is found more often in the second or third trigeminal distributions than in the first. Headaches from brain tumors or subdural hematomas can be bilateral or unilateral.

Quality of Pain

In about 50% of cases, migraine pain is throbbing, pounding, or pulsatile. Tension-type headaches consist of a sensation of pressure, aching, tightness, or squeezing. Cluster headaches are described as boring or burning. Trigeminal neuralgia is often an electrical or stabbing pain. Headaches due to brain tumors can produce a variety of pains, ranging from a dull, steady ache to throbbing.

Severity of Pain

When asking patients about severity, it is very helpful to use a scale of 1 (minimal) to 10 (the worst), even though the ranking may be subjective. For example, a similar headache rated a 7 by a stoic person may be rated a 12 by dramatic patients who want to emphasize the inadequacy of the 10-point scale to express their distress. Migraine pain can vary from mild to severe, and it can change from attack to attack. Severity of pain does not equate with the presence of life-threatening causes. The vast majority of severe headaches are due to migraine or cluster types. However, the new onset of severe headache should be taken very seriously. In contrast, some patients with headaches due to brain tumors or subdural hematomas may report a mild headache similar to a tension type that can be relieved by simple analgesics.

Associated Symptoms and Signs

Before the Headache

About 25% of migraineurs have a prodrome in the hours to days before the headache. Complaints may include changes in the mental state (e.g., irritability, depression, euphoria), neurological symptoms (trouble with concentration; light, noise, and smell hypersensitivity), and general symptoms (diarrhea or constipation, thirst, sluggish feeling, food cravings, or neck stiffness). About 20% of migraines are those with an aura that generally develops over 5 to 20 minutes and lasts less than 60 minutes. The headache can begin before, during, or after the aura. The most common auras in descending frequency are visual, sensory, motor symptoms, and speech and language abnormalities.

Complaints prior to the headache are also very important in diagnosing other causes of headache. For example, low-grade fever and upper respiratory symptoms or diarrhea followed by headache are frequently present in viral meningitis.

During the Headache

Migraine is accompanied by nausea in 90%, vomiting in 30%, and light and noise sensitivity in 80%. These same symptoms are often present in headaches due to subarachnoid hemorrhage or meningitis. Ipsilateral conjunctival injection, tearing, and nasal congestion or drainage typically occur during cluster headaches. Ipsilateral ptosis and miosis are present in about 30% of cases.

After the Headache

After the headache resolves, many migraineurs complain of feeling tired and drained, with decreased mental acuity ("mashed potato brain"). Depression or euphoria is sometimes reported. In some systemic disorders, high fever and headache may be followed by other symptoms or signs.

Aggravating or Precipitating Factors

Trauma

Head and neck trauma are frequently followed by headaches. Headaches beginning after mild head injury are usually benign but raise concerns about a subdural or epidural hematoma present in up to 2%. Paradoxically, about 20% of those with milder degrees of head injuries or whiplash neck injuries may report headaches for months or years after the event, whereas those with more severe injuries may not have persistent headaches.

Medical Conditions

Other medical conditions may be associated with headaches. For example, although migraines often occur postpartum, preeclampsia and cortical venous thrombosis should be considered. During the second and third trimesters of pregnancy, migraines usually decrease in frequency. In 90% of cases, pseudotumor cerebri occurs in obese women. Paroxysmal hypertension with headaches suggests pheochromocytoma. New-onset headaches in someone who is HIV positive could be due to various causes such as cryptococcal meningitis. Headache in a person with a history of cancer (especially lung, breast, melanoma, colorectal, and hypernephroma) raises concern about metastatic disease. Persons with polycystic kidney disease have a 10% risk of having an intracranial saccular aneurysm.

Triggers

Eighty-five percent of migraineurs have one or more triggers. Various triggers include menstruation; stress or periods after stress; alcoholic beverages, especially red wine; foods such as chocolate, aged cheese, those containing monosodium glutamate, nitrates, and aspartame; environmental factors such as glare or flickering lights, loud noise, high altitude, heat and humidity, smoky rooms, and strong odors such as perfumes or cigarette smoke; and a missed meal or hunger. During periods of cluster headaches, alcohol can be a trigger. Tension-type headaches can be triggered by stress.

Trigger Zones

Stimulation of certain areas of the face or mucous membranes of the mouth may trigger pain in trigeminal neuralgia. Washing the face, shaving, eating, speaking, feeling a breeze or cold air, and brushing the teeth may cause an attack. Glossopharyngeal neuralgia may similarly be triggered by swallowing, chewing, talking, coughing, or yawning.

Activity and Posture

A variety of physical activities may trigger benign exertional headaches that can last 5 minutes to 24 hours, and such activities can also cause migraine. Coughing, sneezing, weight lifting, bending, stooping, or straining with a bowel movement can all trigger a bilateral headache of sudden onset that lasts less than 1 minute. Although usually benign, pathology such as chiari malformations and posterior fossa tumors should be excluded (see Chapter 13). When these activities trigger a first, or worst, severe headache (see Chapter 8) lasting hours, subarachnoid hemorrhage should be considered. Exertional headache or jaw pain can occasionally be the presentation of angina. Physical activity and coughing may exacerbate migraine, postlumbar puncture headaches, and those due to brain tumors with mass effect. A severe explosive headache occurring just before or during orgasm can be due to benign orgasmic cephalalgia or subarachnoid hemorrhage. Low-cerebrospinal-pressure headaches can be brought on with sitting or standing and can be relieved by assuming the supine position. Headaches due to raised intracranial pressure may be worse in the supine position. The pain of acute frontal, ethmoid, and sphenoid sinusitis is worse when lying supine and better with the head in the upright position. Pain due to acute maxillary sinusitis is less when supine and worse in the upright position.

Pharmacological

Frequent use of many prescription or over-the-counter drugs can cause rebound headaches in susceptible persons or cause preventive medications to be ineffective. A detailed history of the use of acetaminophen, aspirin, caffeine (in many prescription and over-the-counter medications and beverages), butalbital, narcotics, triptans, ergotamine, and benzodiazepines is important. Acute migraines can be triggered by the use of nitroglycerin and phosphodiesterase inhibitors for erectile dysfunction. Oral contraceptive use can occasionally increase the frequency of migraines.

Relieving Factors

Nonpharmacological Factors

Migraine headaches may resolve with sleep or improve with lying down in a dark, quiet room. Tension-type headaches may improve with relaxation for some people and with exercise in others. Massage or application of ice or heat may improve some headaches.

Pharmacological Factors

Responses to prescription and over-the-counter treatments, including dosages and side effects, should be obtained in detail. Unless specifically asked, some patients will not volunteer use of nonprescription medications. Also ask about the use of herbs such as feverfew and vitamins such as riboflavin.

Evaluation and Treatment History

Other Physicians and Health Care Providers

It is very important to obtain a history of prior evaluations and treatment by physicians and other health professionals, including psychologists, chiropractors, acupuncturists, and physical therapists. In some cases, obtaining the medical records is essential. This can prevent unnecessary repeat testing or not trying a medication previously taken at too low a dose or for an inadequate period of time. Some patients are reluctant or do not disclose this information for various reasons, including their wish to get an independent evaluation or to conceal a history of medication abuse.

Psychosocial History

Substance Use

Ask about use and quantities of tobacco, alcohol, caffeine, and illicit drugs. Rebound headaches commonly occur from drinking as little as two to three cups of coffee daily.

Occupational and Personal Life

A variety of stressors can trigger and contribute to migraine and tension-type headaches. Occupational exposure to toxins should also be considered. The auto mechanic you see in the winter complaining of a headband-pressure-type headache in the afternoon that occurs only at work may have a headache triggered by high levels of carbon monoxide. A school history should be obtained from students.

Psychological History

The treatment of many headaches requires addressing underlying or contributing psychological factors, such as depression, stress, and anxiety.

Sleep History

The obese patient who snores may have sleep apnea that causes headaches in the morning. Sleep deprivation due to restless legs syndrome may contribute to migraine and tension-type headaches. Patients with sleep disturbance and frequent headaches may benefit from sedating tricyclic antidepressants. Sleep difficulties may be due to depression or anxiety.

Impact of Headache

What effect do the headaches have on occupational and personal life? Is the patient missing a lot of work, school, or home activities? Are there many "not tonight, I have a headache" nights damaging a relationship?

Patient's Own Diagnosis

In many cases, patients come to see you with their own diagnosis. You may think you have done a great job of diagnosing migraine correctly. However, the patient or family members think they have a headache due to "sinus," an aneurysm, a brain tumor, or spinal misalignment because their headache education is based on sinus medication commercials, an Internet search, anecdotes (e.g., their cousin had an aneurysm or their aunt had a brain tumor causing headaches), and visits with chiropractors. Patients often go through their differential diagnoses by seeing the ear, nose, and throat physician; optometrist; and chiropractor first. After getting a septoplasty, a new refraction, and manipulation without improvement, they may finally see a neurologist and receive a diagnosis of migraine. Before giving your diagnosis, simply ask what the patient or family members think is the cause. Then explain the basis for your diagnosis and how theirs is unlikely. Inappropriate demands for magnetic resonance imaging (MRI) or computed tomography (CT) scans can be averted and the patient may not shop around for other opinions.

Family History

A history of migraine is also present in perhaps 80% of first-degree relatives. Because more than 60% of those with migraine are not aware of the diagnosis, you may need to ask about a history of bad or sick headaches or perimenstrual headaches in family members. I have diagnosed numerous parents who came for their child's consultation with previously undiagnosed migraine. Perhaps 10% of those with a history of first-degree relatives with intracranial saccular aneurysm(s) have the same disorder. A family history of neurofibromatosis should also raise concern.

Complete Medical and Surgical History

A complete medical and surgical history is crucial not only to consider systemic causes of headache but also to be aware of possible contraindications to medications such as bronchial asthma and nonsteroidal antiinflammatory drugs or beta-blockers or coronary artery disease and triptans. A history of medication allergies or sensitivities is mandatory. You know you are in trouble with some patients who have chronic headaches when their list of so-called drug allergies is longer than the Manhattan telephone directory or they are allergic to all pain pills (except Percodan). Ipsilateral frontotemporal headaches can begin 36 to 72 hours after carotid endarterectomy and can last for months. Postural headaches after a lumbar laminectomy can be due to a dural tear and a cerebrospinal fluid (CSF) leak. A complete review of systems is also important. Galactorrhea and amenorrhea may be present in a woman with a pituitary macroadenoma causing headaches. Progressive weight loss and headaches may be present in cases of metastatic cancer or AIDS. Syncope and headaches could be due to a colloid cyst of the third ventricle.

PHYSICAL EXAMINATION

Abnormal vital signs such as fever or significantly elevated blood pressure may indicate the cause of the headache. A focused general examination may be informative. An erythematous oropharynx and posterior cervical adenopathy in a teenager with new-onset headaches often indicates infectious mononucleosis as the cause. In cases of possible meningitis or subarachnoid hemorrhage, neck stiffness or meningeal signs should be checked for. Findings of cervical region or suboccipital trigger points can suggest a myofascial cause of headaches. Temporomandibular joint (TMJ) tenderness, clicking, or limitation of movement may be seen when the joint is the source of headaches. In headaches due to frontal or maxillary sinusitis, there is usually tenderness to palpation over the affected sinus and nasal drainage.

Examination of arteries may be helpful. In patients with new-onset headaches over the age of 50, the superficial temporal artery should be checked for the presence of induration or a reduced or absent pulse consistent with temporal arteritis. Examining the carotids for pulses and bruits is important in patients at risk for atherosclerotic disease. The carotid bulb may be tender in cases of carotidynia or carotid dissection.

Even the skin exam may be useful. The teenager with acne and papilledema may have pseudotumor cerebri caused by Accutane. The patient with progressive headache and multiple café au lait spots may have neurofibromatosis and an intracranial schwannoma or meningioma. A skin rash, headache, and fever may signify viral meningitis or meningococcal meningitis.

Every patient seen for headaches should have at the least a screening neurological examination, which can be performed within a few minutes (6). Although the exam is usually normal, you do not want to diagnose a patient with tension-type headaches when you might have discovered evidence of papilledema, a mild lateral rectus paresis, unequal pupils, a mild hemiparesis, or a Babinski sign if you had only bothered to perform a brief exam.

SUMMARY OF THE FEATURES OF HEADACHES

Table 1-5 summarizes the features of the three most common primary headaches; Table 1.6 lists those of some secondary headaches.

DIAGNOSTIC TESTING

Indications

For the vast majority of headaches, the diagnosis can be correctly made based on the detailed history and examination without any testing at all. The decision for testing should be made on a case-by-case basis with guidelines suggested in the next section (7–10). Other reasons that physicians order tests include the following: the quest for diagnostic certainty, faulty cognitive reasoning, the medical decision rule that holds it is better to impute disease than to risk overlooking it, busy practice conditions in which tests are ordered as a shortcut, patient expectations, financial incentives, professional peer pressure where recommendations for routine and esoteric tests are expected as a demonstration of competence, and medicolegal concerns. The attitudes and demands of patients and families and the practice of defensive medicine are especially important reasons. A baseball player batting 0.990 could be paid $50 million yearly. However, a physician who is paid $50 for an office visit but has a

Table 1-5. Features of some primary headaches

Feature	Migraine	Episodic tension-type	Episodic cluster
Epidemiology	18% women, 6% men	90% adults	0.4% for men
	4% children before puberty	35% children ages 3–11	0.08% for women
Women/men	3/1 after puberty, 1/1 before	5/4	1/5
Family history	80% of first-degree relatives	Frequent	Rare
Typical age at onset (years)	92% before age 40, 2% after age 50	20–40	20–40
Visual aura	In 20%	No	Occasional
Location	Unilateral, 60%; bilateral, 40%	Bilateral : unilateral	Unilateral
			Especially orbital, periorbital, frontotemporal
Quality	Pulsatile or throbbing in 85%	Pressure, aching, tight, squeezing	Boring, burning, or stabbing
Severity	Mild to severe	Mild to moderate	Severe

Onset to peak pain	Minutes to hours	Hours	Minutes
Duration	4–72 hours; May be less than 1 hour in children	Hours to days	15–180 minutes
Frequency	Rare to frequent	Rare to frequent	1–8 per day during clusters
Periodicity	Menstrual migraine	No	Yes; Average bouts 4–8 weeks; Average 1 or 2 bouts yearly
Associated features	Nausea in 90%, vomiting in 30%, light and noise sensitivity in 80%	Occasional nausea	Ipsilateral conjunctival injection, tearing, and nasal congestion or drainage; Ptosis and miosis in 30%
Triggers	Numerous	Stress, lack of sleep	Alcohol, nitrates
Behavior during headache	Still, quiet, tries to sleep	No change	Often paces
Awakens from sleep	Can occur	Rare	Frequently

similar "diagnosis average" and uses diagnostic testing appropriately could end up as a case on the civil docket.

Indicated testing may not be obtained in some circumstances. Under some managed care plans, physicians may not order appropriate testing because of factors such as at-risk capitation and fear of deselection. Even when they order tests, insurance company reviewers may inappropriately deny certification as "not reasonable and not necessary." For many patients, testing is not obtained because of underinsurance and lack of funds. (At this writing, 40 million Americans are without health insurance.)

Neuroimaging

A CT scan will detect most headaches caused by pathology (Table 1-7 shows causes of headaches that can be missed on a routine CT scan). The use of intravenous contrast may also reveal neoplasms and vascular malformations. The risk of reactions to intravenous contrast is as follows: mild, 10%; moderate, 1%; severe, .01%; and death, .002%. CT scan is superior to MRI for the demonstration of bony pathology, after acute head injury, and acute subarachnoid hemorrhage. However, numerous types of pathology can be missed on a routine CT scan.

MRI is superior to CT scan for evaluating headaches. The costs of CT scan and MRI are often about the same. In addition to general MRI contraindications, such as a pacemaker, about 8% of patients are claustrophobic, with about 2% to the point where they cannot tolerate the study. The yield of MRI may vary, depending on the field strength of the magnet, the use of paramagnetic contrast, the selection of acquisition sequences, and the use of magnetic resonance angiography and venography.

A routine MRI will demonstrate pathology of the paranasal sinuses, pituitary, posterior fossa, cortical veins (such as superior sagittal sinus thrombosis), and cervicomedullary junction (such as a Chiari malformation). In addition, MRI may find evidence of intracranial aneurysms, carotid dissection, infarcts, white matter abnormalities, congenital abnormalities, and neoplasms not seen on CT scan. Spiral CT scan and MRI angiography and venography are almost as sensitive as conventional cerebral angiography in the detection of aneurysms, arteriovenous malformations, arterial dissection, and venous thrombosis.

The yield of CT scan or MRI in patients with any headache and a normal neurological examination is about 2%. A report of the Quality Standards Subcommittee of the American Academy of Neurology (AAN) in 1994 stated, "At this time, there is insufficient evidence to define the role of CT and MRI in the evaluation of patient with headaches that are not consistent with migraine" (7). Table 1-8 provides reasons to consider neuroimaging for headaches. Table 1-9 gives reasons to consider neuroimaging for children with headaches.

Patients who meet IHS criteria for migraine rarely have abnormal neuroimaging findings to explain the headache. The same AAN report stated, "In adult patients with recurrent headaches defined as migraine, including those with visual aura, with no recent change in headache pattern, no history of seizures, and no other focal neurological signs or symptoms, the

Table 1-6. Features of some secondary headaches

Headache type	Epidemiology	Age of onset	Location	Quality and severity	Frequency	Associated features	Comments
Trigeminal neuralgia	4.3/100,000/ year ♀/♂ = 1.6/1	Usually over 40 If <40, consider multiple sclerosis	Unilateral 96% 2nd or 3rd > 1st trigeminal division	Stabbing Electrical bursts Burning Last few seconds < 2 minutes	Few to many/ day	Trigger zone present >90%	Usually due to vascular compression of V. Scan needed to exclude occasional tumor
Brain tumor	Persons/yr in US 24,000 primaries 170,000 with metastases	Any age	Often bifrontal Unilateral or bilateral Any location	Variable, can be pressure or throbbing Mild–severe	Occasional to daily. Usually progressive	Papilledema in 40% At time of diagnosis, headache present in 30% to 70%	Primaries in adults: lung, 64%; breast, 14%; unknown, 8%; melanoma, 4%; colorectal, 3%; hypernephroma, 2%
Pseudotumor cerebri	1/100,000/yr 90% are women 90% are obese	Mean of 30	Often bifronto–temporal but can occur in	Pulsatile Moderate to severe	Daily	Papilledema in 95% Transient visual	MRI scan preferred to better exclude cortical venous

						other locations and unilaterally	obscurations in 70% Intracranial noises in 60% VI nerve palsy in 20%	thrombosis and posterior fossa lesions
Subarachnoid hemorrhage	30,000/yr in US due to saccular aneurysm	Mean of 50	Usually bilateral Any location	Usually severe but can be mild and gradually increasing	Paroxysmal	findings,	Often with nausea, vomiting, stiff neck, focal may be syncope. Stiff neck absent in 36%	CT scan abnormal on first day 95%, third, 74%; 1 week, 50%. Lumbar puncture essential to diagnose
Temporal arteritis	Age >50, annual incidence 18/100,000 ♀/♂ = 3/1	Rare before 50 Mean age of 70	Variable Unilateral or bilateral Often temporo-frontal	Often throbbing May be sharp, dull, burning, or lancinating Mild–severe	Intermittent to continuous		50% have PMR Jaw claudication in 38% 50% have pulse or tender STA	ESR within normal limits (WNL) in up to 36% CRP usually elevated STA biopsy false negative up to 44%

continued

Table 1-6. *Continued*

Headache type	Epidemiology	Age of onset	Location	Quality and severity	Frequency	Associated features	Comments
Acute paranasal sinusitis	More common in children (in whom frontal and sphenoid sinusitis are rare) than in adults	Any age	Frontal—forehead, maxillary—cheek, ethmoid—between eyes, sphenoid—variable	Dull, aching Can be severe	Acute defined as lasting from 1 day to 3 weeks	Fever in about 50%. Nasal congestion and purulent nasal drainage usually present (less often in sphenoid)	Well visualized on routine MRI but not on routine CT scan of head. CT scan of the sinuses is the best study
Subdural hematoma	Occurs in 1% after mild head injury in chronic cases, up to 50% without history of head injury	Any age	Unilateral or bilateral	Mild—severe May be aching, dull, or throbbing	Paroxysmal to constant	50% with normal neurologic exam Alteration in consciousness and local findings may be present	MRI may detect occasional isodense subdural, which can be on missed CT scan

Table 1-7. Causes of headache that can be missed on routine CT scan of the head

Vascular disease
  Saccular aneurysms
  Arteriovenous malformations (especially posterior fossa)
  Subarachnoid hemorrhage
  Carotid or vertebral artery dissections
  Infarcts
  Cerebral venous thrombosis
  Vasculitis (white matter abnormalities)
  Subdural and epidural hematomas
Neoplastic disease
  Neoplasms (especially in the posterior fossa)
  Meningeal carcinomatosis
  Pituitary tumor and hemorrhage
Cervicomedullary lesions
  Chiari malformations
  Foramen magnum meningioma
Infections
  Paranasal sinusitis
  Meningoencephalitis
Cerebritis and brain abscess

Table 1-8. Reasons to consider neuroimaging for headaches

Temporal and headache features
  1. The "first or worst" headache
  2. Subacute headaches with increasing frequency or severity
  3. A progressive or new daily, persistent headache
  4. Chronic daily headache
  5. Headaches always on the same side
  6. Headaches not responding to treatment
Demographics
  7. New-onset headaches in patients who have cancer or who test
      positive for HIV infection
  8. New-onset headaches after age 50
  9. Patients with headaches and seizures
Associated symptoms and signs
  10. Headaches associated with symptoms and signs such as fever,
       stiff neck, nausea, and vomiting
  11. Headaches other than migraine with aura associated with
       focal neurological symptoms or signs
  12. Headaches associated with papilledema, cognitive impair-
       ment, or personality change

Table 1-9.   Reasons to consider neuroimaging for children with headaches

1. Persistent headaches of less than 6 months' duration that do not respond to medical treatment
2. Headache associated with abnormal neurological findings, especially if accompanied by papilledema, nystagmus, or gait or motor abnormalities
3. Persistent headaches associated with an absent family history of migraine
4. Persistent headache associated with substantial episodes of confusion, disorientation, or emesis
5. Headaches that awaken a child repeatedly from sleep or occur immediately on awakening
6. Family history or medical history of disorders that may predispose one to central nervous system (CNS) lesions and clinical or laboratory findings suggestive of CNS involvement

Source: Data from Medina LS, Pinter JD, Zurakowski D, et al. Children with headache: clinical predictors of surgical space-occupying lesions and the role of neuroimaging. *Radiology* 1997;202:819–824.

routine use of neuroimaging is not warranted. In patients with atypical headache patterns, a history of seizures, or focal neurological signs or symptoms, CT or MRI may be indicated." Table 1-10 provides some indications to consider neuroimaging in migraineurs.

Electroencephalography

In the pre-CT-scan era, a skull series and electroencephalography constituted the standard testing for evaluation of headaches. Now, of course, CT and MRI scans are far superior to exclude structural lesions. The report of the Quality Standards Subcommittee of the AAN suggests the following practice parameter: "The electroencephalogram (EEG) is not useful in the routine evaluation of patients with headache. This does not exclude the use of EEG to evaluate headache patients with associated symptoms suggesting a seizure disorder such as atypical migrainous aura or episodic loss of consciousness. Assuming head imaging capabilities are readily available, EEG is not recommended to exclude a structural cause for headache" (11).

Blood Tests

Blood tests are generally not helpful for the diagnosis of headaches. However, there are numerous indications (with examples in Table 1-11) such as the following: erythrocyte sedimentation rate or C-reactive protein, to consider the possibility of temporal arteritis; a mono spot in a teenager with headaches, sore throat, and cervical adenopathy; a complete blood count (CBC), liver function test, HIV test, or Lyme antibody in some patients with a suspected infectious basis; an anticardiolipin antibody and lupus anticoagulant in a migraineur with extensive white matter abnormalities on MRI; a TSH (thyroid stimu-

Table 1-10. Reasons to consider neuroimaging in migraineurs

Unusual, prolonged, or persistent aura

Basilar, confusional, or hemiplegic migraine

Migraine aura without headache

Increasing frequency, severity, or change in clinical features

Migraine status

First or worst migraine

Crash migraine

Onset over the age of 50 years

Late-life migraine accompaniments

Posttraumatic migraine

Patient and/or family request

lating hormone) level because headache may be a symptom in 14% of cases of hypothyroidism; a CBC because headache may be a symptom when the hemoglobin concentration is reduced by one half or more; BUN (blood, urea, nitrogen) and creatinine, to exclude renal failure, which can cause headache; serum calcium because hypercalcemia can be associated with headaches; CBC and platelets because thrombotic thrombocytopenic purpura can cause headaches; and endocrine studies in a patient with headaches and a pituitary tumor.

Additionally, blood tests may be indicated as a baseline and for monitoring certain medications such as divalproex sodium for migraine prophylaxis, carbamazepine for trigeminal neuralgia, and lithium for chronic cluster headaches.

Lumbar Puncture

MRI or CT scan is always performed before a lumbar puncture for the evaluation of headaches except in some cases where acute meningitis is suspected. Lumbar puncture can be diagnostic for meningitis or encephalitis, meningeal carcinomatosis or lymphomatosis, subarachnoid hemorrhage, and high (e.g., pseudotumor cerebri) or low CSF. Table 1-12 provides some presentations where lumbar puncture should be considered. In cases of blood dyscrasias, the platelet count should be 50,000 or greater before safely performing the lumbar puncture. The CSF opening pressure should always be measured when investigating headaches. When measuring the opening pressure, it is important for the patient to relax and at least partially extend the head and legs to avoid recording a falsely elevated pressure.

After neuroimaging as discussed, examples where lumbar puncture is often indicated include the following: the first or worst headache; headache with fever or other symptoms or signs suggesting an infectious cause; a subacute or progressive headache (e.g., an HIV-positive patient or a person with carcinoma); and an atypical chronic headache (e.g., to rule out pseudotumor cerebri in an obese woman without papilledema).

Table 1-11.   Reasons to consider blood tests to evaluate headaches

Indication	Tests
Inflammatory disease (e.g., temporal arteritis or lupus)	ESR, C-reactive protein, ANA, rheumatoid factor
Infectious disease (e.g., HIV, Lyme)	HIV antibody, Lyme antibody
Extensive white matter abnormalities on MR imaging	Lupus anticoagulant, anticardiolipin antibodies
Headaches and a pituitary adenoma	Prolactin level, TSH
Anemia and TTP	CBC with platelets
Metabolic disease	TSH, serum calcium, BUN, creatinine
Baseline and monitoring for drug side effects (e.g., divalproex sodium, NSAIDs, and lithium)	CBC, chemistry profile, TSH

ESR, Erythocyte sedimentation rate; ANA, antinuclear antibody; HIV, human immunodeficiency virus; TSH, thyroid-stimulating hormone; TTP, thrombotic thrombocytopenic purpura; CBC, complete blood count; BUN, blood urea nitrogen; NSAIDs, nonsteroidal antiinflammatory drugs.
Source: Evans RW. Diagnostic testing for headaches. *Med Clin North Am* 2001;85(4):865–885. Used with permission.

MEDICOLEGAL ASPECTS

Because seeing headache patients can be akin to working in a medicolegal minefield, it is appropriate to include a medicolegal section (12,13). Neuroimaging for patients with primary headache disorders is a prototypical example of defensive medicine. (Aside from the cost, you could argue that at least a normal scan may reassure an anxious patient and/or family members and be worthwhile.) Readers in many countries outside the United States may look on this issue as another example of American excess. However, many of the points raised in this section may improve patient care regardless of litigation issues.

There are many reasons for you to be sued for medical malpractice when treating headache patients. Simply stated, medical malpractice is negligent conduct as compared to the standard of care that results in damages as testified to by a medical expert. Then the plaintiffs have to demonstrate, in reasonable medical probability (more likely than not, with a greater than 50% probability) causation that the negligence resulted in damages (harm to the patient, a poor outcome). Your risk of having a successful malpractice suit against you can be significantly reduced by being aware of the many potential areas of exposure and obsessively and compulsively documenting patient encounters, discussions, and telephone calls. Unfortunately, just

Table 1-12. Reasons to consider lumbar puncture to evaluate headaches

Presentation	Possible CSF Diagnosis
First or worst headache	Subarachnoid hemorrhage or meningitis
Headache with fever or other symptoms or signs suggesting an infectious cause	Meningitis or encephalitis
Subacute or progressive headache in a patient with risk factors	Cryptococcal meningitis in HIV-positive patient
	Meningeal carcinomatosis with a history of a primary cancer
	Pseudotumor cerebri in an obese woman without papilledema
Orthostatic headache with diffuse meningeal enhancement on MR imaging	Low CSF pressure syndrome

Source: From Evans RW. Diagnostic testing for headaches. *Med Clin North Am* 2001;85(4):865–885. Used with permission.

because you do the medically correct thing does not protect you from malpractice suits.

Misdiagnosis or failure to diagnose is a potential cause of lawsuits. As discussed earlier in this chapter, most headaches are benign primary disorders where diagnostic testing is not indicated but there are numerous secondary causes that need to be excluded as appropriate such as subarachnoid hemorrhage, meningitis, neoplasms, temporal arteritis, cerebral venous thrombosis, and arterial dissections. Primary care physicians may fail to consider life-threatening secondary pathology and not order appropriate testing because they rarely if ever see serious secondary pathology as a cause of headache with a normal neurological examination. I'm often concerned about missing the subtle or uncommon presentations. Examples include headache presenting due to the following causes: meningeal carcinomatosis with a history of breast cancer many years previously and a normal CT scan; cryptococcal meningitis in a patient without immunosuppression; a sentinel headache seen for the first time weeks after the event in a patient with a background of chronic daily headache; cerebral venous thrombosis in an obese patient with a pseudotumor cerebri type presentation; brief facial pain due to cervical carotid artery dissection; and temporal arteritis with a unilateral nuchal-occipital headache similar to occipital neuralgia in a patient over the age of 50.

The physician has to be familiar with not only atypical presentations but the sensitivity and specificity of diagnostic testing and error in interpretation of the studies. For example, MRI is the preferred neuroimaging study for the evaluation of headaches with the exceptions of acute head trauma and acute subarachnoid hemorrhage. However, a routine MRI of the brain may not be sufficient. In some cases, pathology may be missed without the addition of a magnetic resonance arteriogram (MRA), venogram, postcontrast studies, or additional sections through the area of interest. There are certainly limitations to MR. For example, a high-quality MRA may miss 5% to 10% of intracranial saccular aneurysms detected by cerebral arteriography. As another example, temporal arteritis can rarely be present with a normal or near normal erythrocyte sedimentation rate.

Unless you interpret your own studies, you are also dependent on the skill of the radiologists. The misreading of neuroimages is common. Providing the radiologist with sufficient clinical information can be crucial on the referral form or hospital order. On a nonroutine case, it is often helpful to speak with the radiologist. If you are not sufficiently knowledgeable, obtain a second reading of the study in difficult cases.

A delay in diagnosis can also make you liable. If the inpatient or outpatient scan is not done quickly enough, you may be responsible if you do not demonstrate that you ordered the scan stat, spoke to the radiologist, followed through to see the study was done and that the ward clerk actually sent your request in, and so on. Problems can also arise with managed care plans where a precertification for neuroimaging must be obtained but is turned down. Depending on the criteria used by the insurance company, in some cases, you must use certain "magic words" to get the scan approved.

Let's say that a patient with a normal examination had a thunderclap headache 2 months previously and is just now obtaining a medical opinion for the first time when seeing their primary care physician. Primary care physicians could have liability issues if the patient had a rebleed and their actions were any of the following: they performed no testing; referred the patient to a neurologist who didn't have an opening until 2 months later; obtained a CT scan or even MRI scan with normal findings. The patient now sees a neurologist who opines the headache was probably a migraine but considers the possibility of a sentinel headache. A MRI with MRA of the brain reveals an intracranial saccular aneurysm. However, there can be many sources of delay that can result in a bad outcome if the patient were to have a rebleed in the interim. Examples include the following: the scan was not done for 2 weeks because it took a week to obtain HMO precertification and then a week to schedule the study; the scan was performed on a Friday afternoon and not read until Monday; and a faxed report of the scan comes to your office Friday afternoon after you've already left for the weekend. Or the scan might show a possible neoplasm where the radiologist recommends a contrast-enhanced study. You or your office staff may not appropriately follow up and advise the patient of the finding and obtain additional imaging. Thus delays for which you can be liable can occur in the following areas: obtaining the study; interpretation; communicating with the patient; and taking the next step (e.g., referring to a neurosurgeon).

Informed consent is certainly important to advise the patient of possible adverse events associated with testing or treatment. But do not forget about informed refusal. For example, you may recommend a scan in a new patient with headache and a new-onset seizure where a neoplasm would be found to be present. However, the patient declines, does not follow through, or cannot pay for the study. One year later, the patient and/or family go to an attorney telling them you did not obtain the scan or even though they could not pay for the scan, you did not make arrangements for one. Thus remembering to document is crucial.

Adverse events due to medications are another potential area of exposure. Examples include the following: myocardial infarction in patients with known coronary artery disease or risk factors when given triptans; kidney stones due to topiramate; and a neural tube defect due to valproic acid. It is difficult if not impossible to truly advise patients of all the side effects of medications. Even if you give patients a copy of the package insert and they have a side effect, their attorney could argue you did not adequately explain the risk and that a layperson could not possibly be expected to understand medical terms such as *thrombocytopenia* or *toursade de pointes* without an explanation. Usually we explain the risk of common side effects and rare serious side effects depending on the medication. Patients who become habituated to butalbital and/or opiates may sue you for causing their dependence. Or if a patient who is overusing a butalbital combination is not appropriately withdrawn and has a withdrawal seizure, he or she could hold you responsible. Remember to document and closely follow the amounts of medication you are prescribing. Complications of a procedure done to investigate headaches such as a lumbar puncture or cerebral arteriogram are another area of exposure.

It is also worthwhile to be cognizant of the comorbidity of depression and bipolar disorder and migraine and depression in those with chronic daily headache who might be suicide risks. Depressed patients could take an overdose of their migraine medication such as amitriptyline.

During the last several years, there have been lively debates in many states and in the Congress over medical liability reform and the growing crisis in availability and affordability of insurance. The *Houston Chronicle* ran an editorial on this issue blaming the problem to a significant degree on incompetent drug-addicted physicians and lax enforcement by the state board of medical examiners. My letter to the editor probably expresses the views of many physicians including headache specialists on this issue.

"Bad Medicine/Doctors' malpractice lies at heart of insurance crisis" is a bad editorial (Jan. 12, Editorial Page). I agree with appropriate enforcement by the Texas State Board of Medical Examiners. However, impaired and incompetent physicians are just a small part of the picture. Each year, about 25 percent of physicians in Texas are named in medical malpractice cases. About 85 percent of the cases are closed with no indemnity payment.

Contrary to the implication of the *Chronicle* editorial, I have no impairment or drug addictions, and, in fact, I am listed in the publication *Best Doctors in America.* Yet, I have had three malpractice cases against me in over 20 years of practice after treating more than 40,000 patients. In all three cases, the judge or jury found in my favor but at considerable expense. In the most recent suit, a disgruntled patient sued six physicians, a Texas Medical Center hospital and a large insurance company in a case that was without merit. Yes, we won, but after spending over $1 million for defense attorneys; my bill alone was $175,000. Because of many cases such as this, malpractice premiums are skyrocketing. And guess who really pays? All of us.

Incorrect judgment calls, medication side-effects and complications of surgery are common even when you evaluate the best doctors in Texas. The philosophy that someone has to be responsible is fueling the crisis.

We have two lotteries in Texas. It is time to support Governor Rick Perry's initiative to end the medical malpractice lottery and appropriately compensate those who are truly victims of malpractice. We cannot afford not to. (*Houston Chronicle,* January 13, 2003, Outlook section, p. 2)

The tort reform measure, which places a $250,000 cap per physician on noneconomic damages, passed in Texas in 2003, narrowly, after approval of the legislature and a constitutional amendment that won with 51% of the votes. Although the insurance rates in Texas may go down a bit or stabilize, medical malpractice has hardly gone away. And many states are still in crisis.

REFERENCES

1. Headache Classification Subcommittee of the International Headache Society. The International Classification of Headache Disorders, 2nd ed. *Cephalalgia* 2004;24[Suppl 1]:1–232.
2. Lance JW, Goadsby PJ. *Mechanism and management of headache,* 6th ed. Oxford: Butterworth-Heineman, 1998.
3. Olesen J, Tfelt-Hansen P, Welch KMA (eds). *The headaches,* 2nd ed. Philadelphia: Lippincott Williams & Wilkins, 2000.
4. Silberstein SD, Lipton RB, Dalessio DJ. *Wolff's headache and other head pain,* 7th ed. New York: Oxford University Press, 2000.
5. Silberstein SD, Lipton RB, Goadsby PJ. *Headache in clinical practice,* 2nd ed. London: Martin Dunitz, 2002.
6. Evans RW. The neurologic history and examination. In Evans RW, ed., *Saunders manual of neurologic practice.* Philadelphia: WB Saunders, 2003:1–10.
7. American Academy of Neurology. The utility of neuroimaging in the evaluation of headache in patients with normal neurologic examinations. *Neurology* 1994;44:1353–1354.
8. Frishberg BM. Neuroimaging in presumed primary headache disorders. *Semin Neurol* 1997;17:373–382.
9. Evans RW. The evaluation of headaches. In: Evans RW, ed. *Diagnostic testing in neurology.* Philadelphia: WB Saunders, 1999:1–18.
10. Evans RW. Diagnostic testing for headaches. *Med Clin North Am* 2001;85(4):865–885.

11. American Academy of Neurology. Practice parameter: the electroencephalgram in the evaluation of headache. *Neurology* 1995;45:1411–1413.
12. Saper JR. Medicolegal issues: headache. *Neurol Clin* 1999; 17(2):197–214.
13. Evans RW. Medico-legal headaches: trials and tribulations. In Purdy AR, Rapoport AM, Sheftell FD, Tepper SJ, eds. *Advanced therapy of headache,* 2nd ed. Case Based Strategies for Management. Hamilton, Ontario: BC Decker, 2005.

Migraine

Ninan T. Mathew

INTRODUCTION AND EPIDEMIOLOGY

The last 20 years have witnessed a great deal of advances in our understanding of the pathophysiology, pharmacology, epidemiology, and genetics of migraine. The International Headache Society (IHS) classifies headache into primary headache disorders and secondary headache disorders (Chapter 1) (1). Migraine with and without aura, tension-type headache (episodic and chronic), and cluster headache and other trigeminal autonomic cephalalgias form the majority of primary headache disorders.

Migraine is a primary headache disorder characterized by various combinations of neurological, gastrointestinal, and autonomic changes. The diagnosis is based on the characteristics of headache and associated symptoms.

Epidemiology of Migraine

American Migraine Study I conducted in 1989 revealed that approximately 18% of women and 6% of men in the United States have migraine, resulting in an estimated 23.6 million Americans experiencing migraine (2). The age to gender ratio of migraine is given in Figure 2-1. Migraine prevalence varies with age, the highest being found among persons between 35 and 45 years of age. The prevalence of migraine was found to be higher in households with lowest income, namely, in those earning less than $10,000 annually and was found to be higher in whites than in blacks. American Migraine Study I also revealed that migraine was underdiagnosed and undertreated and associated with substantial disability. Studies in other countries have shown more or less similar prevalence (3–5).

The American Migraine Study II was published in 2001 based on surveys done in 1999, 10 years after the first study (6). This study was based on a validated, self-administered questionnaire sent to a sample of 20,000 households in the United States. A total of 29,727 individuals responded to the questionnaire. Prevalence of migraine was found to be 18.2% among women and 6.5% among men, with an increase between the ages of 8 and about 40 years, declining thereafter in both sexes. Previous studies have shown that migraine prevalence before the age of 12 is more or less equal in both sexes; however, after puberty, there is a female preponderance. The female preponderance, in general, the occurrence of menstrually related migraine in many women, relative relief of migraine during pregnancy in many, and aggravation of migraine with aura in some patients on birth control pills clearly indicate an influence of female hormones in the pathophysiology of migraine. Approximately 23% of households contained at least one member who experienced migraine. Migraine prevalence was higher in whites than in blacks and inversely related to household income as found in the American

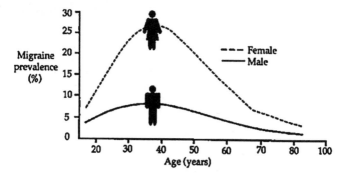

Figure 2-1. Age and gender distribution of migraine in the general population. Reprinted with permission from Stewart WF, et al. Prevalence of migraine headache in the United States in relation to age, income, race and other socioeconomic factors. *JAMA* 1992:267:64–69.

Migraine Study I. In this 10-year period, the prevalence remained about the same as that found in the previous study, but estimated number of migraineurs had increased to approximately 28 million due to population growth.

Both American Migraine Study I and II used the International Headache Society (IHS) criteria for diagnosis (1). A substantial number of people do not meet the full IHS criteria for diagnosis of migraine but do have many features of migraine. This group, referred to as migrainous headaches or probable migraine, may account for another 20 million migraineurs in the United States.

According to studies done in the United States, Spain, Thailand, and France, the prevalence of chronic daily headache, which has been defined as headache occurring more than 15 days each month for 180 days each year, is between 2.9% to 4.7% in the general population (7–10). At least 50% of these are transformed (chronic migraine), which is often associated with considerable medication overuse and comorbidity. Moreover, the quality of life in these patients is extremely poor.

Migraine-Associated Disability

Migraine greatly affects quality of life. WHO ranks migraine among the world's most disabling medical illnesses (11). Eighty-one percent of migraineurs reported functional impairment with the headache in the American Migraine Study II (6). Fifty-three percent reported that severe headache caused extreme impairment in activities and required bed rest. The proportional respondents reporting severe disability was similar in women and men. Duration of migraine associated activity restrictions was greater among women migraineurs. One to 2 days of activity restriction during migraine was experienced by 30.5% of women compared to 22.9% of men.

Approximately 31% of all migraineurs missed more than a day of work or school because of migraine in the 3 months prior to the survey (6). Fifty-one percent reported that work or school activity was reduced by more than 50%. Household and family or social activities were more likely than work or school activity to be disrupted by migraine. Seventy-six percent of respondents reported not doing any household work for more than 1 day in the previous 3 months as a result of headache. Sixty-seven percent reported that household work productivity was reduced by more than 50%. With the exception of household work, which was more frequently disrupted in women than in men, the pattern of results was similar between both sexes. Even though the figures quoted were from surveys done in the United States, similar patterns of disability are seen throughout the world in migraine sufferers.

Many other studies have examined various aspects of headache-related disability. Migraine is not just an episodic disease, but it is also a chronic disorder with episodic exacerbations. Many migraineurs live in fear, knowing an attack will disrupt their ability to work, to take care of their families, or to meet social obligations. Thus there is some disability between attacks as well as during attacks. These more chronic disabling effects generally have not been well studied. Health-related quality of life measurements have shown that compared with such other chronic illnesses as hypertension, diabetes, and coronary artery disease, migraine has lower scores in physical functioning, role functioning (physical), bodily pain, and other health aspects (12). Patients with chronic daily headache have even lower scores in physical functioning, role functioning, bodily pain, and general health as well as mental health measures using the short form 36 (SF 36) instrument. Clinically validated migraine-associated disability scales are available for clinical use. These include the Migraine Disability Assessment Scale (MIDAS) (13) and the Headache Impact Test (HIT) (14).

Data from a population-based sample of about 2,000 migraineurs show that the most disabled, 50% of the migraine sufferers, account for more than 90% of all work loss due to migraine. Because work loss is the principal driver of cost of illness, these findings imply that health care intervention should be directed to the most disabled segment of the migraine population (15).

Economic Impact

A number of studies assessed the economic impact of migraine. Stang and Osterhaus (16) determined that migraineurs in the United States spend more than 3 million days bedridden each month. Employed male migraineurs have approximately 2.7 million days per year of restricted activity, and women experience 18.8 million days of restricted activity. In terms of loss of productivity, the average working male migraineur represents $6,684 and the average female migraineur represents $3,600. The annual cost of labor lost to migraine disability in the United States has been estimated between $5.6 and $17.2 billion (17).

The direct cost of migraine from use of health care facilities is also substantial. National inventory medical care survey conducted from 1976 to 1977 reported that more than 10 million office visits to physicians were for headache. Migraine also results in frequent use of emergency room and urgent care facilities. Many prescriptions and over-the-counter medications are taken for headache disorders.

During the years since American Migraine Study I was conducted in 1989, migraine pharmacotherapy has dramatically improved with the advent of triptans and new preventive therapy. Data from American Migraine Study II suggests that despite the decade of progress, the burden of migraine in the United States remains substantial. Because migraine remains prevalent, disabling, undiagnosed, and untreated in the United States, public health initiatives to improve diagnosis and treatment are needed.

DIAGNOSIS

Physicians should appreciate the fact that primary headache disorders, such as migraine, tension-type headache, and cluster headache, are much more common (about 80% of all headaches) than secondary headache disorders. Headache disorders can exist without any obvious structural or metabolic cause. It is also important to emphasize that recurrent episodic headaches are rarely due to structural lesions.

Positive Diagnosis of Migraine

Migraine is a syndrome of recurrent headaches with a wide variety of neurological and nonneurological manifestations; it is not simply a headache. Diagnosis of migraine is not obtained solely by exclusion of other disorders; *positive diagnosis is possible.* This positive diagnosis should be based on information about the attack profile, on identification of probable triggers, and on understanding of the clinical spectrum, variability, and the natural history of migraine. Positive diagnosis requires a good history of the disorder including family history, accompanying symptoms, and triggers. Also essential are brief physical and neurological examinations, which can provide the most relevant information.

A history of previous recurrent episodes, which is often neglected by physicians, and investigation of any family history are useful. About 70% of migraineurs have a positive family history. Table 2-1 gives the current International Headache Society Classification of migraine.

Migraine can be divided into two major subtypes. *1.1 migraine without aura* is a clinical syndrome characterized by headache with specific features and associated symptoms. *1.2 migraine with aura* is primarily characterized by focal neurological symptoms that usually precede or sometimes accompany the headaches. Table 2-2 gives the International Headache Society Diagnostic Criteria for migraine without aura.

Migraine without aura is the most common subtype of migraine. It has a higher attack frequency and is usually more disabling than 1.2 migraine with aura. Only less than 30% of attacks are migraine with aura. Therefore, it is not necessary to have aura as a symptom to make a diagnosis of migraine.

Very frequent migraine attacks are now distinguished as 1.5.1 chronic migraine. Migraine without aura is the disorder most prone to become chronic, and this chronicity is aided by excessive use of immediate-relief medications and comorbidities.

Table 2-1. IHS classification of migraine

1. Migraine
1.1 Migraine without aura
1.2 Migraine with aura
    1.2.1 Typical aura with migraine headache
    1.2.2 Typical aura with nonmigraine headache
    1.2.3 Typical aura without headache
    1.2.4 Familial hemiplegic migraine (FHM)
    1.2.5 Sporadic hemiplegic migraine
    1.2.6 Basilar-type migraine
1.3 Childhood periodic syndromes that are commonly precursors of
    migraine
    1.3.1 Cyclical vomiting
    1.3.2 Abdominal migraine
    1.3.3 Benign paroxysmal vertigo of childhood
1.4 Retinal migraine
1.5 Complications of migraine
    1.5.1 Chronic migraine
    1.5.2 Status migrainosus
    1.5.3 Persistent aura without infarction
    1.5.4 Migrainous infarction
    1.5.5 Migraine-triggered seizure
1.6 Probable migraine
    1.6.1 Probable migraine without aura
    1.6.2 Probable migraine with aura
    1.6.3 Probable chronic migraine

Table 2-2. Diagnostic criteria for migraine without aura

A. At least 5 attacks fulfilling criteria B–D
B. Headache attacks lasting 4–74 hours (untreated or unsuccess-
    fully treated) (2–4)
C. Headache has at least two of the following characteristics:
    1. unilateral location
    2. pulsating quality
    3. moderate or severe pain intensity
    4. aggravation by or causing avoidance of routine physical
       activity (e.g., walking or climbing stairs)
D. During headache at least one of the following:
    1. nausea and/or vomiting
    2. photophobia and phonophobia
E. Not attributed to another disorder

Migraine with Aura

    The previously used term was classic migraine. These are
recurrent disorders manifesting as attacks of reversible focal
neurological symptoms that usually develop gradually over 5 to

Table 2-3.   IHS diagnostic criteria for migraine with aura

A. At least two attacks fulfilling criteria B–D
B. Aura consisting of at least one of the following, but no motor weakness
   1. Fully reversible visual symptoms including positive features (i.e., flickering lights, spots, or lines) and/or negative features (i.e., loss of vision)
   2. Fully reversible sensory symptoms including positive features (i.e., pins and needles) and/or negative features (i.e., numbness)
   3. Fully reversible dysphasic speech disturbance
C. At least two of the following:
   1. Homonymous visual symptoms and/or unilateral sensory symptoms
   2. At least one aura symptom developed gradually ≥5 minutes and/or different aura symptoms occur in succession ≥5 minutes
   3. Each symptom lasts ≥5 minutes but ≤60 minutes
D. Headache fulfilling the criteria given for migraine without aura in Table 2-2. Headache begins during the aura or follows the aura within 60 minutes
E. Not attributed to another disorder

20 minutes and last for less than 60 minutes. The headache with features of migraine without aura (as already described) usually follows the aura symptoms. Less commonly, headache lacks migrainous features or is completely absent. Typical aura consists of visual and/or sensory and/or speech symptoms. Gradual development, duration no longer than 1 hour, a mix of positive and negative features, and complete reversibility characterize the aura, which is associated with headache fulfilling the criteria described for migraine without aura. Table 2-3 describes the IHS Diagnostic Criteria for migraine with aura. Sometimes, additional loss or blurring of central vision may occur in some patients.

PHASES OF MIGRAINE

Four different phases of migraine recognized are prodrome, aura, headache (during which associated symptoms are experienced), and recovery or resolution phase (Fig. 2-2). However, in a given patient and individual attack, only some of these stages may be present. For example, patients may have aura without headache or headache without any other stages as described earlier. There is still a false impression among some physicians that aura is necessary for the diagnosis of migraine. The same person may have both types of migraine (migraine with aura and migraine without aura) at different times.

Prodrome

Prodromal symptoms may be present in some patients during some attacks but is not universally present. It may be difficult to

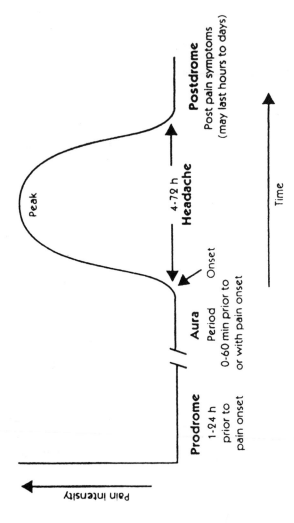

Figure 2-2.   The four phases of migraine attack.

identify, but if the patients are specifically asked about the premonitory symptoms in the 24-hour period before the headache, they often describe symptoms, such as irritability, excitability, hyperactivity, or depression, that they would not otherwise mention and are helpful in the diagnosis. Premonitory symptoms may also include hypoactivity, craving for certain particular foods, repetitive yawning, neck tightness, and so on. These prodromal or premonitory symptoms may indicate central nervous system involvement in the initial phases of migraine attack.

Aura

Migraine with aura is the most common migraine syndrome associated with neurological symptoms. Diagnosis is usually evident by careful history alone, although there are secondary mimics including carotid dissection, arteriovenous malformations, and seizures.

Visual aura is the most common type of aura often presenting as fortification spectrum, that is, a zigzag figure near the point of fixation that may gradually spread right or left and assume laterally convex shape with an angulated scintillating edge leaving variable degree absolute or relative scotoma in its wake (Fig. 2-3). In other cases, scotoma without positive phenomena may occur, and this is often perceived as being of acute onset, but on scrutiny, it usually enlarges gradually. Next in frequency are sensory disturbances in the form of pins and needles moving slowly from the point of origin and affecting a greater or smaller part of one side of the body and face. Numbness may occur in the wake, but numbness may also be the only symptom. Less frequent are speech disturbances, usually dysphasic, but often hard to categorize. If the aura includes motor weakness, it is classified as either familial hemiplegic migraine (1.2.4) or sporadic hemiplegic migraine (1.2.5).

Symptoms usually follow one another in succession beginning with visual, then sensory symptoms and dysphasia, but reverse and other orders have been noted. Patients often find it hard to describe their symptoms, in which case they should be instructed how to time and record them. After such perspective observation, the clinical picture often becomes clearer. Common mistakes are incorrect report of lateralization of headache, of sudden onset when it is gradual, and of monocular visual disturbance when they are homonymous, as well as incorrect duration of aura and mistaking sensory loss for weakness. After an initial consultation, use of an aura diary may clarify diagnosis.

Some patients may have a typical migraine aura with a headache not fulfilling the full criteria for migraine. Others might have a typical aura without headache. More commonly as patients with 1.2.1 typical aura with migraine headache become older, their headache may lose the migraine characteristics or disappear completely even though auras continue. Some individuals, primarily males, may have 1.2.3 atypical aura without headache from the onset.

In the absence of headache fulfilling criteria for migraine without aura (1.1), diagnosis of aura and the distinction from mimics that may signal serious disease (transient ischemic attack) becomes much more important. This distinction may

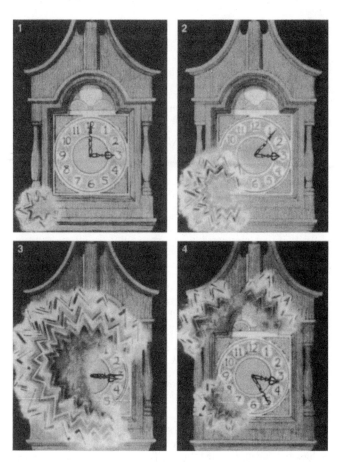

Figure 2-3.   Scintillating, fortification scotoma of migraine appears in one portion of the visual field, typically enlarges to cover central fixation, and then "marches" toward the periphery and breaks apart. Entire phenomena lasts 15 to 30 minutes. Reprinted with permission from Hupp SI, Kline LB, Corbett JJ, Visual disturbances of migraine. *Surv Opthalmol* 1989;33:221–236.

require investigation. Especially when aura begins after the age of 40, when negative features (that is, hemianopsia) are predominant or when aura is prolonged or very short, other causes should be ruled out.

Headache Phase

About 60% of headaches in migraine are predominantly unilateral. It is important to emphasize that headache can switch sides. It can start on one side and go to the other side during the same attack, or it may be on different sides in different attacks.

Although it is important to understand unilaterality and the ability of headache to switch sides to reach a proper diagnosis, a bilateral headache does not exclude the diagnosis of migraine. Approximately 40% to 45% of patients may have bilateral headaches. In some cases, it may start unilaterally and then become all over the head.

A pulsating headache is very characteristic of migraine but not always diagnostic. For example, sometimes fever and associated vasodilatation may cause a pulsating headache as some patients with brain tumors may experience. It may be difficult to get a history of pulsating headache on casual questioning, but most times with careful history taking, the physician may be able to recognize that sometime during the attack, there is some pulsating character to the headache pain of migraine.

Migraine headache is of moderate or severe intensity unlike tension-type headache, which is usually mild. Migraine headaches interfere with a person's ability to function, whereas the majority of tension-type headaches do not.

Migraine headache is aggravated by any activity or posture that increases intracranial pressure, such as coughing or sneezing, bending down, or climbing stairs or physical exercise. Therefore typically a patient with migraine generally does not like to move and prefers to lie down without much movement of the head or the body.

The location of the headache does not help in the diagnosis. Headache, even though typically in the temples, could be frontal, unilateral or bilateral, or occipital or suboccipital. The location of headache may cause some degree of confusion in the diagnosis. When it is bifrontal and around the eye (eyeball pain is very common in patients with migraine), it can be mistaken for sinus headache because of its mere location. When the headache pain is in the occipital and suboccipital regions, including the neck, it can be mistaken for a tension-type headache.

Associated symptoms are also important. Anorexia, nausea, and/or vomiting often accompany migraine headache and are very helpful diagnostic features. Nausea may occur in up to 90% of patients, whereas vomiting occurs in only one third of patients. However, note that nausea and vomiting can accompany any process with increased intracranial pressure or cause meningeal irritation such as meningitis. But the major difference between such disorders and migraine is that migraine is recurrent, whereas in conditions such as meningitis it is usually a onetime occurrence.

There is visually heightened sensory perception manifested by photophobia, phonophobia, and dislike for smells. Patients seek a dark, quiet room. There may also be orthostatic hypertension and dizziness. Behavior of the patient during attacks may be altered; they may be irritable and may seek to be left alone in a dark quiet room. Their verbal expression may be difficult and their memory and concentration poor. Cognitive impairment does occur during migraine attacks. When such behavioral symptoms occur, they may be misdiagnosed as a psychological condition. It is important to recognize that such mental changes can occur during migraine attacks.

Approximately 40% of patients may have nasal or ocular symptoms that are not as prominent as with cluster headache but less severe. When that happens, it may be misdiagnosed as a sinus headache. Depression, fatigue, anxiety, nervousness, irritability, and impairment of concentration are common.

Allodynia in Migraine

Recent research has clearly indicated that a significant percentage of patients with migraine would develop cutaneous allodynia of the scalp or the extracephalic areas of the body such as limbs during a migraine attack (18,19). Allodynia is a phenomenon in which a normally nonpainful stimuli becomes uncomfortable or painful. It is the result of central sensitization of the trigeminal pathways.

Using a semistructured questionnaire, the author has identified that 53.5% of migraineurs may have clinically detectable allodynic symptoms (19). With use of quantitative sensory testing that percentage may increase up to 75% (18). The allodynic symptoms of the scalp include soreness and sensitivity, difficulty brushing/combing the hair, wearing ponytails, and rubber bands, and difficulty lying on the side of headache because of soreness and tenderness of the scalp. The allodynic symptoms in the extracephalic areas include tingling and increased sensitivity as manifested by difficulty wearing neck chains and discomfort on having the blanket touch the body (19).

The practical importance of recognizing allodynia has recently been pointed out by Berstein et al. (20). Central sensitization and resultant allodynia begins its process in the first hour of migraine attack and becomes established by 4 hours or so. The best chance of making a patient pain free with triptan is giving the drug before the allodynic process becomes established (20). Therefore, early treatment with triptan before allodynia develops is extremely important. The lack of consistency of response to triptans and recurrence of headache (found to be fairly common in the initial years of triptan use) may be because of the late use of triptans during the attacks. Therefore it is expected that early treatment will result in (a) early pain-free state, (b) better consistency of response to triptans, and (c) low recurrence of the headache. Now most clinicians feel that assessment of allodynia should become a part of the clinical evaluation.

Apart from the clinical profile, described earlier, the other features that support a diagnosis of migraine are relief after sleep, relief after vomiting, exhaustion when the headache is over, and the history of relief during pregnancy.

Trigger Factors for Migraine

Identification of provocational trigger for a headache is evidence in support of the classification of headache as benign. It is unusual for an organic disorder to show sensitivity to triggers. Physicians should be familiar with the common triggers for migraine listed in Table 2-4. It is important to emphasize that triggers vary between migraine attacks in any given patient, but identification of trigger factors is helpful in the positive diagnosis of migraine. Triggers may also vary according to the physiological state of the person. For example, in and around

Table 2-4. Common provocational triggers for migraine

Hormonal triggers	Menstruation, ovulation, oral contraceptive, hormonal replacement
Dietary triggers	Alcohol, nitrite-laden meat, monosodium glutamate, aspartame, chocolate, aged cheese, missing a meal
Psychological triggers	Stress, period after stress (weekend or vacation), anxiety, worry, depression
Physical/environmental	Glare, flashing lights, visual stimulation, fluorescent lighting, odors, weather changes, high altitude
Sleep-related triggers	Lack of sleep, excessive sleep
Miscellaneous triggers	Head trauma, physical exertion, fatigue
Drugs	Nitroglycerin, histamine, reserpine, hydralazine, ranitidine, estrogen

the menstrual time, patients are more prone to headache with ordinary triggers such as stress.

A history of menstrual headaches or headache during ovulation almost certainly implies migraine as does headache triggered by alcohol, nitrites, and monosodium glutamate–laden food. Weekend headaches or headaches on the first day of vacation is common in migraine. For a person with a history of migraine, relatively minor head or neck trauma can trigger migrainelike episodes, which may respond to antimigraine treatments.

Provocative tests for diagnosis with such agents as reserpine, histamine, or fenfluramine is not reliable and should not be used. Nor are therapeutic tests useful (21). In the past, doctors sometimes considered a positive response to ergotamine to be diagnostic of migraine. Now many physicians falsely believe that if a patient does not respond to a triptan, he or she does not have migraine. It is clear from clinical experience that not all attacks of migraine respond to triptans, and response to drugs should never be a criteria for diagnosis. Other acute vascular headache syndromes such as headache due to rupture of an intracranial aneurysm may temporarily respond to an agent like subcutaneous sumatriptan. Basing the diagnosis on therapeutic response could be dangerous.

Resolution Phase

After the headache, the patient often feels tired, washed out, irritable, or restless and can have impaired concentration, scalp tenderness, or mood changes. Some feel unusually refreshed or euphoric after an attack; others experience depression and malaise.

Migraine Variants

Various migraine variants are recognized and classified in the IHS classification.

Familial Hemiplegic Migraine (FHM)

FHM is characterized by familial occurrence of hemiparesis associated with migrainelike headaches. The aura consists of fully reversible motor weakness and at least one of the following: (a) fully reversible visual symptoms (including flickering lights, spots, or lines) or negative features (i.e., loss of vision); (b) fully reversible sensory symptoms including positive symptoms (i.e., pins and needles) or negative features (i.e., numbness); and (c) fully reversible dysphasic speech disturbances. Usually the auras develop gradually over 5 minutes and different auras occur in succession over a period of 5 minutes or more each. Each aura symptom usually lasts $\geq$ 5 minutes, but $\leq$ 24 hours. The most important diagnostic feature is that at least one first- or second-degree relative has had attacks of similar kind. So the familial occurrence of such attacks with hemiparesis is diagnostic. It may be difficult to distinguish weakness from sensory loss.

New genetic data have allowed a more precise definition of FHM than previously. Specific genetic subtypes of familial hemiplegic migraine have been identified. In FHM1, there are mutations in CACNA1A gene on chromosome 19 (22,23), and in FHM2, mutations occur in ATP1A2 gene on chromosome 1q21-23 (24). If genetic testing is done, genetic subtypes should be specified.

It has been shown that FHM1 very often has basilar type symptoms in addition to the typical aura symptoms and that headache is virtually always present. During FHM1 attacks, disturbances of consciousness (sometimes including coma), fever, CSF pleocytosis, and confusion can occur. FHM1 attacks can be triggered by (mild) head trauma. In approximately 50% of FHM1 families, chronic progressive cerebellar ataxia occurs independently of the migraine attacks. FHM is very often mistaken for epilepsy and unsuccessfully treated as such.

Sporadic Hemiplegic Migraine

In sporadic hemiplegic migraine, attacks occur with a migraine aura including motor weakness usually on one side without a family history of similar illness in first- or second-degree relatives. The main manifestation is fully reversible motor weakness, sometimes associated with visual or sensory or dysphasic aura. Studies have shown that sporadic cases occur with approximately the same prevalence as familial cases. Attacks have the same clinical characteristics as those of familial hemiplegic migraine.

Sporadic cases always require neuroimaging and other tests to rule out other causes. Lumbar puncture is also necessary to rule out pseudomigraine with temporary neurological symptoms and lymphocytic neutrocytosis in the CSF. This condition is more prevalent in males and often associated with transient hemiparesis and aphasia.

Basilar-Type Migraine

In basilar-type migraine, the migraine aura symptoms clearly originate from the brain stem and/or from both hemispheres simultaneously, but there is no motor weakness. The aura in basilar-type migraine consists of at least two of the following fully reversible symptoms, but no motor weakness: (a) dysarthria, (b) vertigo, (c) tinnitus, (d) hyperacusia, (e) diplopia, (f) visual symptoms simultaneously in both temporal and nasal fields of both eyes, (g) ataxia, (h) decreased level of consciousness, and (i) simultaneously bilateral paresthesias. All the auras developed gradually over 5 minutes or more, and different aura symptoms may occur in succession over more than 5 minutes. Each aura symptom lasts usually 5 minutes or more and usually less than 60 minutes. The headaches following these are similar to those seen in patients with migraine without aura. In all these types of migraine, any other cause that could produce similar symptoms have to be ruled out. Basilar-type attacks are mostly seen in young adults. Many patients who have basilar-type attacks also report attacks with typical aura. Differential diagnosis of basilar-type of migraine is anxiety and panic attacks, which may cause some of the symptoms just described. The associated severe headache and the development pattern of the aura symptoms differentiates basilar-type attacks from a panic attack causing similar symptoms.

Childhood Periodic Syndromes: Migraine Precursors

Cyclical Vomiting

Cyclical vomiting occurs in recurrent episodes, usually stereotyped in individual patients, of vomiting and intense nausea. The attacks are associated with pallor and lethargy. There is complete resolution of symptoms between attacks. The clinical features of this syndrome resemble those found in association with migraine headaches. Multiple threads of research over the last years have suggested that cyclical vomiting is a condition related to migraine and may run as a precursor of migraine in children.

Abdominal Migraine

This is an idiopathic recurrent disorder seen mainly in children and characterized by episodic midline abdominal pain manifesting in attacks lasting 1 to 72 hours with normality between episodes. Pain is moderate to severe in intensity and associated with vasomotor symptoms of nausea and vomiting. The abdominal pain has the following characteristics: (a) midline location, periumbilical or poorly localized, (b) dull or just sore quality, and (c) moderate or severe intensity. During the abdominal pain, at least two of the following symptoms may be present: (a) anorexia, (b) nausea, (c) vomiting, and (d) pallor. All other organic conditions have to be ruled out in order to make a positive diagnosis. Pain may be severe enough to interfere with normal daily activities. Children may find it difficult to distinguish anorexia from nausea. The pallor is often accompanied by dark shadows under the eye. In a few patients, flushing is a predominant vasomotor phenomena. Most children with abdominal migraine develop migraine headache later in life.

Benign Paroxysmal Vertigo of Childhood

The probably heterogeneous disorder of benign paroxysmal vertigo of childhood is characterized by recurrent brief episodic attacks of vertigo occurring without warning and resolving spontaneously in otherwise healthy children. Neurological examination and audiometric and vestibular function tests are normal. The attacks are usually short lived. It may be associated with nystagmus or vomiting. Unilateral throbbing headache may occur in some patients.

Retinal Migraine

Retinal migraine manifests as repeated attacks of monocular visual disturbances including scintillations, scotoma, or blindness, associated with migraine headache. These are fully reversible episodes and always confined to the monocular visual field. Headache would meet the criteria for migraine without aura. The ophthalmological examination is usually normal between attacks. Other causes of transient monocular blindness have to be ruled out. One of the confusing issues is that some of the patients who complain of monocular visual disturbances may in fact have hemianopia. Some cases without headache have been reported, but in these cases, their migrainous nature cannot be ascertained. Other causes of transient monocular blindness (amaurosis fugax), such as optic neuropathy or carotid dissection, must be excluded.

COMPLICATIONS OF MIGRAINE

Chronic Migraine

Chronic migraine is defined as migraine occurring for 15 or more days per month for more than 3 months in the absence of medication overuse (1). This entity of chronic migraine is described in detail in Chapter 5, which deals with chronic daily headache. The entity of medication overuse or analgesic rebound headache is also described in detail.

Status migrainosus

Status migrainosus are debilitating migraine attacks lasting more than 72 hours. Usually these occur in patients with migraine without aura who may have unremitting headache for more than 72 hours. They are of severe intensity. These are the type of patients who end up in the emergency room for treatment. Note that status migrainosus can be caused by medication overuse and that factor has to be evaluated. The patients who are in status migrainosus usually are very sick with extreme nausea and vomiting and often dehydrated. Rehydration is an essential part of the treatment.

Persistent Migraine Aura without Infarction

These are patients with aura symptoms persisting for more than 1 week without any radiographical evidence of cerebral infarction. This aura could be visual, sensory, or motor. The visual aura is often bilateral and may last for months or years. It is important to exclude organic conditions like posterior leukoencephalopathy in persistent cases.

Migrainous Infarction

An occasional patient with migraine with aura may develop a cerebral infarction with some persistent neurological symptoms.

Their attacks are typical of previous attacks of migraine with aura, but the difference is that the aura symptoms persist for more than 60 minutes and neuroimaging would demonstrate an ischemic infarction in the relevant areas. Ischemic stroke in migraineurs can only be made if the infarction occurs during a typical attack of migraine with aura. Increased risk for stroke in migraine patients has been demonstrated in women under the age of 45 in several studies. Evidence for association between migraine and stroke in older women and in men is inconsistent. Younger women with migraine with aura, who are heavy smokers and who are on birth control pills, may increase their risk for cerebral infarction. The usual area of cerebral infarction is the posterior occipital lobe and is typically a wedge-shaped infarction. In patients with migrainous infarction, other predisposing causes for cerebral infarctions, such as cardiac abnormalities, anticardiolipin antibody syndrome, and collagen disease, have to be ruled out.

Migraine-Triggered Seizure

A seizure triggered by a migraine aura can occasionally occur. Migraine and epilepsy are paroxysmal brain disorders. Migrainelike headaches are quite frequently seen in the postictal period of an epileptic attack, and sometimes a seizure occurs during or following a migraine attack. This phenomenon, sometimes referred to as migralepsy, has been described in patients with migraine with aura. This is a rare condition.

Probable Migraine

A previously used term was *migrainous disorder* (1). These are attacks and/or headache missing one of the features needed to fulfill all the criteria for a disorder described in the criteria for migraine with aura and without aura. The prevalence of probable migraine is quite high in the clinical population. They should be considered as migraine for all practical purposes and treated as such.

Menstrual Migraine

The International Headache Society recognizes two forms of menstrual migraine (1): pure menstrual migraine without aura and menstrually related migraine without aura.

Pure Menstrual Migraine without Aura

These are migraine attacks in a menstruating woman, fulfilling the criteria for migraine without aura. The attacks should occur exclusively on day 1, plus or minus two, that is, days −2 to +3 of menstruation in at least two out of three menstrual cycles and no other times of the cycle. The first day of menstruation is counted as day 1 and the preceding day as −1. There is no day zero. For the purposes of classification, menstruation is considered endometrial bleeding resulting from either normal menstrual cycle or from withdrawal of exogenous progesterones as in the case of combined oral contraceptives and cyclical hormone replacement therapy.

Menstrually Related Migraine without Aura

In this entity, attacks in a menstruating woman should occur on day 1 plus or minus two, that is, days minus to plus three of the menstruation in at least two out of three menstrual cycles and additionally at other times of the cycle. In other words, these patients have migraines around the menstrual time plus other migraines at other times of the month. The importance of distinguishing between pure menstrual migraine and menstrually related migraine without aura is that the hormone prophylaxis is more likely to be effective for pure menstrual migraine. In order to make a certain diagnosis, a respectively documented evidence by a proper diary is necessary.

Menstrual migraines are mostly migraine without aura in a woman who has migraine both with aura and without aura. Migraine aura does not appear to be associated with menstruation.

Menstrual migraines are usually prolonged, can occur for 4 or 5 days, as long as the menstruation lasts. It is more difficult to treat. Recurrence of headache even with triptans is not uncommon.

Pediatric Migraine

See the details on headaches in the child in Chapter 10. Migraine in children differs to some degree from that of adults. In small children, the attacks are usually short lived, sometimes lasting less than 2 hours. They are predominantly bifrontal. It is rare to have occipital, suboccipital migraine headache in children. If posterior headache is the main manifestation, it needs further work-up to rule out other conditions. Many of the occipital headaches are attributable to structural lesions in children. For young children, photophobia and phonophobia may be inferred from their behavior because they may not report it to the physician. Migraine headache is commonly bilateral in young children; an adult pattern of unilateral pain usually emerges in late adolescence or early adult life.

Differentiating Migraine from So-Called Sinus Headaches

It has been reported that a significant percentage of migraineurs often receive a mistaken diagnosis of so-called sinus headache or tension headache. In one study, 42% of patients with migraine previously received a diagnosis of sinus headaches. The majority of such diagnoses is made by the patient, which is generally accepted by their physicians. The migraine is frequently mistaken for sinus headache because of various reasons and situations. If the migraine pain is situated in the bifrontal, orbital, and infraorbital regions, that is, over the sinuses, it causes confusion with so-called sinus headaches. Migraine is frequently triggered by weather changes, when it can easily be mistaken for a sinus attack. Nasal and ocular symptoms are not uncommon in migraine (occurring in about 40% to 45% of patients). Nasal congestion associated with the headache is often mistakenly thought to be due to sinus. In addition, sinus medications, which contain decongestants, may give patients some relief of their headache pain and thus the diagnosis is attributed to sinus. The majority of patients who are diagnosed as sinus have been found to have migraine with considerable disability and good response to triptans for their acute attacks.

Headache associated with bacterial sinusitis is not a recurrent disorder. It is usually associated with mucopurulent discharge from the nose, fever, tenderness in sinus areas, and radiographical findings of sinusitis. It responds to antibiotics and usually it is not a recurrent disorder. In the so-called sinus headache, the radiographic findings are usually normal.

Differentiating Migraine from Tension-Type Headache

The second major misdiagnosis of migraine is as a tension-type headache. The reasons for these misdiagnoses are as follows: (a) neck pain is very common during migraine attacks, and almost 75% of patients complain of pain, spasm, and tenderness of the neck, which is thought to be a muscle allodynia occurring during migraine; (b) stress is a common trigger of migraine and therefore all headaches that occur under stressful conditions are wrongly attributed as tension headache; (c) 40% of migraine patients have bilateral headache and therefore can easily be mistaken for tension-type headache.

RAPID CLINICAL SCREENING FOR MIGRAINE

A number of research studies have been done to look for the strongest predictors of migraine diagnosis. In an extensive study with validation and revalidation, Lipton et al. (25) found that nausea, disability, and photophobia are probably the best predictors of migraine. They published a rapid screener for migraine (I.D. Migraine) in order to help a busy family practitioner who does not have the luxury of spending a long time taking a detailed history of migraine. They came up with three questions: (a) Nausea: Are you nauseated or sick to your stomach when you have a headache? (b) Disability: Has a headache limited your activities for a day or more in the last three months? (c) Photophobia: Does light bother you when you have a headache? It was found that if two out of these three questions are positive, there is a 93% positive predictive value that one is dealing with a migraine disorder. If three out of three are positive, there is a 98% positive predictive value. I.D. Migraine can be used for rapid screening of migraineurs in a busy practice. Once these positive answers are obtained, further details can be taken to confirm the diagnosis.

Vestibular Migraine or Migrainous Vertigo

This topic is dealt with in detail in the section on migraine and vertigo in Chapter 14.

Differential Diagnosis of Primary Headaches

It is important to make a differential diagnosis among migraine, tension-type headache, and cluster headache because the optimal treatments differ. Distinguishing characteristics are illustrated in Table 2-5, and all these features should be considered together to form the diagnosis. For example, 60% of migraines are predominantly unilateral, whereas all cluster headaches are unilateral, and tension-type headaches are bilateral. It is impossible to make a diagnosis of migraine from the location alone: it could be the back, front, or sides. The pain in tension-type headache is diffuse, whereas for cluster headache it is almost always periorbital or retroorbital.

The frequency of headaches varies greatly between patients. Tension-type headache might occur from once a month to 30 days a month. About 30% of migraineurs in the general population

Table 2-5. Differential diagnosis of primary headaches

Clinical Features	Migraine	Tension-type headache	Cluster headache
Men:women	25:75	40:60	90:10
Laterization	60% unilateral	Diffuse bilateral	100% unilateral
Location	Frontal, periorbital, temporal, hemicranial	Diffuse	Periorbital
Frequency	1–4 per month	1–30 per month	1–3 per day for 3–12 months
Severity	Moderate/severe	Mild/moderate	Extremely severe
Duration	4–72 hours	Variable	15 minutes–3 hours
Pain character	Throbbing, pulsating	Dull	Sharp, boring
Periodicity	±	–	+++
Family history	+++	±	±
Associated symptoms			
Aura	+++	–	–
Autonomic features	±	–	+++
Nausea/vomiting	+++	–	±
Photo/phonophobia	+++	–	±
Exacerbation by movement	+++	–	–

have more than four attacks a month, and clinic patients have even more. Cluster headaches are extremely severe, whereas tension-type headache is normally mild or moderate. The duration of attacks varies, and it is important to emphasize that migraine may vary from the 4 to 72 hours specified in the International Headache Society (IHS) classification (1). Children have shorter headaches, and some adults with chronic headaches may have prolonged migraine lasting for much longer than 72 hours. Cluster headache is of short duration and may be repeated many times a day.

The character of pain may be helpful in differential diagnosis: migraine headache is throbbing and pulsating; tension-type headache is dull; and cluster headache pain is described as sharp, boring, and not throbbing. Periodicity is important. Typically, cluster headache has a characteristic periodicity of 2 to 3 months of headache and remission for a year, whereas there are only rare examples of periodic migraine.

Aura preceding headache is invariably diagnostic of migraine and not seen in the other primary headaches. Such autonomic features as watering from the eyes, redness of the eyes, and runny nose are diagnostic of cluster headache, but occasionally patients with migraine also have some autonomic features in and around the eyes. Vomiting, nausea, and photophobia are seen predominantly in migraine and are rare in other conditions. In migraine, movement often aggravates the headaches, whereas cluster headache patients like to move around: Some run on the spot to get some relief from their pain.

Family history is important in diagnosis. It has been shown that, like migraine, chronic tension-type headache may be familial, whereas episodic tension-type headache is not.

Complicated migraine with neurological symptoms and signs, which is more often seen in the young, is described in Chapter 10.

Differentiation from Organic Disorders

Two particular diagnostic problems are organic conditions that mimic primary headache disorders and organic conditions that coexist with migraine because migraine is such a common disorder. For example, a patient may have a brain tumor or an aneurysm as well as migraine.

Normally, migraines begin gradually and take 3 to 4 hours to peak. Some patients have abrupt headaches that peak in seconds, called *crash migraine* (17). This type of abrupt-onset headache may resemble thunderclap headache (Chapter 5) (18). It is difficult to distinguish this situation from a ruptured intracranial aneurysm. About 25% of thunderclap headaches arise from a rupturing aneurysm, whereas 75% are benign, migrainelike headaches. Sometimes carotid artery dissections cause an acute rapid-onset headache with facial pain, eye symptoms similar to an aura, partial Horner's syndrome, and severe unilateral head pain similar to migraine. Diagnosis is facilitated somewhat because these conditions usually occur in a patient who has not had headaches before.

Table 2-6 lists particular warning signs that a physician should be aware of and investigate carefully (Chapter 1). So-called sudden-onset first headache and the "worst headache ever" should be

Table 2-6. Headache alarms that should alert the physician to the need for further investigation

Sudden-onset "first" headache

"Worst headache ever"

Late-onset new headache

Headache with fever, rash, stiff neck

Progressively increasing headache

Headache with neurological signs and symptoms other than aura

Headache with mental changes

Headache with papilledema

New-onset headache in a patient with cancer or HIV

investigated with neuroimaging. If that is negative, a lumbar puncture should be performed. There are case reports of negative CT scan and lumbar punctures in patients with aneurysms (26), so we recommend doing at least a magnetic resonance angiography to explore subarachnoid hemorrhage and aneurysm.

Late-onset new headache refers to a person who has not had headaches before 55 years of age. Headache with fever, rash, and neck stiffness might arise from meningitis or other conditions. Headache with mental changes, especially in the elderly, might be caused by subdural hematoma. Headache with papilledema must be investigated for signs of intracranial pressure secondary to a brain tumor or idiopathic intracranial hypertension. New-onset headache in a person with cancer or HIV must also be investigated.

Treatment for sufferers of headaches would be greatly improved if doctors were motivated and suitably educated to attempt differential diagnosis of the headache disorders. It should be recognized that secondary headache disorders are not common and usually can be excluded by a simple physical and neurological examination coupled with a good history of previous headaches. The information obtained should then be used to diagnose the primary headache disorder and appropriate treatment programs should be applied. The benefits in avoiding unnecessary delay in adequate relief for the patient, reducing lost productivity, and negating the need for frequent follow-up visits should outweigh any additional time spent in the initial consultation.

Patients with migraine are more prone to tension-type headache in between their acute migraine attacks, leading to a mixed headache syndrome. The tension-type headaches in migraineurs are somewhat different from episodic tension-type headache. They are more frequent and more severe. They may be associated with nausea, photophobia, and phonophobia, unlike episodic tension-type headache. They may be triggered by the same factors that trigger their migraines. So these observations led to the concept of a continuum in primary headache disorders. At one end of the spectrum is the typical migraine with aura and without aura; at the other end of the spectrum is the chronic tension-type headache. But in the middle of the spectrum are mixed forms of migraine and tension-type headaches, which can sometimes become daily or nearly so in many patients.

PATHOPHYSIOLOGY OF MIGRAINE

Migraine can be considered a peculiar response of the central response of the central nervous system (CNS) to a variety of stimuli. Migraineurs have a low threshold for migraine attacks, and this threshold may be genetically determined. The threshold for migraine attacks is modified by many factors, the best example being estrogen, which accounts for the high prevalence of migraine among women, menstrual migraine, amelioration of migraine during pregnancy, and worsening of migraine in some patients taking oral contraceptives. In addition to estrogen, a number of other triggers have already been discussed.

Genetics of Migraine

Genetic epidemiology has shown that risk to first-degree relative of probands with migraine with aura is fourfold, whereas in migraine without aura, it is 1.9 fold, clearly indicating that genetic influence is stronger in migraine with aura (27). A Danish population–based study of twins with migraine showed higher concordance rates for monozygotic twins than some dizygotic twins, notably for migraine with aura (28,29). Recent genetic studies in familial hemiplegic migraine have identified two types of familial hemiplegic (FHM) migraine as discussed earlier.

FHM1 has CACNA1A abnormal mutations on chromosome 19 (22,23), and FHM2 has abnormal mutations of the ATP1A2 gene on chromosome 1q21-23 (24). The FHM1 CACNA1A abnormal mutations are on P/Q calcium channels. These findings may have therapeutic implications in the future because specific P/Q calcium channel antagonists may be developed.

Migraine Aura

Clinical observations, neuroimaging studies, and blood flow measurements clearly indicate that migraine aura originates from the cerebral cortex. The visual aura, which is the most common form of migraine aura, spreads laterally in one hemifield, accelerating and enlarging as it spreads. Disturbance spreading at a steady speed (3 to 6 mm/min) along the primary visual cortex would have these characteristics because the cortical representation of the visual field decreases with distance from the center of vision. The edge of the moving visual disturbance is usually flickering at the rate of 10 to 15 Hz, decreasing in the periphery to 3 or 4 Hz, and it is followed by scotoma, indicating an irritative disturbance at the front followed by a depressed neuronal function (Fig. 2-2). Sensory aura similarly marches at a slow pace, often with tingling at the edge and numbness in its wake. If there is more than one type of aura symptom, such as visual and sensory symptoms, they occur in sequence. The only known disturbance that can explain the slow continuous spread of excitation followed by depression is Leao's cortical spreading depression (CSD) (30A, 30B).

Olesen et al. (31) provided the first evidence in human patients during migraine attacks of slowly spreading cortical hypoperfusion incompatible with spasm of a major artery but fully compatible with the occurrence of CSD. Several later studies of regional cerebral blood flow also support these observations (32–34).

Modern imaging techniques, including functional MRI, do not support ischemia as the cause of migraine aura (35–37). The observation that oxygenation in the visual cortical gray matter—and not the white matter—increases rather than decreases in T2-weighted image intensity argues in favor of a spreading depressionlike event.

Cerebral hypoperfusion is followed by hyperemia in many cases. It is explained by possible release of the calcitonin gene-related peptide (CGRP), which is a potent vasodilator during the aura phase (38).

Regional cerebral blood flow in cerebral hemispheres, apart from nonspecific pain activation, is normal in migraine without aura interictally and during an attack. Thus it appears that migraine aura and the headache of migraine are based on two different mechanisms. The interrelationship between the aura and the occurrence of pain is still not clear. It is possible that CSD induces changes in the cortical perivascular nerve endings and nociceptive systems in the brain stem and, secondarily, activates the trigeminal vascular system, which would account for the pain of migraine.

Brain Stem Changes in Migraine

Various lines of evidence suggest that brain stem nuclei and periaqueductal gray matter (PAG), which are components of ascending and descending pain pathways, are central in the pathophysiology of migraine (39–42). Weiller et al. used positron emission tomography (PET) to monitor changes in regional cerebral blood flow during spontaneous migraine attacks (39). Increased blood flow was detected in portions of the cerebral cortex and in the brain stem. Brain stem activation persisted following the injection of a triptan that relieved migraine symptoms. The authors suggested that a primary dysfunction was localized in the brain stem nuclei ordinarily involved in antinociception. Previous reports suggested that the PAG area and the upper brain stem are important migraine generators. Raskin et al. (43) reported migrainelike attacks in patients in whom electrodes had been implanted in the PAG area for control of back pain (41). These migrainelike attacks were successfully treated by IV administration of dihydroergotamine (41). In addition, dihydroergotamine has been shown in autoradiographic studies to bind to the dorsal raphe area of the upper brain stem (42).

The dorsal raphe nucleus in the PAG area contains 65% of brain 5-HT, whereas the locus ceruleus contains about 96% of brain norepinephrine. It is also interesting that migraine has a comorbid association with a number of psychiatric conditions, including bipolar disorder, anxiety states, and depression, all of which are associated with perturbations in these neurotransmitter substances. Welch et al. (40) reported results of measuring iron homeostasis in PAG of patins with episodic migraine and chronic daily headache. The authors found iron homeostasis to be persistently and progressively impaired in these patients and speculated that this resulted from repeated migraine attacks. Once again, these results strengthen the concept of the upper brain stem being an important area of the brain that is disturbed in migraine. The following is a schematic presentation of the important element in the pathophysiology of migraine.

Genetic predisposition
Channelopathy

$\downarrow$

Central neuronal hyperexcitability
Cortical spreading depression
Brain stem activation

$\downarrow$

Trigeminal vascular activation

Results from other investigative approaches also support the important role of brain stem nuclei in migraine pathogenesis. In cats and nonhuman primates, stimulation of the superior sagittal sinus, which receives trigeminal innervation, results in increased c-Fos expression in the ventral lateral area of the caudal PAG (44). General pain principles suggest that PAG reduces nociceptive input. Normally PAG may inhibit trigeminal firing: in other words, it is part of the normal control system, which may not function appropriately in migraineurs (45).

One functional imaging study demonstrated activation in the dorsal rostral brain stem when a patient with active cluster headache developed a typical migraine without aura during a PET scan (46). This activation overlap with the locus ceruleus appears to be involved in signal-to-noise regulation and selective attention, which corresponds to the clinical experience of migraineurs who report difficulties in concentration and confusion during attacks.

From a pharmacological perspective, antimigraine compounds bind in PAG and around the dorsal raphe nucleus (44–48). In addition, valproate, a prophylactic agent that has been proven clinically effective in migraine, acts on g-aminobutyric acid$_A$ receptors on the dorsal raphe nuclei, resulting in a decreased firing rate of these serotonergic cells (49).

Current research in the neurophysiology of these autonomic loci may begin to explain why acute antimigraine agents are excellent for patients who experience few attacks but less effective in patients with greater attack frequency. Welch et al. (42) observed increased iron deposition in PAG, indicating free radical damage to these areas in chronic daily headache and further supporting the notion that there is dysfunction of these anatomical loci in chronic migraine. Because these areas are dysfunctional, they perhaps lose their natural antinociceptive function, resulting in increased frequency of headache and lack of response to acute medications. Overuse of acute antimigraine agents may also interfere with these brain stem mechanisms and induces rebound (50).

Mechanism of Head Pain in Migraine

Pain can be broadly classified into three types: nociceptive, neuropathic, and idiopathic. Nociceptive pain is the most common and results from tissue injuries (e.g., trauma and postoperative trauma). Opioids are the drugs of choice for nociceptive pain. Neuropathic pain results from pathology of the peripheral or CNS (e.g., diabetic neuropathy and thalamic pain from a brain infarction). For neuropathic pain, anticonvulsants such as carbamazepine and gabapentin are the drugs of choice. In contrast, migraine is an idiopathic pain, with no tissue injury and no detectable pathology. Therefore, it is obvious that the mechanism of migraine pain will be different from that of nociceptive or neuropathic pain and the pharmacology and therapeutic response will be different. None of the specific antimigraine medications, such as the triptans, are useful in nociceptive or neuropathic pain.

For pain to occur anywhere, the primary sensory neuron carrying pain sensation has to be activated. In the case of migraine, the trigeminal nerve anteriorly and the upper cervical nerves C2 and C3 posteriorly carry pain sensation of the head, face, and upper neck. One of the practical implications of this neural circuit (trigeminal in front, upper cervical nerves in the back) is that neck pain, neck muscle tenderness, and spasm are part and parcel of migraine headache. Approximately 75% of migraine attacks are associated with neck pain (51).

The trigeminal nerve supplies not only extracranial tissues but also intracranial structures, particularly the dural and pial blood vessels, the large blood vessels of the brain, the dural sinuses, and the dura mater. The dural and pial blood vessels are richly supplied by trigeminal, sympathetic, and parasympathetic nerve endings. The intracranial blood vessels, particularly, contain 5-HT_1 receptors (52). The 5-HT_{1B} receptors are postsynaptic and found on the blood vessels, whereas the 5-HT_{1D} receptors are presynaptic. 5-HT_{1B} receptors are also found in the central trigeminal system. Activation of the trigeminal vascular system is the primary mechanism of pain in migraine.

How Does Cortical Spreading Depression Excite Trigeminal Vascular Afferents?

Migraine pain is not a direct consequence of cerebral blood flow changes. CSD involves a gross disturbance in the brain's extracellular environment. The potassium level increases to 60 mmol, the extracellular glutamate level increases considerably, and the extracellular calcium level decreases (53). Nitric oxide (NO) is produced both immediately after CSD and as a second prolonged wave lasting for several hours (54). It has been suggested that CSD can excite trigeminal vascular afferents directly because the pial blood vessels are closest to the cortical surface (55). Activation of the extensive network of pial blood vessels and their perivascular nerve endings and subsequent reflex activation of dural may be sufficient to explain migraine pain.

Activation and Sensitization of the Trigeminal Vascular System

Activation and sensitization of the trigeminal vascular system account for head pain and associated symptoms of migraine (Fig. 2-4) (Richard J. Hargreaves, MD, personal communication, 2000). Two changes occur at the neurovascular junction: vasodilation of dural blood vessels and neurogenic inflammatory reaction. The dilated blood vessels stimulate the nerve endings, which release neuropeptides such as CGRP, substance P, and neurokinin A. These are vasoactive polypeptides, which further dilate blood vessels and cause a rapid-onset inflammatory reaction consisting of plasma extravasation and mast cell changes in the perivascular area (56). These changes result in dilated, swollen, and inflamed blood vessels and transduce pain at the trigeminal nerve endings. The pain is then carried through the trigeminal nerve (first-order neuron) into the second-order neurons in the brain stem. Vasodilation and neurogenic inflammation sensitize the first-order neurons rapidly, often within 30 minutes, resulting in a throbbing head pain that is aggravated by non-nociceptive stimuli, including pulsations of the arteries, and activities that increase intracranial pressure, including physical exercise, bending down, coughing, and sneezing (57). This sensitization of the first-order neurons explains why migraine pain is aggravated by physical activity and why migraine patients prefer to stay quiet and not move during a headache.

Activated first-order neurons transmit pain to the second-order neurons in the trigeminal nuclei. C-Fos studies have shown activation of the trigeminal nucleus caudalis. The activated second-order trigeminal neurons have functional connections to other important brain stem centers, particularly to nausea and vomiting centers such as the nucleus tractus solitarius, the activation of which results in nausea and vomiting. Specific antimigraine agents, namely the triptans, have been shown to bind to the trigeminal nucleus caudalis as well as to its functional connections such as the nucleus tractus solitarius; therefore these agents reduce nausea and vomiting in addition to reducing pain (58).

Further activation and sensitization of the trigeminal system occurs involving the third-order neurons from the thalamus to the cortex, which results in other symptoms of migraine, including photophobia, phonophobia, and osmophobia, as well as allodynia (nonnociceptive stimuli producing pain and discomfort). Allodynia can occur during migraine attacks and usually involves the scalp, face, and sometimes the extremities (57). Cutaneous allodynia may manifest as discomfort when combing the hair, scalp tenderness, and difficulty wearing glasses and contact lenses.

In summary, activation and sensitization of the trigeminal vascular system involving the first-, second-, and third-order neurons account for the majority of migraine symptoms, including throbbing pain aggravated by physical activity and movements, nausea and vomiting, photophobia, phonophobia, osmophobia, and allodynia. Difficulty in concentration and impairment of cognitive functions during a migraine attack can also be accounted for by disturbances in the brain stem centers responsible for attention (e.g., the locus ceruleus) (47).

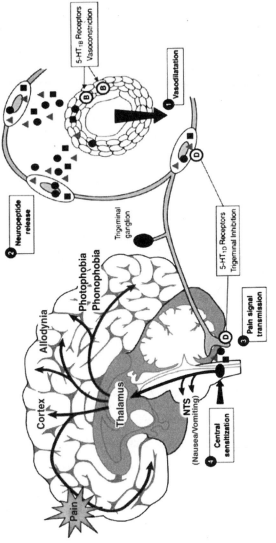

Figure 2–4. Trigeminal vascular pathways involved in the pathogenesis of migraine head pain. Courtesy of R. Hargreaves, MD.

The laboratory correlate of activation of the trigeminal vascular system is the demonstration of elevated levels of CGRP and related peptides in the ipsilateral external jugular venous blood during migraine attacks (38). Sumatriptan reduces CGRP levels and produces clinical improvement. Repeated episodes of migraine result in a chronic sensitized state of the CNS with possible permanent changes in the nociceptive centers of the brain, such as the PAG area, which accounts for daily headache or transformed migraine.

How Specific Antimigraine Medications Work

Specific antimigraine medications such as the triptans, dihydroergotamine, and ergotamine act on the trigeminal vascular system; they are $5\text{-}HT_{1B/1D}$ receptor agonists (59). These agents constrict the dilated extracerebral intracranial blood vessels; reduce neurogenic inflammation around the blood vessels (56); reduce the transmission of pain from outside the brain into the brain; and deactivate the second- and third-order neurons, preventing the progression of the cascade of events that occurs during a migraine attack, which results in the reduction of pain, nausea and vomiting, photophobia, phonophobia, and other associated symptoms. Unlike the triptans, nonspecific medications such as opioids have no vasoconstrictive effect and do not have any specific desensitizing effect on the central trigeminal system.

The Role of Female Hormones in Migraine Pathophysiology

The normal female life cycle is associated with a number of hormonal milestones, including menarche, pregnancy, contraceptive use, menopause, and the possible use of hormone replacement therapy. All these events and interventions alter the level and cycling of sex hormones and may cause a change in the prevalence or intensity of migraine. The menstrual cycle is the result of a carefully orchestrated sequence of interactions among the hypothalamus, pituitary, ovary, and endometrium.

Estrogen and progestins have potent effects on central serotonergic and opioid neurons, modulating both neuronal activity and receptor density. The primary trigger of menstrual migraine appears to be the withdrawal of estrogen rather than the maintenance of sustained high or low estrogen levels (60). However, sustained changes in estrogen levels associated with pregnancy (increased levels) and menopause (decreased levels) also affect headaches. Headaches that occur with premenstrual syndrome appear to be centrally generated and involve inherent rhythms of CNS neurons, including perhaps serotonergic pain-modulating systems.

The basic mechanisms by which fluctuations in female hormones influence the triggering of migraine are not understood at the molecular level. The trigger mechanism may be working through the NO system.

There is still a great deal of unknowns in the pathophysiology of migraine, but modern brain-imaging techniques and advances in molecular biology will help us unravel the mysteries of migraine.

REFERENCES

1. The International Headache Classification of Headache Disorders. *Cephalalgia* 2004;[Suppl 1].
2. Stewart WF, Lipton RB, Celentano DD, et al. Prevalence of migraine headache in the United States in relation to age, income, race and other sociodemographic factors. *JAMA* 1992;267:64–69.
3. Gobel H, Petersen-Braun M, Soyka D. Epidemiology of headache in Germany: a nationwide survey of a representative sample on the basis of the headache classification of the International Headache Society. *Cephalalgia* 1994;14:97–106.
4. Henry P, Michel P, Brochet B, et al. A nationwide survey of migraine in France: prevalence and clinical features in adults. *Cephalalgia* 1992;12:229–237.
5. Rasmussen BK. Epidemiology of headache. *Cephalalgia* 1995;15:45–68.
6. Lipton RB, Stewart WS, Diamond S, et al. Prevalence and burden of migraine in the United States: data from the American Migraine Study II. *Headache* 2001;41:646–657.
7. Scher A, Stewart W, Liberman J, et al. Prevalence of frequent headache in a population sample. *Headache* 1998;38:497–596.
8. Castillo J, Munoz P, Guitera V, et al. Epidemiology of chronic daily headache in the general population. *Headache* 1999;39:190–196.
9. Wang SJ, Fuh JL, Lu SR, et al. Chronic daily headache in Chinese elderly: prevalence, risk factors, and biannual follow-up. *Neurology* 2000;54:314–319.
10. Lanteri M, Minet J, Awiam G, et al. Prevalence and description of chronic daily headache in the general population in France in 2000. *Cephalalgia* 2001;21:468.
11. WHO. World Health Report. www.WHO.INT/WHT/INDEX 2001.
12. Dahlof C. Assessment of health-related quality of life in migraine. *Cephalalgia* 1993;13;233–237.
13. Stewart WF, Lipton RB, Kolodner KB, et al. Validity of the migraine disability assessment (MIDAS) score in comparison to a diary-based measure in a population sample of migraine sufferers. *Pain* 2000;88:41–52.
14. Ware JE, Bjorner JB, Kosinski M. Practical implication of item response theory and computerized-adaptive testing: a brief summary of ongoing studies of widely used headache impact scales. *Med Care* 2000;38:73–82.
15. Stewart WF, Lipton RB. Work-related disability: results from the American Migraine Study. *Cephalalgia* 1996;16:231–238.
16. Stang TE, Osterhaus JT. Impact of migraine in the United States: data from national health interview survey. *Headache* 1992;33:29–35.
17. Osterhaus JT, Gutterman DL, Plachetka JR. Healthcare resource and lost labor: cost of migraine headache in the United States. *Pharmacol Econ* 1992;2:67–76.
18. Burstein R, Yarnitsky D, Goor-Arygh I, et al. An association between migraine and cutaneous allodynia. *Ann Neurol* 2000;47:614–624.
19. Mathew NT, Kailasam J, Seifert T. Clinical recognition of allodynia in migraine. *Neurology* 2004;63.

20. Burstein R, Collins B, Jakubowski M. Defeating migraine pain with triptans: a race against the developing allodynia. *Ann Neurol* 2004;55:19–26.
21. Raskin NH. *Headache,* 2nd ed. New York: Churchill Livingstone, 1988.
22. Joutel A, Bousser MG, Biousse V, et al. A gene for familial hemiplegia migraine maps to chromosome 19. *Nat Genet* 1993;5: 40–45.
23. Ophoff RA, Terwindt GM, Vergouwe MN, et al. Familial hemiplegic migraine and episodic ataxia type-2 are caused by mutations in the Ca2+ channel gene CACNL1A4. *Cell* 1996;87:543–552.
24. DeFusco M, Marconni R, Silvestori L, et al. Halpo insufficiency of ATP1A2: encoding the Na(+)/K (+) pump alpha 2 subunits associated with familial hemiplegic migraine type 2. *Nat Genet* 2003;33:192–196.
25. Lipton RB, Dodick D, Sadovsky R, et al. A self-administered screener for migraine in primary care: the ID Migraine validation study. *Neurology* 2003;61:375–382.
26. Day JW, Raskin NH. Thunderclap headache: symptom of unruptured cerebral aneurysm. *Lancet* 1986;2:1247.
27. Russell MB, Olesen J. Increased familial risk and evidence of genetic factor in migraine. *Br Med J* 1995;311:544.
28. Ulrich V, Gervil M, Kyvik KO, et al. Evidence of a genetic factor in migraine with aura: a population-based Danish twin study. *Ann Neurol* 1999;45:242–246.
29. Gervil M, Ulrich V, Kyvik KO, et al. Migraine without aura: a population-based twin study. *Ann Neurol* 1999;46:606–611.
30A. Lauritzen M. Pathophysiology of migraine aura: the spreading depression theory. *Brain* 1994;117:199–210.
30B. Leao AAP. Spreading depression of activity in cerebral cortex. *J Neurophysiol* 1944;7:359–391.
31. Olesen J, Larsen B, Lauritzen M. Focal hyperemia followed by spreading oligemia and impaired activation of rCBF in classic migraine. *Ann Neurol* 1981;9:344–352.
32. Woods RP, Iacoboni M, Mazziotta JC. Bilateral spreading cerebral hypoperfusion during spontaneous migraine headache. *N Engl J Med* 1994;331:1689–1692.
33. Anderson AR, Friberg L, Olesen TS, et al. SPECT demonstration of delayed hyperemia following hypoperfusion in classic migraine. *Arch Neurol* 1988;45:154–159.
34. Anderson AR, Muhr C, Valind S, et al. Regional cerebral blood flow and oxygen metabolism during migraine with and without aura. *Cephalalgia* 1997;17:570–579.
35. Cutrer FM, Sorensen AG, Weisskoff RM, et al. Perfusion-weighted imaging defects during spontaneous migraine aura. *Ann Neurol* 1998;43:25–31.
36. Friberg L, Olesen J, Larsen NA, et al. Cerebral oxygen extraction, oxygen consumption and regional cerebral blood flow during aura phase of migraine. *Stroke* 1994;25:974–979.
37. Functional MRI (MRI) of visually triggered headache. Activation, suppression and propagation of "bold" effect. *J Cereb Blood Flow Metab* 1997;17[Suppl]:S176.
38. Goadsby PJ, Edmundson L, Ekman R. Vasoactive peptide release in extracerebral circulation of humans during migraine headache. *Ann Neurol* 1990;28:183–187.

39. Weiller C, May A, Limmroth V, et al. Brain stem activation in spontaneous human migraine attacks. *Nat Med* 1995;1:658–660.
40. Night YE, Kaube H, Bartsch T, et al. Effect on trigeminal firing of PQ-type calcium channels in the periaqueductal grey. *Cephalalgia* 2001;21:285.
41. Tajti J, Uddman R, Edvinsson L. Neuropeptide localization in the "migraine generator" region of the human brainstem. *Cephalalgia* 2001;21:96–101.
42. Welch KM, Nagesh V, Aurora S, et al. Periaqueductal grey matter dysfunction in migraine: cause or burden of illness? *Headache* 2001;41:629–637.
43. Raskin NH, Hosobuchi Y, Lamb SA. Headache may arise from perturbation of brain. *Headache* 1987;27:416–420.
44. Goadsby PJ, Gundlach AL. Localization of $_3$H-dihydroergotamine binding sites in the cat central nervous system: relevance to migraine. *Ann Neurol* 1991;29:91–94.
45. Hoskin KL, Bulmer DC, Lasalandra M, et al. Fos expression in the midbrain periaqueductal grey after trigeminovascular stimulation. *J Anat* 2001;198:29–35.
46. Knight YE, Bartsch T, Kaube H, Goadsby PJ. P/Q type calcium channel blockade in the PAG facilities trigeminal nociception: a functional genetic link for migraine. *Neuroscience* 2002;22 (RC213):1–6.
47. Bahra A, Matharu MS, Buchel C, et al. Brain stem activations specific to migraine headache. *Lancet* 2001;357:1016–1017.
48. May A, Goadsby PJ. The trigeminal vascular system in humans: pathophysiologic implications for primary headache syndromes of the neural influences on the cerebral circulation. *J Cereb Blood Flow Metab* 1999;19:115–127.
49. Nishikawa T, Scatton B. Inhibitory influence of GABA on central serotonergic transmission. Raphe nuclei as the neuroanatomical site of GABA-ergic inhibition of cerebral serotonergic neurons. *Brain Res* 1985;331:91–103.
50. Mathew NT, Kurman R, Perez F. Drug-induced refractory headache: clinical features and management. *Headache* 1990;30:634–638.
51. Kaniecki RG, Totten J. Cervicalgia in migraine: prevalence, clinical characteristics and response for treatment. *Cephalalgia* 2001;21:296–297.
52. Ferrari MD, Saxena PR. On serotonin and migraine: a clinical and pharmacological review. *Cephalalgia* 1993;13:151–165.
53. Olesen J, Goadsby PJ. Synthesis of migraine mechanisms. In: Olesen J, Tfelt-Hansen P, Welch KMA, eds. *The headaches,* 2nd ed. Philadelphia: Lippincott Williams & Wilkins, 2000;331–336.
54. Read SJ, Smith MI, Hunter AJ, et al. Enhanced nitric oxide release during cortical spreading depression following infusion of glyceryl trinitrate in the anaesthetized cat. *Cephalalgia* 1997;17:159–165.
55. Moskowitz MA, Nozaki K, Kraig RP. Neocortical spreading depression provokes the expression of c-Fos protein-like immunoreactivity within trigeminal nucleus caudalis via trigeminovascular mechanisms. *J Neurosci* 1993;13:1167–1177.
56. Moskovitz MA. Basic mechanisms in vascular headache. *Neurol Clin* 1997;45:27–31.

57. Burstein R, Yarnitsky D, Goor-Aryeh I, et al. An association between migraine and cutaneous allodynia. *Ann Neurol* 2000; 47:614–624.
58. Goadsby PJ. Current concepts of the pathophysiology of migraine. *Neurol Clin* 1997;15:27–42.
59. Humphrey PPA, Feniuk W. Mode of action of the antimigraine drug sumatriptan. *Trends Pharmacol Sci* 1991;12:444–446.
60. Somerville BW. The role of estradiol withdrawal in the etiology of menstrual migraine. *Neurology* 1972;22:355–365.

Treatment of Acute Attacks of Migraine

Ninan T. Mathew

Aims of treating acute episodes of migraine are (a) to make the patient headache free as soon as possible, (b) to reduce the associated symptoms such as nausea, vomiting, photophobia, or sonophobia, which contribute to disability or impairment, and (c) to reduce the disability from acute attacks so the overall quality of life improves. In addition, growing evidence indicates that the effective treatment of individual attacks, by achieving pain free as soon as possible, before central sensitization and allodynia develops, may reduce the chances for development of transformed or chronic migraine. Therefore, with early effective treatment of individual attacks, we might be able to modify the disorder (1).

MEDICATIONS USED FOR ACUTE ATTACKS OF MIGRAINE

Medications for acute attacks can be divided into nonspecific and specific. Commonly used classes of nonspecific medications are given on Table 3-1. Table 3-2 lists specific acute antimigraine medications. Rescue medication, which can be used in the emergency room or physician's office or by the patient as self-administration (using intramuscular or subcutaneous injections), are given in Table 3-3.

Nonspecific medications are widely used because they are effective in mild to moderate attacks of migraine. They are relatively less expensive and many of them are available without prescription. However, many issues are associated with use of nonspecific medications, which include low efficacy rate, higher recurrence of headaches, higher potential for analgesic rebound, addictive potential with frequent use, and gastric, hepatic, or renal adverse events.

OPTIMIZING TREATMENT WITH NONSPECIFIC MEDICATIONS

Use of Effective Dose

One of the reasons why many patients do not obtain adequate headache relief with nonspecific agents is the inadequate dosing. Normally patients tend to take 200 mg of ibuprofen first and keep repeating 200 mg every 4 to 6 hours, which generally does not help them obtain a pain-free state. If ibuprofen is taken at the dose of 600 to 800 mg initially, however, it may have a better chance of inducing the pain-free state. Soluble preparation of ibuprofen is found to be more effective than regular tablets. Similarly, naproxen sodium 550 to 750 mg is a more effective dose.

Early Treatment

Early treatment with adequate dose should apply to all acute migraine treatments because of development of relative

Table 3-1. Nonspecific medications used for treatment of acute migraine attacks

A. Acetaminophen
B. Prostaglandin inhibitors
   - Aspirin
   - Nonsteroidal inflammatory agents (NSAIDs)
     - Oral
     - Suppositories
     - Injectable
   - COX^2 inhibitors
C. Combination analgesics
   - Isometheptene combinations
D. Combination analgesics with high potential for rebound headaches
   - Aspirin/acetaminophen/caffeine combination
   - Butalbital/caffeine/aspirin/acetaminophen combinations with or without codeine
E. Opioids
   - Oral
   - Transmucosal
   - Nasal spray
   - Injectable

Table 3-2. Specific antimigraine agents Serotonin (5-ht$_{1b/1d}$) agonist

Selective Triptans
Almotriptan (Axert)
Eletriptan (Relpax)
Frovatriptan (Frova)
Naratriptan (Amerge, Naramig)
Rizatriptan (Maxalt)
Sumatriptan (Imitrex, Imigran)
Zolmitriptan (Zomig)
Nonselective Triptans
Ergotamine (Cafergot)
Dihydroergotamine (DHE)—nasal, injectable

gastroparesis and subsequent poor absorption of oral agents from the intestines, development of nausea and vomiting, and most definitely development of central sensitization and cutaneous allodynia. It is clinical common sense to treat migraine head pain before it becomes severe.

Avoid Medications with High Analgesic Rebound Potential

Medications with high potential of analgesic rebound are caffeine/acetaminophen/aspirin combinations. All such combinations

Table 3-3. Pharmacokinetics of oral triptans

Triptans	T-Max	Half-life T$\frac{1}{2}$(h)	Bioavailability	Lipophilicity	Metabolism
Almotriptan (Axert)	1.5–1.9	3.5	70	−0.35	MAO CYP-3A4
Eletriptan (Relpax)	1.5	4–5	50	+0.5	CYP-3A4
Frovatriptan (Frova)	3.3	26	30	−1.5	CYP-1A2
Naratriptan (Amerge, Naramig)	3	6	74	−0.2	MAO CYP1A2 P450
Rizatriptan (Maxalt)	1.5	2	42	−0.75	MAO
Sumatriptan (Imitrex, Imigran)	2 2	15 −1.2	MAO		
Zolmitriptan (Zomig)	2.25	3	40	−0.7	MAO

are available over the counter without prescription. Excedrin Migraine has 65 mg of caffeine in each tablet. Double-blind placebo-controlled studies using caffeine and recent epidemiological studies have clearly shown that caffeine is a major risk factor for rebound headache and chronic migraine (2,3). In addition, excess amounts of caffeine causes other symptoms of caffeinism such as nervousness, tremor, sleeplessness, and anxiety. Many patients with high caffeine intake may have to resort to sleeping pills on a regular basis. Inability to relax because of excess caffeine adds an additional factor that may perpetuate the headache.

Patients may not volunteer the information about their caffeine-containing over-the-counter medication intake because many believe them to be insignificant. Therefore, during history taking, it is critical to ask the patient specifically about nonprescription over-the-counter medication use.

Efficacy for acetaminophen/aspirin/caffeine combinations (Excedrin) has been reported (4). However, these studies have excluded patients with severe migraine, particularly those needing bed rest or having vomiting, and have not collected data beyond 6 hours. Because of the latter, there is no data on the recurrence rate of headaches when using these combination analgesics. Recurrence rate is expected to be very high with their use. Moreover, pain-free rate at 2 hours, which is now accepted as the gold standard primary end point, is low with combination analgesics.

Butalbital/Caffeine/Acetaminophen/Aspirin Combination with and without Codeine

These prescription medications unfortunately are too widely used in the headache population. Note that hardly any well-designed placebo-controlled double-blind trials use these combinations in migraine. Common experience is that these combinations containing butalbital and caffeine, if taken frequently, result in both escalation of headache frequency and intake of medications. Addictive potential of butalbital, a short-acting barbiturate, is well recognized. Sudden withdrawal of these medications may result in a number of withdrawal symptoms such as restlessness, sleeplessness, diarrhea, increased sweating, tremor, and, most disturbingly, generalized seizures.

Concomitant frequent use of medication that causes rebound results not only in increased frequency of headache and escalation of doses but also relative ineffectiveness of preventive medication as well as specific abortive medication such as triptans. Therefore, it is imperative to discontinue the analgesic rebound-producing medications before preventive treatment is prescribed. It is also advised not to combine triptans with combination analgesics. The best combination in the acute therapy is triptans and NSAIDs.

Opioids

Opioids such as codeine, hydrocodone, or OxyContin, if taken frequently, also may result in escalation of headache frequency resulting in eventual excessive use and habituation. Presence of opioids in the system may reduce the effectiveness of preventive and specific antimigraine drugs.

Indications for opioids in acute treatment is very limited. The best indications is in a patient with ischemic heart disease and migraine and migraine in pregnancy, where triptans are contraindicated. There may be an occasional patient who may not respond to triptans, ergotamine, or dihydroergotamine, requiring an opioid as a rescue. A major disadvantage of injectable opioids like morphine or meperidine is their sedating effect, which prolongs the disability of migraine attacks. Transmucosal Fentanyl Citra may be a reasonable alternative, which can be used as a rescue medication at home, avoiding expensive and time-consuming visits to the emergency rooms for attacks that are unresponsive to other agents (5,6).

Apart from the few limited indications just described, opioids have no place in the routine management of migraine attacks. A recent report indicates that daily scheduled opioids (DSO) have not only a low percentage of efficacy but also a high prevalence of misuse (7). Agents like butorphanol nasal spray should be avoided because of their high addictive potential with frequent use.

Stratify Treatment

The two approaches to treatment of acute migraine attacks are step care and stratified care.

Step Care

The mainstream approach to acute treatment of migraine in many countries might be termed *step care* across attacks. Patients are started at the bottom of the therapeutic pyramid, and if the treatments fail, the therapy is escalated. This is the approach recommended in some of the published treatment guidelines. The patient consults, migraine is diagnosed, and the patient starts at the bottom of the therapeutic pyramid. If patients are satisfied with the first-line treatment (usually simple analgesics), they continue it. If not, they may have a follow-up consultation and are prescribed treatment a second time (usually combination analgesics), or all too often they conclude the doctor has nothing to offer and they lapse from care. If second-line treatment works, the patient is satisfied and continues on that treatment; if it does not work, either the patient lapses from care or, if the patient is highly motivated and the doctor allows it, the patient may receive a third-line treatment (specific antimigraine drugs). If this also fails, further options may be explored, such as injectable or nasal rather than an oral triptan, or a different triptan therapy or DHE. At some stage in this sequence of stepwise care, there may be a referral from a primary care to specialist tertiary care.

The fundamental assumption of step care is that all patients have the same treatment needs. This is a useful cost-effective methodology if the patient responds favorably to first-line therapy. The disadvantages of stepwise care are that successful treatment may be delayed, resources may be wasted on follow-up visits and failed prescriptions, patients and physicians may become discouraged, and patients may lapse from care (8).

Stratified Care

Stratified care, in contrast, stratifies attacks and patients according to their therapeutic need. Heterogeneity of migraine demands a stratified approach. Those with severe episodes, which are disabling, would then be assigned specific medications that have proven efficacy, and patients with mild or low disability, whose therapeutic needs are less, may be treated with simple analgesics. Patients and physicians should be flexible in using medications according to need. Patients and their attacks must be stratified. Patient education is highly essential in this respect. Not every attack needs high-end therapy and therefore some flexibility in the treatment approach is essential. Because of the high cost of specific medications like triptans and poor accessibility to obtain them because of managed care restrictions, the following approach is recommended by the French Agence Nationale d'Accréditation et d'Evaluation en Santé (ANAES), October 2002. The author finds this a reasonable guideline, which in essence is a step-care written plan.

ANAES Guidelines

Therapeutic Strategy for Patients Already Treated with Nonspecific Medications

During the first consultation, evaluate the efficacy and tolerability of current nonspecific therapy by ascertaining the following:

- Is the headache significantly relieved within 2 hours of taking the medication?
- Is the patient taking this medicine only once?
- Does the treatment allow this patient to return quickly to normal social, family, and professional activities?
- Is the treatment well tolerated?

If the answer is "yes" to all four questions, no change in the treatment is indicated. If the answer is "no" to one or more out of four questions, prescribe both an NSAID and a triptan.

- Instruct the patient to treat first with the NSAID.
- Use a triptan, if relief is not achieved in 2 hours with the NSAID.
- If the NSAID is not efficacious or not well tolerated, treat with triptan alone.

The French recommendations take into account the heterogeneity of migraine and combine both nonspecific treatment (NSAIDs) and specific agents (triptans).

Using these guidelines, patients should still treat the headache when the pain is mild.

Specific Antimigraine Medications for Acute Attacks

Specific medications used in the treatment of acute attacks of migraine are given in Table 3-2. Selective agents have affinity only to 5-HT$_{1B/1D}$ receptors. In contrast, the nonselective agents have affinity to other serotonin receptors and noradrenergic and dopaminergic receptors as well. Triptans are therefore cleaner drugs with less side effects than ergotamine and dihydroergotamine, which cause more nausea and vomiting because of their affinities to dopaminergic receptors.

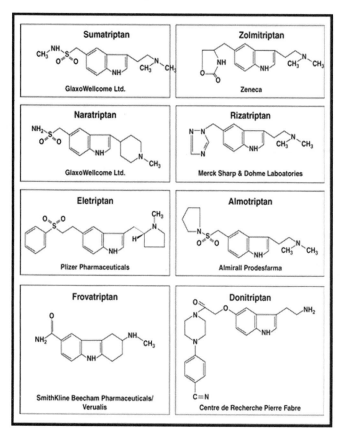

Figure 3.1

TRIPTANS

Triptans are a family of specific serotonin (5-HT$_{1B}$ and 5-HT$_{1D}$ and in some cases 5-HT$_{1F}$) receptor agonists. They are designer drugs obtained by modifying the serotonin molecule. Even though the currently available seven triptans belong to the same family and all have a basic indole ring in their structure, the side chains of each one of them are different (Fig. 3-1). Therefore, the pharmacokinetic properties are also different, which translates into obvious differences in the clinical efficacy. For example, some of them have low T-max (accounting for more rapid onset of action and better efficacy), some have longer half-life (accounting for lower recurrence rate), some are more lipophilic (accounting for better absorption from the intestines and better CNS penetration), and some have poor bioavailability (accounting for inconsistency in response) (9). Therefore, not all triptans are the same in their clinical efficacy and tolerability.

Table 3-4. Available triptan preparations

Triptan	Oral tablet to be swallowed	Rapidly disintegrating over the tongue tablets	Nasal spray	Subcutaneous injection
Almotriptan (Axert)	✓			
Eletriptan (Relpax)	✓			
Frovatriptan (Frova)	✓			
Naratriptan (Amerge, Naramig)	✓			
Rizatriptan (Maxalt)	✓	✓		
Zolmitriptan (Zomig)	✓	✓	✓	
Sumatriptan (Imitrex, Imigran)	✓		✓	✓

Table 3-3 summarizes the pharmacokinetics and metabolic pathways of the seven oral triptans available. Table 3-4 shows the different preparations of triptans available.

Mechanisms of Action of Triptans in Migraine

The mechanisms of action of triptans are multiple (10). Here are the foremost known mechanisms:

1. Normalization of the dilated intracranial arteries (mostly dural) because of their selective cranial vascular constriction effect.
2. Reduction of neurogenic inflammation by reducing the release of vasoactive peptides such as calcitonin gene-related peptide (CGRP) at the perivascular space.
3. Inhibitory effect on the central trigeminal system (trigeminal nucleus caudalis).

At present, it is difficult to say which one of these modes of action has the most import. Central effects may be equally important as their peripheral (first sensory neuron) effects.

Nonoral Preparations of Triptans

Although all seven triptans are available as oral (swallowable) tablets, only a few nonswallowable preparations are marketed. These include rizatriptan wafer (Maxalt MLT), zolmitriptan rapid-dissolving tablets (Zomig ZMT), sumatriptan nasal spray, zolmitriptan nasal spray, and subcutaneous sumatriptan.

Pharmacokinetics and clinical effects of melt preparations (Maxalt MLT and Zomig ZMT) are essentially the same as regular tablets, but convenience of use without having to take water is the main advantage. This may prompt early use of the preparation, which patients can carry with them and use anywhere, any time without water as soon as the headache starts.

Nasal sprays of zolmitriptan and sumatriptan have shorter T-max and therefore more rapid onset of action. The elimination kinetics are the same as that of oral preparation. Even though there are no direct comparative trials, zolmitriptan nasal spray has distinct advantages over sumatriptan nasal spray, which include more rapid onset of action, as early as 10 minutes, and definitely better taste.

Subcutaneous sumatriptan has the shortest T-max of all triptans and the best effects, and it is the preparation of choice when very rapid effect is desired. Therefore, it becomes the primary triptan preparation in the treatment of cluster headache attacks and in migraine attacks of abrupt onset ("crash migraine"). But it has the disadvantage of being an injection and is associated with more side effects such as chest tightness, rush feeling, paraesthesias, and so on. In addition, recurrence rate is also high. The next best preparation for rapid effect is zolmitriptan nasal spray.

Clinical Trials of Triptans

In the traditional triptan trials, patients were asked to wait until the headache was moderate or severe before they took the medication. The primary end point in all the studies was 2-hour headache response, which was defined as moderate or severe head pain becoming mild or no pain in 2 hours after the medication. Secondary end point was 2 hours pain free. Two-hour pain free is the new recommended end point by the International Headache Society. Other secondary end points include relief of nausea, vomiting, photophobia, phonophobia, and improvement in disability. Recurrence of headache (headache returning to moderate or severe after it has been reduced to mild or no pain) within 24 hours was also recorded.

Another important secondary end point was introduced for later studies, namely sustained pain free, which is defined as pain-free response in 2 hours, no recurrence for 24 hours, and no rescue medications for 24 hours. This is the most desirable end point and is being adopted in many new clinical trials. Intrapatient consistency of response and patient acceptability or preference are also evaluated routinely.

NEW PARADIGM IN MIGRAINE THERAPY: EARLY TREATMENT WITH TRIPTANS

Early treatment with triptans when the pain is mild is the current approach to migraine therapy. Early treatment has clinical rationale because most migraine attacks start out as mild headache and progress to moderate or severe in a few hours, and therefore it is clinically logical to treat at the mild stage. Physiological rationales are twofold. First, early treatment with a triptan before the central sensitization and resultant allodynia develops ensures better pain-free response (11). Late treatment after allodynia develops may result in a response that is relatively less satisfactory than the robust pain-free response obtained by early treatment. Central sensitization sets the stage for recurrence of headache and may be responsible also for inconsistent response. Second, a relative gastroparesis develops during untreated migraine attacks, resulting in poor passage of oral medication to the intestines and subsequent poor absorption (12). Early treatment before the gastroparesis sets in, therefore, is important. Early treatment, when the pain is mild, results in early pain-free, less recurrence of headache, less need for multiple medications, less disability, and fewer side effects.

Almotriptan (Axert)

Almotriptan has nanomolecular affinity for 5-HT_{1B}, 5-HT_{1D}, and 5-HT_{1F} receptors, micromolecular affinity of 5-HT_{1A} and 5-HT_7 receptors, and negligible affinity for most other relevant receptors (13). Almotriptan has the highest reported oral bioavailability of 70% among the triptans, with a T-max of 1.5 to 1.9 hours and elimination half-life of 3 to 4 hours. There are no gender-related differences in pharmacokinetics (13). Up to 55% of orally absorbed almotriptan is eliminated unchanged in urine (45%) and stool (10%). Approximately 45% is metabolized (27% through MAO-A and 12% through CYP 3A4 and 2D6) (13). This explains why almotriptan has no significant interactions with other medications. Because the renal elimination route is so important, the dose should not exceed 12.5 mg in 24 hours in patients with severe renal impairment. After double-blind placebo-controlled trials in more than 3,000 migraine patients, 12.5 mg almotriptan was selected as the best dose, considering optimum efficacy and tolerability.

In the meta-analysis of 2,294 patients, 2-hour pain response in traditional trials was 61% compared to 35% with placebo. Almotriptan shows significant onset of efficacy in 30 minutes. Two-hour pain-free response is 39%.

Two randomized controlled trials (RCTs) comparing almotriptan 12.5 mg and sumatriptan (one using 50 mg and another using 100 mg) showed comparable 2-hour headache response. Two-hour pain-free responses for 12.5 mg almotriptan and 100 mg sumatriptan were 39% and 37%, respectively, in one study (13). In addition, fewer patients experienced migraine recurrence with almotriptan 12.5 mg than with sumatriptan 100mg (18.0% vs 24.6 %). Thus 82% of patients treated with almotriptan 12.5 mg maintained pain relief over 24 hours (13a). Finally, Diener and Gebert found that migraineurs who were nonresponders to sumatriptan 50 mg were likely to respond to almotriptan 12.5 mg with a placebolike adverse event profile (13b).

Based on Ferrari meta-analysis (14), almotriptan 12.5 mg, rizatriptan 10 mg, and eletriptan 80 mg showed the highest pain-free response at 2 hours compared to sumatriptan 100 mg. Sustained pain free was also high for almotriptan, along with rizatriptan 10 mg and eletriptan 80 mg.

Safety and Tolerability of Almotriptan

Almotriptan has the best tolerability data of all triptans. Ferrari meta-analysis (14) showed placebo subtracted all adverse events to be lowest for almotriptan and naratriptan (Frova triptan was not included in the meta-analysis).

CNS-adverse events for almotriptan is similar to that of place-bo. Chest symptoms (chest pressure, heaviness, throat symptoms, etc.) are lowest for almotriptan. Sumatriptan produces more chest symptoms than any other triptan.

Consistency of Response

Almotriptan consistency data is one of the best among triptans, 75% responding in two out of three attacks (14). The only other oral triptan with higher consistency data is rizatriptan.

Early Treatment with Almotriptan While the Pain is Still Mild

Since the treatment paradigm has shifted to early treatment with triptan, although the pain is still mild, new studies have been done using almotriptan. Using almotriptan 12.5 mg as early as possible at the onset of migraine headache resulted in a 2-hour pain-free response of 77% and a sustained pain-free response (2–24 hours) of 67% in patients whose pain was treated while pain was mild, compared to 44% and 37% while the pain was treated when it was moderate or severe (15). Recurrence rate after early intervention while the pain was mild was 13% compared to 27% with moderate or severe pain. Need for rescue medication was 9% versus 17%, respectively (15).

Therapeutic Summary of Almotriptan

Overall, almotriptan exhibits the best balance between efficacy and tolerability. Efficacy parameters of significance for almotriptan include speed of onset of action within 30 minutes, high 2-hour headache-free response, high sustained pain-free response, and very good consistency of response. Almotriptan has a tolerability profile that is similar to placebo with the lowest incidence of CNS and chest symptoms among the triptans.

Eletriptan (Relpax)

Eletriptan binds rapidly and selectively to 5-HT_{1B} and 5-HT_{1D} receptors with a four- to eightfold higher affinity than sumatriptan (16). It also has affinity for 5-HT_{1F} receptors. Eletriptan is more lipophilic than other triptans, allowing more rapid and better absorption after oral administration and better penetration into the CNS, even though it is a substrate for the active p-glycoprotein (P–GP) efflux system (17). High lipophilicity more than compensates for the effect of P–GP efflux (17). T-max is 1.5 hours with an elimination half-life of approximately 4 to 5 hours. Thus oral eletriptan is an oral triptan with a low T-max and a long half-life, accounting for its rapid speed of onset and low recurrence rate. Plasma binding of eletriptan is high. Oral bioavailability is 50% compared to sumatriptan with 15%. This accounts for higher consistency of response for eletriptan. Ninety percent of the dose is metabolized through CYP3A4 pathways in the liver. The available dose of eletriptan in the United States is 40 mg, whereas 40 and 80 mg are available in Europe.

Eletriptan has been studied in approximately 11,000 patients, in 74,000 migraine attacks. Combining data from seven pivotal trials revealed a clear dose-response relationship, with 2-hour response rates of 50%, 60%, and 66% for 20, 40, and 80 mg doses, respectively, compared with 24% for placebo ($P < 0.0001$).

Eletriptan 80 mg was also statistically superior to the 40 mg dose (P <0.01) (17).

Two-hour pain-free response and sustained pain-free response showed a similar trend as 2-hour headache response. Three direct comparative trials of eletriptan with 100 mg sumatriptan were done. In a large study involving approximately 2,100 patients, Mathew et al. reported highly statistically significant superiority of 40 mg eletriptan over 100 mg of sumatriptan in all end points studied, including sustained pain free (18). Even though encapsulated sumatriptan was used in direct comparative trials, there was no impact of encapsulation on the efficacy of sumatriptan. *In vitro* dissolution rates and bioequivalence were equal to nonencapsulated sumatriptan. Moreover, the 2-hour response of encapsulated sumatriptan was essentially the same as that of nonencapsulated sumatriptan. Direct comparison with 2.5 mg naratriptan and 40 mg eletriptan, as well as 40 mg eletriptan and 2.5 mg of zolmitriptan, showed that 40 mg eletriptan had significantly a higher sustained pain-free response. Patients who had previously reported inadequate relief from rizatriptan responded to eletriptan very well (19).

Headache Recurrence Rate with Eletriptan

Clinical trials revealed that the recurrence rate of eletriptan is one of the lowest among the triptans. Placebo subtracted recurrence rate is low for 40 mg and 80 mg eletriptan, other triptans with similar low recurrence rates being almotriptan, naratriptan and frovatriptan. But the essential difference between triptans with low recurrence rates, is that eletriptan and almotriptan also demonstrate an initial good response and rapid onset of action.

Data from seven trials showed that a subgroup of patients who were treatment failures with sumatriptan showed a 2-hour headache response rate of 39%, 37%, and 49%, for eletriptan 20, 40, and 80 mg versus 19% for placebo. In switch studies involving patients who failed sumatriptan or NSAIDs treatment, eletriptan 40 mg was found to be significantly effective. Two-hour headache response of eletriptan was reported to be almost double that of ergotamine caffeine combination (Cafergot).

Safety and Tolerability of Eletriptan

Because eletriptan is metabolized through the CYP3A4 system, theoretically there can be interaction with agents metabolized through the same system. Plasma levels of eletriptan may go up in the presence of concomitant CYP3A4 inhibitors (20). An analysis and review of adverse events in eletriptan when combined with CYP3A4 inhibitors has revealed that adverse events were essentially the same whether the patients were on or off CYP3A4 inhibitors, including very potent agents like ketoconazole (20). Although the physician has to be aware of drug interactions and respect the warnings, undue alarm about them is not warranted. Recent coronary angiogram studies in patients with relatively normal coronary arteries, using very high doses of intravenous (IV) eletriptan, did not show any higher reduction of coronary artery diameters compared to 6 mg subcutaneous sumatriptan and placebo. This study, in general, reassures that triptans are relatively safe in patients with normal coronary arteries and points out that even high doses of IV eletriptan were not associated with any increased cardiovascular risk. However, like any other triptans, eletriptan is contraindicated in patients with known coronary artery disease and should be used only after appropriate work-up in those with significant risk factors for vascular disease.

Early Treatment with Eletriptan While the Pain Is Still Mild

A recent placebo-controlled trial by Brandes et al. clearly showed very high 2-hour pain-free response of 71%, 69%, and 67% when eletriptan was used before 30 minutes, between 30 and 60 minutes, and after 60 minutes, respectively, while the pain is still mild (21). The 24-hour sustained pain-free response was 56% compared to 18% with placebo when the medication was taken while the pain is mild.

Therapeutic Summary of Eletriptan

Desirable combination of pharmacokinetics such as a low T-max, longer half-life, and high lipophilicity ensures a rapid onset of action within 30 minutes, high efficacy, very low recurrence rate, and higher sustained pain-free response, which results in having to take only one dose, especially when taken early in the attack when the pain is mild. Among the rapid-acting oral triptans, eletriptan has one of the lowest recurrence rates. Lack of increased reduction in the coronary artery diameter even in the presence of high doses of IV eletriptan and the lack of increased clinical adverse events in the presence of CYP3A4 inhibitors are reassuring.

Frovatriptan (Frova)

Frovatriptan has a terminal half-life of 25 hours, the longest among triptans. It is not metabolized by MAO or by CYP3A4; therefore concerns about drug interaction are almost absent. Preclinical studies have shown a functional selectivity of frovatriptan for cerebral arteries compared to coronary arteries (22). Two-hour response of 2.5 mg frovatriptan in placebo-controlled studies was 37% to 46% compared to 21% to 27% for placebo (P <0.001). Time of onset of action is 1 hour, and median time to headache relief is 3.3 hours. These two facts generally indicate slower onset of action and longer time for relief compared to other agents such as oral almotriptan, eletriptan, rizatriptan, sumatriptan, and zolmitriptan. In long-term trials, median time to relief was 4 hours, which in general is not an acceptable time frame in the majority of patients.

A subset of approximately one third of patients tried on frovatriptan 2.5 mg showed 85% headache response in 2 hours compared to 37% for the total population. Thus there appears to be individual variation to the response of frovatriptan. Recurrence rate of frovatriptan is low. Approximately 17% are probably related to its long half-life.

The best niche for frovatriptan in clinical practice is for "miniprophylaxis" of menstrual migraine. Frovatriptan 2.5 mg twice daily starting a day before the expected day of headache in the perimenstrual time and taken for 5 or 6 days every month has been shown to reduce the chances of menstrually related migraine significantly (23).

The tolerability profile is excellent for frovatriptan. Patients with higher risk for coronary vascular disease tolerated frovatriptan equally well as that without cardiovascular risk. In a randomized double-blind placebo-controlled study of 75 patients, who had previously documented coronary artery disease or were at high risk, frovatriptan was well tolerated without an increase in cardiovascular abnormalities (24). In direct comparison trials with 100 mg sumatriptan, significantly fewer triptan-adverse events including throat tightness were noted with frovatriptan (24). Frovatriptan has been shown to have no significant interactions with ergotamine and propranolol, the two commonly used medications by migraine patients.

Therapeutic Summary of Frovatriptan

Slower onset of action and longer time to get relief offsets the low recurrence rate. Therefore Frova is not the drug of choice for those migraine attacks in which rapid relief is desired. The best area for use of frovatriptans may prove to be in the "miniprophylaxis" for menstrual migraine. Excellent tolerability, particularly less cardiovascular events, is a positive feature. It may prove to be useful in habitually slow-onset prolonged migraine, especially when the use of other triptans is associated with high recurrence, resulting in multiple doses.

Naratriptan (Amerge, Naramig)

Naratriptan in recommended dose of 2.5 mg has been a slower onset of action and poorer 2-hour efficacy than many other triptans. Thus, whereas naratriptan is not the best therapeutic choice for a patient requiring rapid relief, it may be an optimal choice for patients suffering long duration migraine of slow onset or for a patient for whom tolerability is especially important. Like frovatriptan, naratriptan also has excellent tolerability and a low recurrence rate.

Two-hour headache response for naratriptan is approximately 52%, compared to most other triptans, which are in the range of 60% or more (25). In a large open-label study lasting for 1 year in 15,301 migraine attacks, 84% of migraine attacks treated with naratriptan had no adverse events (26). Direct randomized double-blind comparison of 2.5 mg naratriptan with 10 mg rizatriptan showed that naratriptan was better tolerated than rizatriptan, although naratriptan had less efficacy than rizatriptan. In open-label trials, patients cite longer duration of action and fewer side effects as the main reason for preferring naratriptan over other triptans.

Naratriptan has been successfully used in the prodrome phase of migraine with resultant reduction in the severity of subsequent headache phase. Naratriptan has also been shown to be effective in miniprophylaxis of menstrually associated migraine (27). Naratriptan taken twice daily for 5 days beginning 2 days before the expected onset of menstrually related migraine is a useful approach.

Therapeutic Summary of Naratriptan

With relatively longer half-life and low recurrence rate, naratriptan has more or less the same therapeutic features as frovatriptan. Therefore, one of its better indications will be miniprophylaxis of menstrually related migraine. As with frovatriptan, naratriptan may also be considered for patients with habitually slow-onset prolonged migraines.

Rizatriptan (Maxalt)

Rizatriptan has a T-max of approximately 1 hour and a half-life of approximately 2 hours, with an oral bioavailability of 40% to 45%. This pharmacokinetic profile is superior to sumatriptan, which has a T-max of 2.5 hours and bioavailability is around 14%. Rizatriptan has a good dose-response profile. Unlike sumatriptan, rizatriptan is available in 10 mg and 5 mg tablet as well as in a wafer form (Maxalt MLT). The Maxalt wafer form has a distinct advantage of being very user friendly. It can be taken anywhere, anytime without the use of water; therefore the convenience factor is very high with the wafer form compared to the tablet, even though efficacy is no different.

Efficacy of Rizatriptan

Rizatriptan has a high 2-hour pain-free response. In direct randomized double-blind placebo-controlled comparative trials of rizatriptan with sumatriptan, naratriptan, and zolmitriptan, more patients on 10 mg rizatriptan were pain free in 2 hours compared to 100 mg of sumatriptan (40% vs. 33%, P = 0.019), naratriptan 2.5 mg (45% vs. 21%, P = 0.001), zolmitriptan 2.5 mg (43% vs. 26%, P = 0.041) (28). Similar superiority of rizatriptan over sumatriptan, naratriptan, and zolmitriptan has been shown in relieving associated symptoms of migraine. Sustained pain-free response was numerically higher for rizatriptan 10 mg compared to 100 mg sumatriptan (27% vs. 23%) and significantly higher compared to naratriptan 2.5 mg (29% vs. 17%, P = 0.004) and zolmitriptan 2.5 mg (32% vs. 24%, P = 0.013) (28).

In 19,987 migraine attacks treated with 10 mg rizatriptan in an open-label trial, 86% had headache response in 2 hours compared to 56% in 2,240 migraine attacks treated with usual treatments, which include NSAIDs, acetaminophen, ergotamine, indomethacin, opioids, and barbiturate compounds (28). A prospective randomized open-label study in 358 migraine patients that compared rizatriptan 10 mg and sumatriptan 100 mg showed that 57% of patients preferred rizatriptan, whereas 43% preferred sumatriptan.

Meta-analysis of triptans by Ferrari et al. (14) showed that 10 mg of rizatriptan had higher absolute and placebo-subtracted 2-hour headache response, 2-hour pain-free response, 24-hour sustained pain free, and higher consistency of response. In fact, rizatriptan has the best consistency rate compared to other triptans (86%) of patients responded in two out of three attacks.

Early Treatment with Rizatriptan When the Pain Is Still Mild

In one study, it was reported that 70% of patients who took rizatriptan when the pain is still mild became pain free in

2 hours compared to a placebo response of 22% (P = >0.01) (29). Because rizatriptan has a short T-max and rapid onset of action, it is an ideal triptan for early use. In open-label trials, it has been shown that compared to other triptans such as sumatriptan, zolmitriptan, and naratriptan, patients who took rizatriptan needed the least number of tablets per attack for adequate control of their migraine. Those patients who were unresponsive to sumatriptan have been shown to respond significantly to rizatriptan and zolmitriptan, the response to rizatriptan being superior (30).

Therapeutic Summary of Rizatriptan

The low T-max and the rapid onset of action results in one of the best 2-hour pain-free responses with rizatriptan. In addition, the best consistency data makes rizatriptan a very desirable agent for the treatment of acute attacks of migraines. Tolerability is not as good as that of almotriptan. Recurrence rate is higher than that of sumatriptan and much higher than eletriptan. Overall, patient satisfaction is high with rizatriptan, and the number of tablets used to treat individual attacks is lower with rizatriptan compared to sumatriptan, naratriptan, and zolmitriptan. Rizatriptan wafer has the distinct advantage of convenience of use without water and can be taken anywhere anytime. The 5 mg tablets or wafers may be useful for children.

Sumatriptan (Imitrex, Imigran)

Sumatriptan, the first triptan to be introduced, is available in three forms, rapidly dissolving tablet (25 mg, 50 mg, 100 mg), nasal spray (5 mg and 20 mg), and 6 mg subcutaneously.

Subcutaneous sumatriptan with a 95% bioavailability is the most efficacious of all triptans with a 82% efficacy in 2 hours. The recommended dose is 6 mg. Onset of action is extremely rapid—within 10 minutes—and most appropriate for patients with a rapidly peaking headache condition such as cluster headache and nocturnal severe crash migraine. Subcutaneous sumatriptan can be used as a rescue medication when oral triptans fail. In patients with habitually severe attacks, subcutaneous sumatriptan can be prescribed. It has recently been shown that subcutaneous sumatriptan may be effective even in the presence of cutaneous allodynia (31). Subcutaneous sumatriptan may be associated with more triptan symptoms, which include chest discomfort, heaviness of the chest and throat, paresthesias involving the head, neck, and extremities, anxious feeling, and mild difficulty breathing. Some patients get adequate relief with a smaller dose of 3 mg and prefer them over 6 mg. Fewer of these symptoms occur with the use of sumatriptan tablets and sumatriptan nasal spray. In general, chest symptoms occur more commonly with the use of sumatriptan than with other triptans, particularly with almotriptan and eletriptan. Sumatriptan is generally not associated with central nervous systems unlike the newer triptans, which may cause such symptoms as somnolence, asthenia, and dizziness.

Note that the newly released sumatriptan rapid dissolving tablet is still an oral tablet that needs to be swallowed. It dissolves in the stomach more rapidly than the old conventional sumatriptan tablets with resulting reduction of T-max by approximately 10 minutes. There is no evidence that the 2-hour efficacy of the new rapidly dissolving tablet is significantly different from the conventional sumatriptan tablet. The data published so far is not comparable to the original sumatriptan tablets because the study with new rapid dissolving tablets was done while the pain was still mild.

The starting dose for tablets is 100 mg. Up to two tablets can be allowed in 24 hours. Tablets have slower onset of action than subcutaneous sumatriptan. The time of onset of action is around 30 minutes, which is comparable to agents like rizatriptan, eletriptan, and almotriptan. Average 2-hour headache response is 59%.

The recommended dose of sumatriptan nasal spray is 20 mg for adults. Efficacy of sumatriptan nasal spray is intermediate compared to tablets and subcutaneous injections. The time of onset of action after sumatriptan nasal spray is about 15 to 20 minutes. Here again, when rapid onset of action is important, sumatriptan nasal spray is a good option.

Recurrence of headache is a problem with many of the triptans including sumatriptan. Recurrence rate for sumatriptan is about 30%. Recurrence can be treated with a second dose with most patients; however, some have multiple recurrences, which may lead to overuse of medications, resulting in rebound phenomenon. If that happens, patients should be switched to a triptan with low recurrence rate such as almotriptan, eletriptan, naratriptan, or frovatriptan and be started on preventive medications.

Sumatriptan has also been shown to be effective in special subgroups of migraine patients such as women with menstrual migraine, migraineurs with asthma, those with early morning migraine, and in children. In children, appropriate smaller doses are used. Sumatriptan nasal spray has been shown to be useful in the pediatric population, particularly in adolescents.

Early Treatment with Sumatriptan

Recent prospective trials as well as retrospective analysis have shown that early use of sumatriptan tablets including the currently available rapidly dissolving tablets have superior 2-hour pain-free response when used early in the attack while the headache is still mild, compared to when used while the headache is moderate or severe. With early treatment while the pain is still mild, 2-hour pain-free response rate using rapidly dissolving tablets is 66% (32).

Therapeutic Summary of Sumatriptan

Undoubtedly, subcutaneous sumatriptan is the most effective triptan preparation, most useful in rapid-onset disabling migraine and cluster headache attacks where rapid relief is desired. However, its side effect profile may prevent frequent use of sumatriptan injection. Subcutaneous sumatriptan is the drug of choice for cluster headache attack.

The 100 mg sumatriptan tablets are inferior to rizatriptan 10 mg, almotriptan 12.5 mg, and eletriptan 40 mg and 80 mg. It is equal to zolmitriptan and superior to naratriptan and frovatriptan (14).

Sumatriptan nasal spray is more rapid in onset of action than tablets but less than that of subcutaneous preparation. Adolescents may prefer nasal spray. Taste of sumatriptan nasal spray is more unpleasant than that of zolmitriptan nasal spray.

Zolmitriptan (Zomig)

Zolmitriptan (Zomig) is available in three forms at the present time, which include tablets 2.5 mg and 5 mg, rapidly dissolving tablet (zolmitriptan ZMT) 2.5 mg and 5 mg, as well as nasal spray 5 mg. Zolmitriptan has a T-max of 2 hrs with a half-life of 2.5 to 3 hours. The bioavailability is 40% to 48%. The lipophilicity is intermediate between sumatriptan and eletriptan. It has an active metabolite, which itself may have some therapeutic benefit. It has been shown to penetrate the brain and bind itself to brain stem centers such as trigeminal nucleus caudalis and monoaminergic areas.

Zolmitriptan nasal spray is rapidly absorbed. Almost 70% of the absorption in the first hour is through the nasopharynx. Plasma drug levels are noticed early at 5 minutes. Brain levels are noticed very rapidly. Clinical effects begin in 10 minutes, and there is a statistically significant response in 15 minutes in patients with migraine. Because of its rapid absorption, it may become very useful in the acute treatment of cluster headaches. The best indications for zolmitriptan nasal spray would be in migraine patients who need rapid relief including those who wake up early morning or in the middle of the night with a headache, those with crash migraine, and those who cannot afford to spend significant time waiting for the relief of headache such as migraine attacks occurring at work or in school. It may also be the preparation of choice in patients who have nausea and vomiting from the onset and those who find it difficult to swallow tablets. Adolescents and children seem to like nasal spray compared to tablets. The 2-hour headache response, 2-hour head pain-free rate, sustained pain-free and recurrence rates are no different with zolmitriptan tablets compared to sumatriptan. However, the nasal spray has distinct advantages.

Zolmitriptan rapidly dissolving tablets (Zomig ZMT) has the same convenience as rizatriptan wafer (Maxalt MLT). It can be taken without water and used anywhere, anytime. The ZMT tablets have not been shown to be superior in efficacy to regular tablets as in the case of rizatriptan wafer and rizatriptan tablets.

Therapeutic Summary of Zolmitriptan

The main advantage of zolmitriptan is its availability in nasal spray form, which has clearly been shown to have very rapid onset of action. Therefore, zolmitriptan nasal spray is useful in situations where rapid relief is desired. Zolmitriptan nasal spray has the advantage of better taste and may become a very effective agent in cluster headache attacks. Zolmitriptan tablets and ZMT are not superior to sumatriptan tablets and definitely inferior in their efficacy to rizatriptan, eletriptan, and not as well tolerated as almotriptan.

Contraindication for Triptans

Because triptans are known to cause some degree of vasoconstriction of the coronary arteries due to their affinity for 5-HT_{1B} receptors, the following are stipulated as contraindications for triptan use: (a) Ischemic heart disease manifesting as angina at rest or angina on exertion and myocardial infarction. Other cardiac disorders such as arrhythmias are also relative contraindications. (b) Uncontrolled hypertension: However, hypertension that is treated and controlled should not be considered as a contraindication. (c) Hemiplegic and basilar migraine. This is a controversial area and not every headache specialist agrees with this contraindication because neurological complications of migraine are now considered due to neuronal events rather than ischemia. The contraindications were stipulated initially because it was assumed neurological complications of migraine are due to ischemia of the brain. However, for practical purposes, it is prudent not to use triptans in patients with hemiplegic or basilar migraine on a routine basis. (d) Concomitant use of other 5-HT_1 agonists including ergotamine and 5-HT_2 antagonists like methysergide are to be avoided because of the cumulative effect on coronary constriction. (e) Patients with multiple risk factors for coronary disease such as heavy smokers, those with uncontrolled hypertension, untreated hypercholesterolemia, and diabetes should be relative contraindications until a work-up is done to exclude occlusive coronary artery disease.

Tolerability and Safety of Triptans

Triptan Sensations

Sensations of tightness, pain, pressure and heaviness of the chest and throat can occur after treatment with triptans. They are most commonly seen with injectable sumatriptan. Among the rapidly acting oral triptans, sumatriptan has the highest incidence of triptan sensations compared to almotriptan with placebolike side effects. In general, triptans with slow-onset action such as frovatriptan and naratriptan cause less triptan sensations. According to the meta-analysis, by Ferrari et al., almotriptan has an overall tolerability profile superior to sumatriptan and similar to that of raratriptan (14).

Prescribers' concern about cardiovascular safety is one of the major reasons why triptans are still not used very widely in clinical practice. In June 2002 the American Headache Society convened the triptan cardiovascular safety expert panel, whose report was published in 2004 (33). Review of all available data by the panel demonstrated that triptans are generally well tolerated. Chest symptoms occurring during the use of triptans are usually nonserious and usually not attributed to ischemia of the heart. Incidence of triptan associated serious cardiovascular adverse events in both clinical trials and clinical practice appears to be extremely low. When they do occur, serious cardiovascular events have most often been reported in patients at significant cardiovascular risk or those with overt cardiovascular disease. Adverse cardiovascular events have also occurred, however in patients without evidence of cardiovascular disease. Several lines of evidence suggest that nonischemic mechanisms are responsible for triptan-associated chest symptoms, although the precise mechanism of chest symptoms have not been adequately determined to date. The nonischemic mechanisms mentioned are changes in esophageal function, direct effect of the triptan on the pulmonary vasculature, and alteration in energy metabolism of muscle of the chest wall. Importantly, most of the clinical trials and clinical practice data on triptans are derived in patients without cardiovascular disease. Therefore, the conclusion of the panel cannot be extended to patients with cardiovascular disease. The cardiovascular safety profile of triptan favors their use in the absence of contraindications. Based on a review of the cardiovascular tolerability and safety of triptans, the American Headache Society experts panel recommended that risk factors for coronary heart disease be assessed before triptans are prescribed.

Major Risk Factors for Coronary Heart Disease (CHD)

The following are risk factors for CHD: cigarette smoking, hypertension, high (LDL) cholesterol, more than 159 mg per dl, low high-density (HDL) cholesterol (less than 40 mg per dl), family history of premature coronary artery disease (less than 55 years of age in males with first-degree relative or less than 65 years of age in females with first-degree relative), and age: men 45 years or more, women 55 years or more. The current guidelines for cardiovascular risk prediction, although not strongly predictive of acute coronary events, allow stratification of patients according to whether they are at low, intermediate, or high risk for coronary disease and associated sequelae. This frame for risk assessment can be applied to decisions for prescribing triptans. Patients with low risk for coronary artery disease (one or no risk factors) can be prescribed triptans without a need for a more intensive cardiovascular evaluation. Conversely, patients with coronary artery disease or coronary heart disease risk equivalents should not be prescribed triptans according to the current prescribing recommendations. Patients with an intermediate risk of coronary heart disease (two or more risk factors) require more intensive cardiovascular evaluation before triptans can be prescribed.

Practical Issues with Triptan Use

1. *Recurrence is common with many triptans.* If the headache recurs, a second dose of the same triptan can be used effectively in the majority of situations. If the patients have habitual recurrence, an effective triptan with a lower recurrence rate such as almotriptan and eletriptan should be considered. Recurrence can be reduced by early intervention when the pain is still mild, before the allodynia sets in. Recurrence can also be reduced by combining the triptans with a NSAID or a COX2 inhibitor (34).

2. *Partial response.* If the patient responds only partially when a lower dose of a particular triptan dose is used, a second dose can be used within 2 hours or double the dose of the same triptan can be used next time. Sumatriptan 50 mg or zolmitriptan 2.5 mg are examples.

3. *Early-onset nausea and vomiting.* Even though, in the majority of patients, nausea and vomiting occur after the headache

reaches moderate or severe stage, some patients may develop them early in the attacks. Using a nasal or subcutaneous preparation is the most logical choice for this situation. However, patients who dislike nasal spray or injection can combine oral triptan with oral metoclopramide and use them early in the attack.

4. *Lack of response to triptan.* Lack of response to a particular triptan does not mean the whole class has to be given up. It has been shown that those who do not respond to a particular triptan may respond to a different triptan tablet. There are data to show that people who do not respond to sumatriptan may respond to zolmitriptan (35), almotriptan, rizatriptan (35), and eletriptan.

5. *Inconsistency of response.* Inconsistencies are usually due to poor bioavailability of the compound. If a particular triptan is inconsistent in its effectiveness, another triptan with more consistency may be tried.

6. *Tachyphylaxis.* If a triptan loses its effect over a period of time, another triptan should be tried.

7. *Multiple recurrences and rebound.* Rebound may be seen occasionally with the use of triptans (36). If one sees escalation of the frequency of episodes of migraine and escalation of triptan use in a given patient, rebound from triptan may be suspected. In that situation, discontinuing that triptan may result in reduction of the frequency of migraine approximately within 2 weeks. Those patients may need prophylactic therapy and they should be switched to a triptan with a low recurrence rate such as almotriptan and eletriptan.

8. *Enhancing the effect of triptans.* Apart from early treatment, combination of triptan with nonsteroidal naproxen or a COX2 inhibitor is becoming the trend in the treatment of acute migraine.

CLINICAL USE OF NONSELECTIVE 5-HT$_1$ AGONISTS

Ergotamine

The oral and rectal absorption of ergotamine is erratic, displaying great interindividual variation. Bioavailability is less than 5% for the oral dosage form but is considerably higher after rectal dosing (37). Peak plasma concentrations are reached about 1 hour after oral and rectal dosing, but plasma levels after rectal administration are as much as 20 times higher (38,39). The biological effects of the drug last much longer than the drug's short elimination half-life of 2 to 3 hours would suggest. This is probably explained by the actions of one or more of its metabolites. The elimination half-life of its metabolites (20 hours) conforms closely to the duration of peripheral vasoconstriction after ergotamine administration.

Powerful and selective constriction of the external carotid artery and its branches is produced by ergotamine. Only slight alphaadrenergic blockage occurs at doses used clinically, and the vasoconstrictor effect is mediated by a direct effect on arterial serotonin receptors (40). Because ergotamine is a 5HT$_{1B}$/5HT$_{1D}$ receptor agonist, the mode of action in migraine is essentially the same as that of triptans. Ergot alkaloids have been found to depress the firing rate of serotonergic neurons of the brain stem raphe (41), so stabilization of serotonergic neurotransmission may be the major action of ergotamine, as appears to be the case for the preventive antimigraine drugs (42).

Early treatment has been a long tradition with ergotamine. An adequate dose should be taken as soon as possible and should *not* be divided into half-hourly or hourly supplements; if the initial dose fails, subsequent doses usually fail also. A sub-nauseating dose, if possible, should be determined. A dose that provokes nausea—probably a centrally mediated side effect—is too high and may even intensify a migraine attack. The appropriate dosage of ergotamine is best arrived at by titrating the patient's capacity to tolerate ergotamine during a headache-free period. The average dose of the suppository is one half (1 mg), so that if encountering a patient for the first time during a headache attack, it is common to give 1 mg immediately and if there is no improvement within 45 minutes, another 1 mg. Rectal administration is more effective. Nausea and vomiting are limiting side effects. Ergotamine is also contraindicated in coronary and peripheral artery disease.

Dihydroergotamine (DHE)

About 10 years after the introduction to clinical medicine of ergotamine, DHE was studied for its effectiveness in aborting attacks of migraine and found to be as good as ergotamine, if not better (43). It was further noted in early studies that despite the close similarities in chemical structure, unlike ergotamine, DHE had minimal to no effects on peripheral arterial constriction. Modern studies have affirmed that DHE has only modest arterial effects but is a potent venoconstrictor, allowing for its usefulness in the treatment of orthostatic hypotension (44). Like ergotamine, idiosyncratic hypersensitivity to the drug occasionally occurs, and rare instances of severe peripheral arterial spasm and coronary spasm have been reported.

DHE is presently available as a parenteral preparation and as a nasal spray. A major advantage of DHE over ergotamine is that the former can be given IV with far less nausea, and thus it can terminate an acute attack quickly even when the attack is at its peak and attended by profuse vomiting and prostration (45). Therefore, IV DHE is the most useful recommendation in an emergency room setting. A further advantage is that it does not result in physical dependence (46).

DHE for Acute Migraine

Following parenteral administration, peak plasma levels of DHE are rapidly achieved: 15 to 45 minutes after it is given subcutaneously, 30 minutes after intramuscular (IM) administration, and 2 to 11 minutes following IV dosing. Plasma levels obtained after subcutaneous dosing are 40% lower than those after IM administration of 1 mg. Therefore, IM administration of 1 mg is preferable to subcutaneous administration. Patients can be taught to self-administer IM injection. After DHE nasal spray administration, plasma levels ware achieved in 30 to 60 minutes. Nasal DHE (Migranal) is slower in onset of action than triptans, and the currently available preparation is not very user friendly. However in patients who do not respond to triptan or are not able to tolerate them, DHE nasal spray is a good alternative. Recurrence rate is less with DHE nasal spray than with triptans.

For attacks that have already climaxed, the accepted protocol includes prochlorperazine, or metoclopramide 5 mg IV, followed immediately by 0.5 mg DHE given IV slowly, over 2 to 3 minutes. If the attack has not begun to subside in 30 minutes, another 0.5 mg DHE is given IV (with or without prochlorperazine or metoclopramide). Using this protocol in a prospective controlled study with patients entering a hospital emergency department because of headache, 85% were treated successfully, without the need for narcotic analgesics (46).

DHE in Intractable Migraine

Mathew et al. have documented that episodic migraine may become incessant and refractory to standard therapy (47). For many of these patients, drug dependence cycles have become established; for others, disabling headaches continue unabated, seemingly indefinitely. The use of DHE 0.5 ml given IV every 8 hours has revolutionized the therapeutic approach to this segment of the patient population, 90% of whom become headache free within 2 days of treatment (46). Metoclopramide 5 mg is used adjunctly with DHE. In order for IV DHE to be successful to break the cycle of status migrainosus or chronic migraine, the following conditions have to be met: (a) Patients should be taken off drugs, which cause rebound such as caffeine containing analgesics, butalbital combination analgesics, and opioids. (b) Opioids such as meperidine should not be given concomitantly with DHE.

ANTIEMETIC AND PROKINETIC AGENTS

Metoclopramide

Nausea and vomiting are common symptoms of migraine. Even though triptans reduce nausea and vomiting along with the reduction of headache, some patients may still require an antiemetic agent in addition. Gastric stasis and subsequent delayed absorption of medications occurs during migraine. Metoclopramide, because of its antiemetic properties and its ability to promote gastric emptying (gastric prokinetic agent), is most suitable for migraine patients. It is a dopamine and 5-HT$_3$ receptor antagonist with no antipsychotic or sedative effect. It is rapidly absorbed from the gastrointestinal tract and has a half-life of 4 to 6 hours. It easily crosses the blood–brain barrier.

Metoclopramide is usually combined with oral agents including NSAIDs and triptans. Oral dose is 10 to 20 mg, rectal suppository is 20 mg, or an IM dose of 10 mg may be used. If there is risk for vomiting, metoclopramide can be administered 10 to 20 minutes before the acute antimigraine medication is given. Metoclopramide (5 mg IV) can be combined with DHE IV in patients with status migrainosus.

Akathisia and restlessness occurs as side effects with IV use. Dystonic reactions can occur, but rarely.

Domperidone

Domperidone, a related compound available in Europe, is also effective in treating nausea of migraine. It has the advantage of not producing any extrapyramidal side effects. Domperidone

(30 mg) has been shown to abort a migraine attack if given in the prodromal phase.

Neuroleptics

Prochlorperazine

Prochlorperazine 10 mg IV has been shown to be effective in treating not only the nausea and vomiting of migraine, but the pain itself (48). Prochlorperazine may be a useful alternative to opioids in the emergency room. Ten milligrams can be repeated in 30 minutes if necessary.

Dystonic reaction may occur, but it is less sedating than chlorpromazine. Orthostatic hypotension is not common as a side effect of prochlorperazine unlike chlorpromazine.

Chlorpromazine

A 12.5 mg IV dose is an effective agent for treating migraine attacks in the emergency room. Orthostatic hypotension is a common side effect. Therefore, patients should be asked to lie down for at least 2 hours after the drug is given. A dose can be repeated in 30 minutes if necessary. Sedation is a common side effect.

Droperidol

Droperidol, an anesthetic adjunct, has been shown to be a useful antimigraine agent in an emergency room setting (49). The recommended dose would be 2.5 mg IV or IM. Sedation is a prominent side effect.

TREATMENT OF ACUTE MIGRAINE IN SPECIAL CIRCUMSTANCES

Menstrually Associated Migraine (MAM)

There are two approaches to treatment of menstrually associated migraine, which typically starts a day or two before the menstruation, on the first day of menstruation, or toward the end. Untreated menstrual migraine may last 4 or 5 days. The first approach is *abortive treatment,* using a triptan or an NSAID or a combination of the two at the very onset of headache and repeating them if the headache recurs. Menstrually related migraines do respond to triptans equally well as nonmenstrual migraine. Triptans with good efficacy and a low recurrence such as eletriptan are preferred for this approach. The second approach is *miniprophylaxis.* Those who have regular menstruation and predictable onset of headache in relation to menstrual flow may be given a triptan with a low recurrence rate twice daily starting a day before the expected day of headache 4 or 5 days every month, so the headache can be prevented. There is some good data with frovatriptan 2.5 mg twice a day and reasonable data with naratriptan 1 mg twice a day with this kind of approach. Eletriptan with its low recurrence rate may also be a good candidate for such an approach.

Early Morning Headache

Some patients habitually wake up very early in the morning with migraine episodes. If that is a pattern, it may be worthwhile using a longer acting triptan just before they go to bed to see whether one could prevent such an attack. (This approach is still anecdotal.)

Headache in High Altitudes

Migraineurs who go to high altitude for vacation or skiing may develop severe episodes of migraine on arrival. In order to prevent such episodes, miniprophylaxis with a triptan may be worthwhile considering.

Headache in the Emergency Room

Patients with status migrainosus (migraine that lasts for more than 72 hours associated with nausea, vomiting, photophobia, and sometimes dehydration) may not respond to oral medications at that state. The following are the options in the emergency room when such a patient arrives for treatment: (a) IV DHE 1 mg combined with metoclopramide 5 mg given slowly. This could be repeated after 6 hours. (b) IV sodium valproate (Depacon) 500 mg diluted in 20 cc normal saline IV push may be a good alternative (50). (c) Those who cannot tolerate DHE or do not get adequate relief from Depacon may be given neuroleptics such as IV prochlorperazine, IV chlorpromazine, or IV or IM droperidol as already described.

Is there a place for opioids in the emergency room? In the majority of patients with migraine in the emergency room, opioid treatment is not necessary because they do respond to one of the medications just listed. The opioids should be used only as a last resort as a rescue medication, and it is also important to emphasize that specific medications like DHE should not be mixed with opioids.

REFERENCES

1. Loder E, Biondi D. Disease modification in migraine: a concept that has come of age? *Headache* 2003;43(2):135–143.
2. Silverman K, Evans SM, Strain EC, et al. Withdrawal syndrome after double blind cessation of caffeine consumption. *N Engl J Med* 1992;327:1109–1114.
3. Scher AI, Lipton RB, Stewart W. Risk factors for chronic daily headache. *Curr Pain Headache Rep* 2002;6:486–491.
4. Lipton RB, Stewart WF, Ryan RE. Efficacy and safety of acetaminophen, aspirin, and caffeine in alleviating migraine headache pain: three double-blind, randomized, placebo-controlled trials. *Arch Neurol* 1998;55(2):210–217.
5. Singer RS. Oral transmucosal fentanyl citrate in the outpatient treatment of severe pain from migraine headache. *Pain Clinic* 2004;6:10–13.
6. Landy S. Oral transcutaneous fentanyl citrate (OTFC) for the treatment of migraine headache pain: a case series in outpatients. *Headache* 2003;43:529.
7. Saper JS, Lake AE, Hamel RL, Lutz TE, et al. Daily scheduled opioids for intractable head pain: long term observations of a treatment program. *Neurology* 2004;25 62(10):1687–1694.
8. Lipton RB, Stewart WF. Clinical application of zolmitriptan. *Cephalalgia* 1997;17(Suppl 18):53–59.
9. Goadsby PJ. A triptan too far? *J Neurol Neurosurg Psychiatry* 1988;64:143–147.

10. Hargreaves R, Shepheard SL. Pathophysiology of migraine—new insights. *Can J Neuro Sci* 1999;26(Suppl 3):S12–S19.
11. Burstein R, Collins B, Jakubowski M. Defeating migraine pain with triptans: a race against the development of cutaneous allodynia. *Ann Neurol* 2004;55(1):19–26.
12. Volans GN. The effect of metoclopramide on the absorption of effervescent aspirin in migraine. *Br J Clin Pharmacol* 1975;2:57–63.
13. Pascual J. Almotriptan. In: Humphrey P, Ferrari M, Olesen J, eds. *The triptans: novel drugs for migraine.* New York: Oxford University Press 2001;247–252.
13a. Dowson AJ, Massiou H, Lainez JM, Cabarrocas X. Almotriptan is an effective and well-tolerated treatment for migraine pain: results of a randomized, double-blind, placebo-controlled clinical trial. *Cephalalgia* 2002;22:453–461.
13b. Diener HC, Gebert I. A double-blind, randomized, parallel-group trial of almotriptan 12.5 mg vs placebo in migraine patients who respond poorly to sumatriptan 50 mg. *Neurology* 62(5, Suppl 7):A151–A152.
14. Ferrari MD, Roon KI, Lipton RB, et al. Oral triptans (serotonin 5-HT(1B/1D) agonists) in acute migraine treatment: a meta-analysis of 53 trials. *Lancet* 2001;358(9294):1668–1675.
15. Mathew NT. Early intervention with almotriptan improves sustained pain-free response in acute migraine. *Headache* 2003;43(10):1075–1079.
16. Bradsley-Elliott A, Noble S. Eletriptan CNS. *Drugs* 1999;12:325–333.
17. Jackson N. Experience with eletriptan. In: Humphrey P, Ferrari M, Olesen J, eds. *The triptans: novel drugs for migraine.* New York: Oxford University Press 2001;247–252.
18. Mathew NT, Schoenen J, Winne P, et al. Comparative efficacy of eletriptan 4 mg versus sumatriptan. *Headache* 2003;43(3);214–222.
19. Goldstein J, Tiseo P, Denaro J, et al. Eletriptan for acute treatment of migraine in patients with unsatisfactory response to rizatriptan. *Headache* 2004;44:473.
20. Mathew NT. Tolerability and safety of eletriptan in the treatment of migraine: a comprehensive review. *Headache* 2003;43:962–974.
21. Brandes JL, Roberson S, Hilliard B, et al. Early treatment of migraine: a prospective double-blind placebo-controlled trial of eletriptan in the early stages of attack. *Headache* 2004;44:467–468.
22. Parsons AA, Raval P, Smith S, et al. Effects of the novel high-affinity 5-HT(1B/1D) receptor legend frovatriptan in human isolated basilar and coronary arteries. *J Cardiovasc Pharmacol* 1998;32:220–224.
23. Frovatriptan in menstrually associated migraine: On file. Vernalis.
24. Elkind AH, Satin LZ, Nila A, Keywood C. Frovatriptan use in migraineurs with or at high risk of coronary artery disease. *Headache* 2004;44:403–410.
25. Mathew NT, Asgharnejad M, Webester C, et al. Naratriptan is effective and well tolerated in the acute treatment of migraine: results of a double-blind placebo-controlled crossover study. *Neurology* 1997;49:1485–1490.

26. Heywood J, Bomhof MA, Pradalier A, et al. Tolerability and efficacy of naratriptan tablets in the acute treatment of migraine attacks for 1 year. *Cephalalgia* 2000;20:470–474.
27. Newman LC, Mannix L, Landy S, et al. Naratriptan as prophylaxis for menstrually associated migraine: a randomized, double-blind placebo controlled study. *Cephalalgia* 2000;20:424.
28. Allen C. Rizatriptan: clinical update. In: Humphrey P, Ferrari M, Olesen J, eds. *The triptans: novel drugs for migraine.* New York: Oxford University Press 2001:199–205.
29. Mathew NT, Kailasam J, Meadors L. Early treatment of migraine with rizatriptan—a placebo controlled study. *Headache* 2004;44:669–673.
30. Mathew NT, Kailasam J, Gentry P, et al. Treatment of nonresponders to oral sumatriptan with zolmitriptan and rizatriptan: a comparative open trial. *Headache* 2000;40:464–465.
31. Freitag F, Diamond S. Does sumatriptan 6 mg subcutaneous override the effects of allodynia in acute migraine outcome? *Headache* 2004;44:476–477.
32. Carpay J, Schoenen J, Ahmad F, et al. Efficacy and tolerability of sumatriptan tablets in a fast-disintegrating formulation for acute treatment of migraine: results of a multicenter, randomized, placebo-controlled study. *Clin Ther* 2004;26:214–223.
33. Dodick DW, Martin VT, Smith T, et al. Cardiovascular tolerability and safety of triptans. A review of clinical data. *Headache* 2004 (Suppl 1):S20–S30.
34. Krymchantowski AV, Bigal ME. Rizatriptan versus rizatriptan plus rofecoxib versus rizatriptan plus tolfenamic acid in the acute treatment of migraine. *Headache* 2004;44:465–466.
35. Mathew NT, Kailasam J, Gentry P, et al. Treatment of nonresponders to oral sumatriptan with zolmitriptan and rizatriptan. A comparative open trial. *Headache* 2000;40:464–465.
36. Katsarava Z, Fritsche G, Muessig M, et al. Clinical features of withdrawal headache following overuse of triptan and other headache drugs. *Neurology* 2001;57:1694–1698.
37. Perrin VL. Clinical pharmacokinetics of ergotamine in migraine and cluster headache. *Clin Pharmacokinet* 1985;10:334–352.
38. Ibraheem JJ, Paalzow L, Tfelt-Hansen P. Low bioavailability of ergotamine tartrate after oral and rectal administration in migraine sufferers. *Br J Clin Pharmacol* 1983;16:695–659.
39. Sanders SW, Haering N, Mosberg H, et al. Pharmacokinetics of ergotamine in healthy volunteers following oral and rectal dosing. *Eur J Clin Pharmacol* 1986;30:331–334.
40. Muller-Schwelnitzer E. Studies on the 5-HT receptor in vascular smooth muscle. *Res Clin Stud Headache* 1978;6:6–12.
41. Muller-Schwelnitzer E. Pharmacological actions of the main metabolites of dihydroergotamine. *Eur J Clin Pharmacol* 1984;26:699–705.
42. Aghajanian GK, Wang RY. Physiology and pharmacology of central serotonergic neurons. In: Lipton MA, Dimascio A, Kollan KF, eds. *Psychopharmacology: a generation of progress.* New York: Raven Press, 1978:171–183.
43. Horton BT, Peters GA, Blumenthal LS. A new product in the treatment of migraine: a preliminary report. *Mayo Clin Proc* 1945;20:241–248.

44. Aellig WH. Investigation of the venoconstrictor effect of 8'hydroxydihydroergotamine, the main metabolite of dihydroergotamine in man. *Eur J Clin Pharmacol* 1984;26:239–242.
45. Callaham M, Raskin NH. A controlled study of dihydroergotamine in the treatment of acute migraine headache. *Headache* 1986;26:168–171.
46. Raskin NH. Repetitive intravenous dihydroergotamine as treatment for intractable migraine. *Neurology* 1986;36:995–997.
47. Mathew NT, Stubits E, Nigam MP. Transformation of episodic migraine into daily headache: Analysis of factors. *Headache* 1982;22:66–68.
48. Jones J, Sklar D, Dougherty J, et al. Randomized double-blind trial of intravenous prochlorperazine for the treatment of acute headache. *JAMA* 1989;261:1174–1176.
49. Silberstein SD, Young WB, Mendizaleal JE, et al. Acute migraine treatment with droperidol: a randomized double blind placebo controlled trial. *Neurology* 2003;60:315–321.
50. Mathew NT, Kailasam J, Meadors L, et al. Intravenous valproate sodium (Depacon) aborts migraine rapidly. A preliminary report. *Headache* 2000;40:720–723.

Preventive Treatment of Migraine

Ninan T. Mathew

Treatment of individual attacks of migraine generally does not prevent the next attack coming on. However, frequent use of acute medications, whether they are over-the-counter nonprescription agents or prescription drugs, may result in increased numbers of headache, leading to medication overuse. A significant number of patients with migraines, therefore, require preventive treatment. Preventive treatment can be divided into pharmacological and nonpharmacological approaches. Many chronic migraine patients may require a combination of the two.

GOALS OF PREVENTIVE TREATMENT

Goals of preventive treatment of migraine are (a) reduction in the frequency, severity, and duration of migraine attacks, (b) reduction of disability and improvement of the quality of life, and (c) improvement of the responsiveness of acute attacks to abortive therapy.

INDICATIONS FOR PHARMACOLOGICAL PREVENTIVE TREATMENT

The following is a modified list from the U.S. Headache Consortium Guidelines (1):

1. Migraine that substantially interferes with patient's daily routine despite acute treatment. Missing work, being ineffective at work, or interference with routine household tasks and activities or inability to plan and enjoy social and leisure activities are considerations for prophylactic treatment.
2. High frequency of migraine attacks (usually more than two per week). High frequency results in increased disability and higher chances of increased acute medication overuse.
3. Chronic migraine.
4. Failure of acute medications.
5. Contraindications to acute medications, especially those with ischemic heart disease.
6. Troublesome adverse events from acute medications.
7. Acute medications overuse (more than two times a week).
8. Special circumstances such as hemiplegic or basilar migraine with risk of neurological injury.

Table 4-1 lists the currently used medications for migraine prevention.

HOW DO PREVENTIVE MEDICATIONS WORK?

Ample evidence suggests there is a central neuronal hyperexcitability in patients with migraine (2–9). Agents that reduce frequency and severity of migraine may be acting by decreasing

Table 4-1. Currently used medications for migraine prevention

Beta-Adrenergic Blockers
Propanolol[a]
Timolol[a]
Nadolol
Metoprolol

Tricyclic Antidepressants
Amitriptyline
Nortriptyline
Protriptyline
Doxepin

Other Antidepressants
SSRIs[b]
SNRIs (e.g., Venlafaxine)

Antiepileptic Agents
Divalproex sodium[a]
Topiramate[a]
Gabapentin
Lamotrigine
Levetiracetam
Zonisamide

Calcium Channel Blockers
Verapamil
Flunarizine
Diltiazem

5-HT$_2$ Antagonists
Methysergide
Methylergonovine
Cyproheptadine
Pizotifen

Neurotoxins
Botulinum Toxin Type A (Botox)

NSAIDs and COX$_2$ Inhibitors
Atypical Antipsychotics
—Naproxen, Fenamate
—Valdecoxib

Angiotensin Inhibitors
—Angiotensin-converting enzyme (ACE) inhibitor: Lisinopril
—Angiotensin II Type 1 (AT1) receptor blocker: Candesartan

continued

Table 4-1. *Continued*

Miscellaneous Agents

Riboflavin

Coenzyme Q10

Feverfew

Magnesium

[a]Approved by the FDA in the United States.
[b]Migraine-preventive efficacy of SSRIs has not been shown.

central hyperexcitability, thereby raising the threshold for cortical spreading depression. They may reduce activation of "migraine generators" and enhance central antinociception.

A number of biochemical and neurophysiologic observations suggest that mobilization of serotonin (5-HT) may precipitate a migraine attack (10–13). The preventive medications have diverse modes of action centrally in the brain. They may involve one or many of the following mechanisms: 5-HT_2 antagonism, regulation of voltage gated ion channels, modulation of central neurotransmitters (norepinephrine, serotonin, and dopamine), enhancement of GABAergic inhibition, and alteration in neuronal oxidative metabolism. None of the migraine preventive agents are specific for migraine, and none of them are effective in more than 60% to 65% of patients. They all have other primary indications.

DRUG SELECTION FOR PREVENTION

Factors determining the selection of agents depend on (a) patient profile, age, frequency and severity of migraine attacks, and the degree of disability, (b) relative efficacy of the drug, (c) comorbidity, (d) side effect profile of the drug, and (e) risk-to-benefit ratio.

FACTORS THAT INTERFERE WITH THE EFFECT OF PREVENTIVE MEDICATIONS

1. Concomitant frequent use of analgesics, particularly combination analgesics containing caffeine, butalbital, and opioids.
2. Concomitant overuse of 5-HT_1 agonist, including ergotamine and triptans.
3. Vasodilatory drugs such as nitroglycerin and nifedipine.
4. Oral contraceptives (in some patients).

REASONS FOR FAILURE OF PREVENTIVE THERAPY

The reasons of failure of preventive therapy include incorrect diagnosis, failure to recognize comorbidities, concomitant use of analgesic rebound-producing agents, inadequate doses, inadequate treatment period, not adopting strategic copharmacy (described later), and unrealistic expectations. Because none of the preventive medications are more than 60% to 65% effective, chronic frequent migraines are difficult to control fully. These facts should be explained to the patient before treatment is begun, so the patient will have realistic expectations about the outcome of the treatment. Not addressing behavioral and lifestyle issues (nonpharmacological treatments) while on medication is another major reason for treatment failure.

PRACTICAL CONSIDERATIONS IN PREVENTIVE PHARMACOTHERAPY

The following are some of the practical considerations while using preventive therapy:

1. *Start small, go slow.* It is extremely important to start with small doses of prophylactic medication initially and to build up the dosage gradually because patients tolerate the medication better with this strategy. For initial therapy, choose the most effective agent with fewer side effects. Large doses of any agents on the first day may cause significant side effects and the patient may hesitate to continue the medication. This is particularly true of medications such as amitriptyline and topiramate. Migraine patients frequently require a lower dose of a preventive medication than needed for other conditions. For example, migraine patients require amitriptyline generally in the dose of 25 to 50 mg, whereas larger doses are used for patients with depression. Similarly, the topiramate dose for migraine is around 100 mg per day, whereas patients with epilepsy may require 400 mg or more per day. Gradual building up of the dose to therapeutic level cannot be overemphasized.

2. *Give adequate trial with optimum dose.* Try medication for at least 3 months before pronouncing it ineffective.

3. *Withdraw medication gradually.* This is particularly important in beta-blockers, calcium channel blockers, and selective serotonin uptake inhibitors (SSRIs). If headaches are well controlled, a drug holiday can be undertaken following a slow taper program. Many patients experience continual relief after discontinuing medications or may not need the same dose. Dose reduction may provide better risk-to-benefit ratio. However, a significant number of patients with frequent or chronic migraine may need to continue their medications for a long time.

STEPS BEFORE PREVENTIVE THERAPY IS INITIATED

Steps before preventive therapy is initiated include recognition of medical comorbidities such as hypertension and asthma and psychiatric comorbidities such as depression, panic attacks, anxiety, and bipolar illness. Analgesic/ergotamine and triptan rebound must be recognized. Such patients must be detoxified from the offending medications before preventive treatment is prescribed. Always combine pharmacotherapy with nonpharmacological approaches including dietary adjustments, physical exercise, and relaxation using any suitable technique, particularly biofeedback and behavioral counseling. Lifestyle changes such as regular sleep habits and avoiding unnecessary stressful routines are essential. Adequate contraception for women with the potential to become pregnant is extremely important.

Whenever possible, use one agent at a time. There is a place for rational strategic copharmacy, discussed later.

LENGTH OF TREATMENT

There is no set rule for the length of treatment using preventive medications. Generally, preventive treatment is given for at least 6 months. Patients must understand that preventive medications take a number of weeks to show the desired effect. Premature discontinuation and frequent switching of medications should be discouraged. Many patients with chronic migraine need continuous prophylactic therapy.

TACHYPHYLAXIS TO PREVENTIVE THERAPY

Clinical experience has indicated that tachyphylaxis becomes a problem in long-term management with preventive agents. Even very effective medications such as methysergide may produce tachyphylaxis after a while; therefore, it is important to monitor the patient over a period of time and adjust the dosage or change medication if necessary. Overall, assessment of success of prophylactic therapy may become difficult because of spontaneous improvement in migraine, unpredictable cycles of worsening in some patients, and high placebo response.

BETA ADRENERGIC BLOCKING AGENTS

Table 4-2 lists the usual dosages of the commonly used beta adrenergic blocking agents that are effective in migraine prevention (14). The biological basis of the effect of beta-blockers in migraine may include 5-HT_{2B}, reduction of the amplitude of contingent negative variation (CNV), and blockage of the nitric oxide activity. Clinical efficacy of beta-blockers has been shown to have no correlation to its ability to enter the central nervous system, membrane stabilizing properties, 5-HT_2 blocking properties, or beta receptor selectivity.

Beta-blockers are particularly effective for patients with migraine associated with stress, hypertension, and angina. The antianxiolytic property of beta-blockers help particularly for people under stress who cannot relax and have frequent migraines.

Beta-blockers are generally fairly tolerated by healthy young adults. However, they can produce fatigue, lethargy, depression, and mild cognitive impairment. Nocturnal hallucinations are not uncommon with agents like propranolol, whereas it is rare with nadolol. Fatigue is also more commonly seen with propranolol than with nadolol. Beta-blockers generally should be avoided in patients with severe depression. Decreased exercise tolerance may be a problem and may restrict their use by athletes. Decreased exercise tolerance has to be explained to the patient before it is prescribed. Less common adverse events include male impotence, orthostatic hypotension, and bradycardia. Beta-adrenergic agents are contraindicated in patients with congestive cardiac failure, asthma, Raynaud's disease, and insulin-dependent diabetes. Beta-blockers should be avoided in asthenic patients with no energy levels.

For comparison purposes, Pfelt-Hansen and Welch (15) developed a scheme of rating clinical efficacy, scientific proof of

Table 4-2. Beta adrenergic blocking agents

Medication	Dosages
Propranolol (Inderal)[a]	40–240 mg per day in divided doses
Propranolol Long-Acting (Inderal LA)[a]	60–160 mg once daily
Nadolol (Corgard)	40–160 mg once daily
Timolol (Blocadren)[a]	Up to 20 mg twice daily
Metoprolol (Lopressor)	50–100 mg per day
Atenolol (Tenormin)	50–100 mg per day

[a]FDA approved for migraine in the United States.

efficacy, and potential for side effects rated from a scale from 1+ to 4+++. Table 4-3 gives a rating modified from Pfelt-Hansen and Welch. Beta-blockers in general are rated high in clinical efficacy.

ANTIEPILEPTIC DRUGS

Normally, a balance exists between GABAergic inhibition and amino acid–mediated excitation in the central nervous system. It is possible that there is a disinhibition due to decreased GABAergic inhibition that results in central neuronal hyperexcitability in migraine patients. This situation is similar to what one might see in epilepsy. GABA is highly concentrated in the visual cortex and periaquaductal area of the brain stem. GABA receptor subunits are expressed in cerebral blood vessels as well (16).

Valproate

A dual action of valproate results in reduction of migraine frequency and severity. The central action in the brain includes an elevation of brain GABA levels, reduction of the firing rates of serotonergic cells in the dorsal raphe (17), and reduction of c-Fos activation in the trigeminal nucleus caudalis (18). The peripheral effects include reduction of experimental neurogenic inflammation in the trigeminal vascular system, an effect mediated through $GABA_A$ receptor agonism (19). A number of randomized double-blind placebo-controlled clinical trials have been done on valproate in migraine that proved efficacious (20–22). Divalproex sodium (Depakote) 500 to 1,000 mg and sodium valproate are effective as is the extended-relief formulation (Depakote ER). The comparative study with propranolol has shown that the efficacy of valproate is more or less equal to that of propranolol for the frequency of reduction and reduction of headache days per month (23).

The most common initial side effect of valproate is nausea and/or vomiting, but as treatment continues, this side effect gradually lessens. It appears that the extended-release divalproex sodium (Depakote ER) has fewer side effects compared to

Table 4-3. Clinical efficacy,[a] scientific proof of efficacy, and potential for side effects,[a] rated on a scale from + to ++++ for some drugs used in migraine prophylaxis

Drug	Clinical efficacy	Scientific proof of efficacy	Side effect potential	Examples of side effects (examples of contraindications)
Beta-blockers				
Propranolol Nadolol Timolol Metoprolol Atenolol	++++	++++	++	Fatigue, cold extremities, vivid dreaming, depression (asthma, brittle diabetes, atrial ventricular conduction defects)
Antiepileptic Drugs				
Valproate	++++	++++	++	Nausea, asthenia, tremor, weight gain, and hair loss (liver disease)

Topiramate	++++	++++	++	paresthesias, cognitive impairment (glaucoma, kidney stones)
Gabapentin	+++	+++	+	drowsiness
Antiserotonin Drugs				
Methysergide	++++	++	++++	chronic use, fibrotic disorders (cardiovascular disease)
Pizotifen	+++	++	+++	weight gain, sedation (obesity)
Tricyclic Antidepressants				
Amitriptyline	+++	++	++	sedation, dry mouth, weight gain (glaucoma)
SSRIs	++	+	++	sexual dysfunction
Calcium Channel Blockers				
Flunarizine	+++	++++	+++	sedation, weight gain, depression, parkinsonism (depression, parkinsonism)

continued

Table 4-3. *Continued*

				Side effects (contraindications)
Verapamil	++	+		Constipation, water retention (bradycardia, AV conduction defects)
NSAIDs				
Naproxen	++	+++		Dyspepsia, peptic ulcer (active peptic ulcer, renal disease)
Tolfenamic acid	++	+++		Dyspepsia, peptic ulcer (active peptic ulcer, renal active peptic ulcers, renal disease)
Neurotoxins				
Botulinum toxin type A	++++	++	+	(myasthenia gravis, patients on aminoglycosides)

Source: Modified from Pfelt-Hansen P, Welch KMA. Migraine; prioritizing prophylactic treatment. In: Olesen J, Pfelt-Hansen P, Welch KMA eds. *The headaches*, 2nd ed. Philadelphia: Lippincott Williams & Wilkins, 2000:500 (15).

[a]Rating is based on a combination of published literature and personal experience of the authors cited and the present author.

the original preparation. Gradually increasing small doses over a period of 2 to 3 weeks is recommended. Most patients benefit at doses of 500 to 1,500 mg per day. Other adverse effects include tremor, weight gain, asthenia, and loss of hair, which makes valproate less acceptable to many. Fear of hepatotoxicity is unfounded in healthy individuals. Hepatitis and other hepatic dysfunctions are contraindications. There is no correlation between the blood levels of valproate and its clinical effects; therefore estimation of blood levels is not absolutely necessary. However, it is recommended that blood count and liver enzymes be tested periodically, possibly once every 3 months to monitor any change in the profile. The divalproex is definitely contraindicated during pregnancy because of the teratogenic effects, particularly neural tube abnormalities. Interaction with barbiturates should be kept in mind, and it is better to avoid barbiturate (butalbital) containing immediate-relief medications in patients receiving valproate. Valproate is now approved for three different indications: epilepsy, migraine, and mania.

A rare complication such as pancreatitis has to be kept in mind. If a person receiving valproate complains of persistent upper abdominal pain, the possibility of pancreatitis has to be considered even though it is a rare adverse event. It is controversial whether long-term valproate therapy produces ovarian dysfunction as a result of multiple ovarian cyst formation, which may lead to menstrual irregularities. Overall, the author tries to avoid valproate in young women because of that reason as well as the inherent tendency of weight gain with valproate.

Topiramate

Topiramate, a D-fructose derivative, has been found to be effective in two large double-blind placebo-controlled multicenter trials (24–26). Topiramate, both 100 mg and 200 mg, is effective in reducing migraine attack frequency by 50% in half the patients. It is recommended to titrate the dose gradually, starting at 25 mg of topiramate daily for a week, increasing to 50 mg on the second week, 75 mg the third week, and 100 mg the fourth week. The efficacy difference between 100 mg and 200 mg is not significant. However, the side effects are more with 200 mg. If a patient cannot tolerate 100 mg, it may be reduced to 75 or 50 mg (to a tolerable dose). Many patients may respond to as little as 25 or 50 mg of topiramate a day.

The immediate side effects are paresthesias involving the extremities and lips and face in some patients. The gradual titration of the dose usually will avoid this problem, and a prior explanation of the possible side effect will also help patients. They should be reassured that the paresthesias will disappear as they continue to use the medication. If the paresthesias are bothersome, they can be reduced by drinking orange juice, eating bananas, or by taking 20 to 40 mEq of potassium (KCL) per day. Another important, but less common, adverse event is cognitive impairment, which results in difficulty finding the right word and difficulty concentrating and focusing. This may also be explained to patients beforehand, so they can adjust the dose according to the tolerable levels. In patients who have significant cognitive side effects, the medication may have to be discontinued.

Weight Loss with Topiramate

One of the desirable side effects of topiramate is weight loss, unlike valproate where weight gain is a major problem. Weight loss is welcomed by patients and therefore becomes an ideal drug for young women with frequent migraine. The topiramate may alter the taste for certain items, particularly for soft drinks, which is a very welcomed adverse event. In the clinical trials, an average weight loss was 4% to 5% of body weight. In clinical practice, we see some patients losing up to 30% of their body weight.

Rare adverse events include renal stone formation, which occurs in about 1% of patients, and the rare development of acute myopia and secondary angle-closure glaucoma. If a patient on topiramate complains of eye pain or blurred vision, it is imperative that an ophthalmological examination to rule out glaucoma be done. This is an acute event with complete resolution when topiramate is discontinued.

Oral Contraceptives and Topiramate

It has been determined that up to 200 mg of topiramate per day does not interfere with the effectiveness of oral contraceptives. The majority of patients with migraine do not need more than 200 mg of topiramate.

The exact mode of action of topiramate in migraine is not known. It has multiple effects, which include increase in GABA levels in the brain, effects on voltage gated ion channels including calcium channels, and carbonic hydrase inhibition. Because of the latter, topiramate may be an effective agent for the treatment of idiopathic intracranial hypertension with headache because it helps reduce the increased intracranial pressure as well as reduce the weight in patients with that condition. Topiramate may also be a good choice for diabetic patients with migraine because it was initially developed as an antidiabetic agent.

Gabapentin

Gabapentin has been shown to be effective in a randomized double-blind placebo-controlled trial for prophylaxis of migraine (27). Gabapentin increases the GABA levels in the brain, but its precise mechanism of action is unknown. Gabapentin is a fairly well-tolerated medication, and a dose up to 2,400 mg per day is tried. An initial open-label study showed efficacy of gabapentin in migraine and transformed migraine (28). Gabapentin has been shown to have a beneficial effect on neuropathic pain states such as diabetic neuropathy (29), postherpetic neuralgia, trigeminal neuralgia, and complex regional pain syndrome. It has also been shown to be as effective as propranolol in the treatment of essential tremor (30). The low side effect profile of gabapentin is a distinct advantage over valproate and topiramate, even though the clinical efficacy is not as good.

Other antiepileptic drugs such as levetriacetam, zonisamide, and lamotrigine have not been proven to be useful in double-blind placebo-controlled trials. However, certain physicians use them, and there may be some usefulness for these agents in some patients.

Clinical Use of Antiepileptic Drugs

Although beta-blockers are widely used as an initial drug in migraine prevention, antiepileptics may be considered the first-line drug under many circumstances. When beta-blockers are contraindicated in such conditions as asthma, congestive cardiac failure, low blood pressure, orthostatic hypotension, and cardiac conduction defects, anticonvulsants become first-line drugs. Beta-blockers are known to produce depression in some patients; therefore they can be replaced by an anticonvulsant. Patients with migraine who are on immunotherapy for allergy treatments should not take beta-blockers concomitantly, and therefore they may be switched to an antiepileptic drug. Beta-blockers are known to reduce exercise tolerance in those who exercise regularly. Antiepileptic drugs have no effect on exercise tolerance. When there is comorbid epilepsy and migraine or epilepsy and bipolar illness, antiepileptics may be considered first-line drugs.

Among the antiepileptic drugs currently used, topiramate should be the first choice because of its proven efficacy and the ability of the compound to cause weight loss. Gradual titration of the dose and adjustment according to the tolerability is important. There is no interaction between antiepileptic drugs and 5-HT_1 agonists such as ergotamine and triptans.

Antidepressants

Tricyclic Compounds

Antidepressants, particularly tricyclic compounds, are widely used in the prophylaxis of migraine and tension-type headache. Amitriptyline (Elavil) in doses ranging from 10 to 200 mg per day is probably the most commonly used antidepressant in migraine prevention (31). Biological basis of its action includes modulation of 5-HT and norepinephrine. Amitriptyline has been shown to inhibit trigeminal neuronal activation experimentally. Antidepressant effect adds to the clinical benefit even though the antimigraine effect of amitriptyline has been shown to be independent of the antidepressant effect (31).

Tricyclic antidepressants are particularly effective in patients with frequent migraine attacks, migraine with medication overuse, migraine with insomnia, migraine with interictal tension-type headache, chronic daily headache, and migraine with depression. Combination therapy of tricyclic antidepressants, particularly amitriptyline, with beta-blockers is a very practical way of treating patients with frequent migraine, particularly those associated with depression, stress, anxiety, and sleep problems (32).

Amitriptyline causes more anticholinergic side effects such as dry mouth and dysuria than nortriptyline. The latter is a good choice for those with the side effects just described with amitriptyline.

SSRIs

In one trial, fluoxetine, an SSRI antidepressant, was not found to be more effective than placebo for migraine prophylaxis (33). The same study reported that fluoxetine is useful in treating chronic daily headaches. However, SSRIs are used extensively in patients with chronic migraine, particularly because of the comorbid depression and anxiety. F-fluoxetine was found to produce statistically significant improvement of attack frequency, headache days per month, and patients' global satisfaction of its usefulness (34).

The major disadvantage of SSRIs is the sexual dysfunction side effects and the withdrawal effects on the patient when medication is discontinued. Withdrawal is worse for paroxetine. In general, tricyclic antidepressants are preferred over SSRIs in the preventive treatment of migraine.

Venlafaxine (Effexor), the first specific serotonin and norepinephrine uptake inhibitor, may be effective in migraine prophylaxis, and it is used by many physicians even though there are no double-blind placebo-controlled trials. The author uses venlafaxine more often than SSRIs. The anxiety-reducing property of this compound is an added advantage.

CALCIUM CHANNEL BLOCKERS

The agency for health care policy and research analyzed 45 controlled trials (14). Flunarizine was found to be most effective, nimodipine had mixed results, and nifedipine was difficult to interpret. Verapamil was more effective than placebo in two of three trials, but those two trials had high dropout rates, rendering the findings uncertain (35).

However, the most commonly used calcium channel blocker for prophylaxis of migraine is verapamil, even though it has lesser clinical efficacy compared to flunarizine. It is a well-tolerated medication; therefore many physicians are comfortable using it long term. Verapamil is the drug of choice in the prophylaxis of cluster headache where larger doses like 480 mg or more may be used. For migraine prophylaxis, the average dose is 180 mg to 240 mg per day. Sustained release formulations are available, making it convenient for use one dose a day. Patients with complicated migraine, with neurological symptoms (prolonged aura), may benefit from verapamil preventive therapy. However, there are no studies to support that clinical impression. Many physicians use verapamil to treat late life transient migraine accompaniments, described by Fisher (36). Verapamil is especially useful in patients with comorbid hypertension or in those with contraindications for beta-blockers such as asthma or Raynaud's disease. The most common adverse events of verapamil are constipation and water retention.

Flunarizine is the most effective calcium channel blocker; however, it is not available in the United States. Adverse events include Parkinsonism, depression, and weight gain.

It is interesting to note that many of the prophylactic agents for migraine affect voltage gated ion channels, particularly calcium channels. These include calcium channel blockers, valproate, topiramate, and propranolol through its membrane-stabilizing effect.

Developing the specific antagonist that acts on P/Q type calcium channel (based on recent data of specific P/Q calcium channel chromosome 19 abnormality—CACNA 1A—in familial hemiplegic migraine) (37,38) may improve preventive therapy of migraine.

5-HT₂ ANTAGONISTS

Methysergide has remained one of the most effective antimigraine prophylactic agents. However, as shown in Table 4-3, the potential side effects might be viewed as less than attractive.

Methysergide may cause weight gain and peripheral edema. With more than 6 months of use, retroperitoneal, pericardial, and subendocardial fibrosis may occur, a rare complication (1 in 2,500). It appears to be an idiosyncratic reaction because the great majority of patients do not develop these complications. Major vessel constriction, mesenteric vascular fibrosis, and small bowel infarctions have been reported rarely. Concurrent use with other ergots alkaloids, beta-adrenergic blockers, dopamine, erythromycin, or troleandomycin may increase the risk for arterial spasms and occlusion. Methylsergide should not be combined with triptans. Methylsergide should be reserved for very refractory severe migraine patients. Many clinicians recommend an interval without the drug for 4 weeks every 6 months, but whether this practice decreases the toxicity is unclear. If one were to use methylsergide over a long term, periodic checkups for fibrotic reactions—including chest X-ray, echocardiogram, and CT of the abdomen—are recommended. Methylsergide is not easily available at the present time. Compounding pharmacies in various cities might be able to dispense it.

Cyproheptadine appears to be an effective agent in the preventive treatment of migraine in children and may be the drug of choice in the pediatric age group, even though there are no controlled trials to support this practice. It has no major side effects except increased appetite, weight gain, and slight drowsiness. Best indication is in smaller children in the age range of 7 to 10 who have very frequent migraine episodes.

Pizotifen, a benzocycloheptathiophene derivative, is also effective. Adverse events include drowsiness, increased appetite, and weight gain. It is not available in the United States, but it is available in Canada and many other countries.

NSAIDS AND COX₂ INHIBITORS

Naproxen (39) and tolfenamic acid are two agents that have been tried for migraine prevention. Clinical efficacy of both is not as good as that of beta-blockers, valproate, topiramate, or methylsergide. The gastric and renal side effect potential prevents them from being long-term drugs. However, for short-term prophylaxis, particularly around the menstrual time, agents like naproxen sodium may be very effective.

NSAIDs act in multiple ways, producing prostaglandin inhibition, reducing neurogenic inflammation perivascularly, and influencing central serotonin neurotransmission. There is no correlation between the degree of platelet inhibition and the prophylactic restrictiveness of NSAIDs.

COX$_2$ inhibitors are gaining a great deal of use in migraine, both in acute treatment and also for short-term preventive treatment. Long-term safety of these agents are still under investigation.

MISCELLANEOUS AGENTS

Even though magnesium deficiency in the brain is implicated in the pathophysiology of migraine, there is still no proof that magnesium replacement is of any benefit in migraine prophylaxis. The only double-blind placebo-controlled study in patients with migraine without aura (69 patients) reported negative results (40), even though a previous small study in menstrual migraine reported magnesium to be effective (41). Mauskop et al. (42) emphasized the importance of serum ionized magnesium measurements in determining the magnesium state in migraine patients and have used IV magnesium in patients found to have low ionized magnesium levels (42). These observations have not been confirmed yet.

Riboflavin

Based on theoretical considerations of possible altered mitochondrial energy metabolism in migraine (43,44) and the striking link between mitochondrial encephalomyopathy, lactacidosis, and strokelike episodes (MELAS) and migraine (45,46), riboflavin 200 mg twice daily was studied in a double-blind placebo-controlled trial (47). Riboflavin reduced the frequency of migraine significantly compared to placebo (47).

Riboflavin (vitamin B$_2$) is the precursor of flavin mononucleotide and flavin adenine dinucleotide, coenzymes required for the activity of flavoenzymes in the transfer of electrons in oxidation-reduction reactions. The beneficial clinical response to high dose of riboflavin has been observed in some patients with mitochondrial myopathies (48) and encephalomyopathies (49) associated with mutation of mitochondrial DNA. If deficient mitochondrial energy metabolism is a casual factor in migraine, logistically, riboflavin might have some beneficial effect. The author has not found riboflavin to be significantly effective in migraine prevention.

Coenzyme Q10

Coenzyme Q10, which acts in a similar fashion influencing mitochondrial oxidative metabolism, has been reported to be effective as a prophylactic agent in migraine in a double-blind, placebo-controlled trial (50). Further confirmation is needed before it can be recommended as an effective treatment.

Melatonin

In an open label study of 34 migraineurs, 78.1% had at least a 50% reduction in headaches 3 months after starting melatonin 3 mg 30 minutes before bedtime (50a). A complete response was reported by 25% and a greater than 75% reduction was reported by 21.8%. These dramatic findings certainly warrant a placebo controlled study.

Natural Products

Feverfew (Tanacetum parthenium) is a medicinal herb, the effectiveness of which has not been established (51). Feverfew may be acting through nitric oxide mechanism, which is implicated in the pathophysiology of migraine. Because there is no definite evidence-based efficacy determination, feverfew cannot be recommended at the present time.

Petasites hybridus root (butterbur) is a perennial shrub. A standard extract (75 mg twice daily) was effective in a double-blind placebo-controlled study (52). The most common adverse event was belching. Until confirmatory studies are done or extensive clinical experience with this agent is available, it cannot be advocated as an effective preventive treatment for migraine.

ANGIOTENSIN INHIBITORS

An association has been reported between migraine and the angiotensin-converting enzyme (ACE)-DD gene. One randomized, double-blind, placebo-controlled crossover trial involving 47 patients (60 enrolled) with episodic migraine suggested that lisinopril in doses of 20 mg is effective in reducing hours with headache and headache pain, headache days, migraine days, and severity index by 20%, 17%, 21%, and 20%, respectively, compared with placebo (53). Cough is one of the main side effects associated with angiotensin-converting enzyme inhibitors. Further studies are needed.

Angiotensin 2 Receptor Blocker: Candesartan

In a similar study to the one with lisinopril, the same group demonstrated that 16 mg of candesartan led to a reduction in the number of headache days (13.6 vs. 18.5 with placebo, P = 0.001) (54). This again was a small study involving 60 patients with episodic migraine with two 12-week periods. As with lisinopril, further large-scale studies are needed before recommendation can be made about the use of angiotensin inhibitors in migraine prophylaxis.

NEUROTOXINS: BOTULINUM TOXIN TYPE A (BOTOX)

Pain relief associated with use of botulinum toxin type A (Botox) for treatment of cervical dystonia and spasticity has been frequently reported (55–58). Botulinum toxin type A is a novel prophylactic headache treatment that through its action on neuromuscular junction has muscular effects without vascular and systemic effects. In addition, there may be direct antinociceptive effects as well (59). Botulinum toxin type A has shown promise for treatment of headache in several clinical trials, but uncertainty remains as to how botulinum toxin type A ultimately should be used for frequent headache and which patients are best suited for treatment.

Botulinum toxin has been used in several different headache types. The initial observation was rather serendipitous, when Dr. William Binder, a plastic surgeon, observed that many of his patients who had undergone Botox injections for treatment of glabellar lines reported substantial improvement in headache frequency and severity. After making these initial observations, he helped design and complete a multicenter open-label trial of botulinum toxin type A in patients with migraine (60). Of 77 patients studied, 36 patients with migraine reported complete relief of the headaches. The mean duration of effect of Botox was found to be 4.1 months, and 27 of the 77 (38%) reported partial response. Site of injections was determined based on particular needs of the patient but generally included frontalis, temporalis, corrugator, procerus muscles, and, in a few patients, suboccipital muscles as well. The dose used also varied from patient to patient. Except for brow ptosis, no significant adverse effects were experienced.

The first multicenter double-blind placebo-controlled trial involved 123 patients with IHS-defined migraine who experienced between two and eight severe migraine headaches in each month (61). The patients were randomized to one of three groups, placebo, 25 units Botox, or 75 units Botox. Eleven standard injection sites were used including frontalis, temporalis, corrugator, and procerus muscles. Bilateral injections were performed. Compared with placebo, patients receiving 25 units of Botox A experienced the following effects after Botox injection: (a) significantly fewer and less severe migraine headaches each month, (b) reduction in the amount of acute medications used, and (c) lower incidence of emesis. There was no difference between those receiving 75 units of Botox and those receiving placebo. No adverse events were reported except diplopia in two cases and transient ptosis in 13 cases. Brin et al. (62) in a separate study presented the results of a randomized placebo-controlled multicenter study of Botox in migraine prophylaxis. In this study, several injection site patterns were used. Those patients who received Botox injections in the temporal and frontal regions experienced significantly greater pain relief than the placebo group.

In a study of 30 patients with IHS-classified migraine headache experiencing between two and eight attacks each month, patients were randomized to receive 50 units or placebo injections (63). The fifteen injection sites included temporalis, frontalis, corrugator, procerus, trapezii, and splenius capitis muscles bilaterally. Patients were observed for 90 days. Compared with placebo-treated patients who did not experience any significant change of headache frequency and severity, those who received Botox injections had significant reduction of the headache frequency at 90 days (2.5 vs. 5.8) (P = <0.01) as well as severity. No significant adverse events were reported.

In an open-label study evaluating the effects of botulinum toxin type A on disability in episodic and chronic migraine, treatment with 25 units of Botox resulted in decreased migraine associated with disability in 54% of patients (64). In a large prospective study undertaken by Mathew et al. (65), the migraine-associated disability scale (MIDAS scale) was used. Patients who responded were shown to have significant reduction in their MIDAS scale, and the reduction of MIDAS scale was maintained with repeated injections of Botox (65). In that particular study, botulinum toxin type A injections were given up to 4 years. In addition to reduction in the MIDAS scale, these patients exhibited many fewer headache attacks and reduced use of acute medications such as triptans and nonsteroidals. It was pointed out that botulinum toxin may have a "disease-modifying effect" in chronic migraine.

Many of the reports concluded that there may be an increase in benefit experience with repeated treatment with botulinum type A for patients with chronic migraine (66–68). These observations, although not derived from randomized controlled studies, are important to consider because many injectors indicate, some empirically discovered, that for maximum benefit to be realized from Botox, the patient may need treatment at least several times.

From extensive experience, the author feels Botox has a place in the management of chronic migraine with significant disability for patients who are resistant to prophylactic pharmacotherapy. It is ideal for those migraineurs who have contraindications for triptans and ergotamine and those who have significant adverse events from prophylactic pharmacotherapy. It is also probably a good choice in patients with chronic migraine in the older age group because it is not associated with any adverse events such as sedation and disorientation. Botulinum injections are not recommended for episodic infrequent migraine patients or as a first-line therapy.

In those who get adequate response, the headache may start relapsing after 3 to 4 months and repeat treatments may be necessary. No long-term adverse events have been reported except atrophy of the muscles in the anterior areas of the temples.

STRATIFICATION OF MIGRAINE PROPHYLAXIS

Migraine prophylaxis could be continuous, intermittent, or episodic. Continuous daily treatment with prophylactic medications is necessary when migraines are frequent and when migraines are associated with interictal nondescript tension-type headache. Patients with severe menstrual migraine or those who get headaches when visiting high altitudes may require medication for a limited time. Intermittent prophylaxis in menstrual migraine is usually given 2 or 3 days before the menstruation and through the period. Episodic prophylaxis may be instituted when there is a known trigger for headache. For example, exercise-induced headache can be partially prevented by using medications like beta-blockers or indomethacin. The same applies to headache induced by sexual activity where the patient may take a prophylactic agent prior to the event.

THE ROLE OF COMORBIDITY IN PROPHYLACTIC TREATMENT OF MIGRAINE

Comorbidity may result in certain therapeutic opportunities. Table 4-4 shows therapeutic opportunities provided by comorbid conditions. However, comorbidity may impose therapeutic limitations in using certain medications. Table 4-5 lists the therapeutic limitations because of comorbidity. Therapeutic limitations due to side effects are also a problem. Table 4-6 shows the therapeutic limitations as a result of side effects.

Table 4-4.   Comorbidity and therapeutic opportunities

Disorders	Medication
Migraine + hypertension	Beta-blockers
Migraine + angina	Calcium channel blockers
Migraine + stress	Beta-blockers
Migraine + depression	Tricyclic antidepressant (TCA), Selective serotonin reuptake inhibitor (SSRI), Venlafaxine
Migraine + insomnia	TCA
Migraine + underweight	TCA
Migraine + epilepsy	Divalproex, Topiramate
Migraine + mania	Divalproex, Topiramate

Table 4-5.   Comorbidity and therapeutic limitations

Migraine + epilepsy	Tricyclic antidepressant (TCA)
Migraine + depression	Beta-blockers
Migraine + obesity	TCA, Divalproex

Table 4-6.   Therapeutic limitations due to side effects

Asthma	Beta-blockers
Elderly with cardiac disease	Tricyclic antidepressant (TCA) Calcium channel blockers Beta-blockers
Athlete	Beta-blockers
Professions requiring quick recall and sharp cognitive ability	Beta-blockers TCAs, Topiramate
Liver dysfunction	Valproate

A primary antimigraine prophylactic agent can be combined with compatible agents for treating comorbidity (depression, anxiety, panic disorder, hypertension, sleeplessness). As long as the antimigraine drug and the drug used for comorbidity do not interact with each other, it is certainly logical to use combinations. Table 4-7 shows certain examples of rational copharmacy in migraine.

Drug combinations are commonly used for patients with

Table 4-7. Rational copharmacy

Suggested	Antidepressants + Beta-blocker
	Calcium channel blocker
	Divalproex, Topiramate
	Methylsergide
	Methylsergide + Calcium channel blocker
	Selective serotonin reuptake inhibitor (SSRI) + Tricyclic antidepressants
Caution	Beta-blocker + Calcium channel blocker
	Methylsergide
	Monoamine oxidase + Amitriptyline or inhibitor (MAOI) nortriptyline
Contraindications	MAOI + SSRI
	Most tricyclic antidepressants (except amitriptyline or nortriptyline)
	Carbamazepine

Rational or Strategic Copharmacy

refractory headache disorders. Some combinations, such as antidepressants and beta-blockers, are suggested; others, such as beta-blockers and calcium channel blockers, should be used with caution; and some, such as monoamine oxidase inhibitors (MAOIs) and SSRIs, are contraindicated because of potentially lethal interactions (Table 4-7). Many clinicians find the combination of an antidepressant (such as a tricyclic antidepressant or SSRI) and a beta-blocker act synergistically. Lance has advocated combining methysergide with a vasodilator such as a calcium channel blocker to decrease side effects. Divalproex or topiramate used in combination with antidepressants is a logical choice to treat refractory migraine complicated by depression or bipolar illness.

USE OF ABORTIVE MEDICATIONS ALONG WITH PREVENTIVE TREATMENT

Even though preventive agents reduce the frequency and severity of migraine attacks, many patients have breakthrough migraine or tension-type headache while on them. Menstrual migraine is a good example of the breakthrough headache. In general, preventive medications make acute agents more effective.

While using the acute medications, one should make sure they are not overused. A limit of use two times a week is recommended to prevent secondary failure of preventive treatment. Table 4-8 shows the potential drug interactions between abortive and preventive agents.

Table 4-8. Caution and contraindications for combining abortive and prophylactic antimigraine therapy

Agent	Caution	Contraindicated
Methlysergide	Ergotamine, Dihydroergotamine, Triptans	
Monoamine oxidase inhibitors	Oral Sumatriptan Zolmitriptan Rizatriptan	Meperidine Sympathomimetics (Midrin)
Divalproex	Overuse of short-acting barbiturates	
Propranolol	Rizatriptan Zolmitriptan	
Antifungal agents	Eletriptan	

REFERENCES

1. Ramadan NM, Silberstein SD, Freitag FG, et al. Evidence-based guidelines of the pharmacological management for prevention of migraine for the primary care provider. www.Neurology.org., 1999.
2. Golla FL, Winter AL. Analysis of cerebral responses to flicker in patients complaining of episodic headache. *Electroencephalogr Clin Neurophysiol* 1959;11:539–549.
3. Schoenen J, Maertens de Noordhout A. Contingent negative variation and efficacy of beta-blocking agents in migraine. *Cephalalgia* 1986;6:229–234.
4. Nyrke T, Kangasniemi P, Land AH. Difference of steady-state visual evoked potentials in classic and common migraine. *Electroencephalogr Clin Neurophysiol* 1989;73:285–294.
5. Blin O, Azulay J, Masson G, et al. Apomorphine-induced yawning in migraine patients: enhanced responsiveness. *Clin Neuropharmacol* 1991;14:91–95.
6. Welch KMA, D'Andrea G, Tepley N, et al. The concept of migraine as a state of central neuronal hyperexcitability. *Neurol Clin* 1990;8:817–828.
7. Aurora SK, Ahman BK, Alsayed F, et al. Cortical stimulation silent period is shown in migraine with aura. *Neurology* 1998;50(Suppl 4):351–352.
8. Mathew NT, Mullani N. Migraine with persistent visual aura measured by PET. *Abstract Neurol* 1998;50(Suppl 4):A350–A351.
9. Ramadan NM, Halvorson H, Vande-Linde A, et al. Low brain magnesium in migraine. *Headache* 1989;29:416–419.
10. Curran DA, Hinterberger H, Lance JW. Total plasma serotonin, 5-hydroxyindoleacetic acid and p-hydroxy-m-methoxymandelic acid excretion in normal and migrainous subjects. *Brain* 1965;88:997–1010.
11. Anthony M, Hinterberger H, Lance JW. Plasma serotonin in migraine and stress. *Arch Neurol* 1967;16:544–552.
12. Kimball RW, Friedman AP, Vallejo E. Effect of serotonin in migraine patients. *Neurology* 1960;10:107–111.

13. Peatfield RC, Olesen J. Migraine: precipitating factors. In: Oleson J, Tfelt-Hansen P, Welch KMA, eds. *The headaches.* New York: Raven Press, 1993:243.

14. Gray RN, Goslin RE, McCrory DC, et al. Drug treatments for prevention of migraine headache prepared for the agency for healthcare policy and research. Contract No. 290-94-2025. Available from national technical information service accession no. 127953 (Technical Review 2-3), February 1999.

15. Tfelt-Hansen P, Welch KMA. Migraine: prioritizing prophylactic treatment. In: Olesen J, Tfelt-Hansen P, Welch KMA, eds. *The headaches,* 2nd ed. Philadelphia: Lippincott Williams & Wilkins, 2000:499–505.

16. Limmroth V, Lee WS, Cutrer FM, et al. Meningeal $GABA_A$ receptors located outside the blood brain barrier mediate sodium valproate blockade of neurogenic and substance P-induced inflammation: possible mechanisms in migraine. *Cephalalgia* 1995;15:102.

17. Nishikawa T, Scatton B. Inhibitory influence of GABA on central serotoninergic transmission: raphi nuclei as the neuroanatomical site of GABAergic inhibition of cerebral serotoninergic neurons. *Brain Res* 1985;341:331–391.

18. Cutrer FM, Limmroth V, Ayata G, et al. Valproate reduces c-Fos expression in trigeminal nucleus caudalis (TNC) after noxious meningeal stimulation. *Cephalalgia* 1995;15(Suppl 14):96.

19. Cutrer FM, Moskowitz MA. Actions of valproate and neurosteroids in a model of trigeminal pain. *Headache* 1996;36:285.

20. Hering R, Kuritzky A. Sodium valproate in the prophylactic treatment of migraine: double-blind study versus placebo. *Cephalalgia* 1992;12:81–84.

21. Jensen R, Brinck T, Olesen J. Sodium valproate has a prophylactic effect on migraine without aura: a triple-blind, placebo-controlled crossover study. *Neurology* 1994;44:647–651.

22. Mathew NT, Saper JR, Silberstein SD, et al. Migraine prophylaxis with divalproex. *Neurology* 1995;52:281–286.

23. Kaniecki RG. A comparative study of propranolol and divalproex sodium in the prophylaxis of migraine. *Arch Neurol* 1997;54:1141–1144.

24. Mathew NT, Schmitt TJ, Neto W, et al. Topiramate in migraine prevention: MIGR 001. *Neurology* 2003;60(Suppl 1):A336.

25. Silberstein SD, Neto W, Schmitt J, et al. For MIGR-001 Study Group. Topiramate in migraine prevention. Results of a large controlled trial. *Arch Neurol* 2004;61:490–495.

26. Brandes JL, Saper JR, Diamond M, et al. Topiramate for migraine prevention. A randomized controlled trial. *JAMA* 2004;291:965–973.

27. Mathew NT, Rapoport A, Saper J, et al. Efficacy of gabapentin in migraine prophylaxis. *Headache* 2001;41:119–128.

28. Mathew NT. Gabapentin in migraine prophylaxis. *Cephalalgia* 1996;16:367.

29. Gorson KG, Schott C, Rand WM, et al. Gabapentin in the treatment of painful diabetic neuropathy: a placebo controlled double-blind, crossover trial. *Neurology* 1998;50:A103.

30. Girowell A, Kulisevsky J, Barbanog M, et al. A double-blind placebo controlled comparative trial of gabapentin and propranolol in patients with essential tremor. *Neurology* 1988;50:A71–A72.

31. Couch JR, Ziegler DK, Hassaneur R. Amitriptyline in the prophylaxis of migraine: effectiveness and relationship of antimigraine and antidepressant effects. *Neurology* 1976;26: 121–127.

32. Mathew NT. Prophylaxis of migraine and mixed headaches. *Headache* 1981;20:105–109.

33. Saper JR, Silberstein SD, Lake AE, et al. Double-blind trials of fluoxetine: chronic daily headache and migraine. *Headache* 1994;34:497–502.

34. Steiner TJ, Ahmed F, Findley LJ, et al. S-fluoxetine in the prophylaxis of migraine: a phase II double-blind randomized placebo-controlled study. *Cephalalgia* 1998;18:289–296.

35. Silberstein SD, Saper JR, Freitag F. Migraine diagnosis and treatment. In: Silberstein SD, Lipton RB, Dalessio DJ eds. *Wolff's headache and other head pain,* 7th ed. New York: Oxford University Press, 2003: 121–237.

36. Fisher CM. Late life migraine accompaniments, further experience. *Stroke* 1986;17:1033–1042.

37. Joutel A, Bousser MG, Biousse V, et al. A gene for familial hemiplegia migraine maps to chromosome 19. *Nat Genet* 1993;5:40–45.

38. Ophoff RA, Terwindt GM, Vergouwe MN, et al. Familial hemiplegic migraine and episodic ataxia type-2 are caused by mutations in the $Ca2+$ channel gene CACNL1A4. *Cell* 1996;87: 543–552.

39. Welch KMA, Ellis DJ, Keenanpa. Successful migraine prophylaxis with naproxen sodium. *Neurology* 1985;35:1304–1310.

40. Pfaffenrath V, Wessely P, Meyer C, et al. Magnesium in the prophylaxis of migraine: a double-blind placebo controlled study. *Cephalalgia* 1996;16:436–440.

41. Facchinetti F, Sances G, Borella P, et al. Magnesium prophylaxis of menstrual effects on intracellular magnesium. *Headache* 1991;31:298–310.

42. Mauskop A, Altura BT, Cracco RQ, et al. Intravenous magnesium sulfate relieves migraine attacks in patients with low serum ionized magnesium levels: a pilot study. *Clin Sci* 1995;89:633–636.

43. Barbiroli B, Montagna P, Cortelli P, et al. Abnormal brain and muscle energy metabolism shown by 31P magnetic resonance spectroscopy in patients affected by migraine with aura. *Neurology* 1992;42:1209–1214.

44. Welch KMA, Levine SR, D'Andrea G, et al. Preliminary observations on brain energy metabolism in migraine studied by in vivo 31-phosphorus NNMR spectroscopy. *Neurology* 1989;39: 538–541.

45. Dvorkin GS, Aderman F, Carpenter S. Classical migraine, intractable epilepsy and multiple strokes: a syndrome related to mitochondrial encephalopathy. In: Anderman F, Lugaresi E, eds. *Migraine and epilepsy.* Boston: Butterworth-Heineman, 1987; 203–232.

46. Mosewich RK, Donat JR, DiMauro S, et al. The syndrome of mitochondrial encephalomyopathy, lactic acidosis, and stroke-like episodes presenting without stroke. *Arch Neurol* 1993;50: 275–278.

47. Schoenen J, Jacquy J, Lemaerts M. Effectiveness of high dose riboflavin in migraine prophylaxis: a randomized controlled trial. *Neurology* 1998;50:466–469.

48. Arts WFM, Scholte HR, Boggard JM, et al. NADH-CoQ reductase deficient myopathy: successful treatment with riboflavin. *Lancet* 1983;2:581–582.

49. Penn AMW, Lee JWK, Thuillier P, et al. MELAS syndrome with mitochondrial tRNA[LeulUURI] mutation: correlation of clinical state, nerve conduction, and muscle[31]P magnetic resonance spectroscopy during treatment with nicotinamide and riboflavin. *Neurology* 1992;42:2147–2152.

50. Sandor PS, Diclemende L, Coppola G, et al. Co-enzyme Q10 for migraine prophylaxis: a randomized controlled trial. *Cephalalgia* 2003;23:577.

50a. Peres MF, Zukerman E, da Cunha Tanuri F, et al. Melatonin, 3 mg, is effective for migraine prevention. Neurology. 2004;63 (4):757.

51. Vogler BK, Pittler MH, Ernst E. Feverfew as a preventive treatment for migraine: a systemic review. *Cephalalgia* 1998;18:421–435.

52. Lipton RB, Gobel LH, Wilks K, et al. Efficacy of petasites (an extract from petasites rhizome) 50 and 75 mg for prophylaxis of migraine: results of a randomized double-blind, placebo-controlled study. *Neurology* 2002;58(Suppl 1):A472.

53. Schrader H, Stovner LI, Helde G, et al. Prophylactic treatment of migraine with angiotensin connecting enzyme inhibitor (lisinopril): Randomized placebo controlled crossover study. *BMJ* 2001;322:19–22.

54. Tronvik E, Stovner LJ, Helde G, et al. Prophylactic treatment of migraine with angiotensin II receptor blocker: a randomized controlled trial. *JAMA* 2003;289:65–69.

55. Greene P, Kang LJ, Fahn S, et al. Double-blind, placebo-controlled trial of botulinum toxin injections for the treatment of spasmodic torticollis. *Neurology* 1990;40:1213–1218.

56. Jankovic J, Schwartz K. Botulinum toxin injections for cervical dystonia. *Neurology* 1990;40:277–280.

57. Naumann M, Yakovleff A, Durif F, for the BOTOX® Cervical Dystonia Prospective Study group. A randomized double-masked, crossover comparison of the efficacy and safety of botulinum toxin type A produced from the original bulk toxin source and current bulk toxin source for the treatment of cervical dystonia. *J Neurol* 2002;249:57–63.

58. Brashear A, Gordon MF, Elovic E, et al. Intramuscular injection of botulinum toxin for the treatment of wrist and finger spasticity after a stroke. *N Engl J Med* 2002;347:395–400.

59. Cui M, Khanijou S, Rubino J, et al. Botulinum toxin A inhibits the inflammatory pain in the rat formalin model. In: *Abstracts of the 30th Annual Meeting of the Society for Neuroscience,* November 4–9, 2000, New Orleans, LA. Available at: http://sfn. scholarone.com/itin2000/main.html. Accessed October 25, 2002. Abstract 246.2.

60. Binder WJ, Brin MF, Blitzer A, et al. Botulinum toxin type A for treatment of migraine headaches: an open-label study. *Otolgolaryngol Head Neck Surg* 2000;123:669–676.

61. Silberstein S, Mathew N, Saper J, et al. Botulinum toxin type A as a migraine preventive treatment. *Headache* 2000;40:445–450.

62. Brin ME, Swope DM, O'Brien C, et al. Botox for migraine: double blind, placebo-controlled, region-specific evaluation [abstract]. *Cephalalgia* 2000;20:421.

63. Barrientos N, Chana P. Efficacy and safety of botulinum toxin type A in the prophylactic treatment of migraine. Paper presented at the American Headache Society 44th Annual Scientific Meeting, Seattle, WA; June 21–23, 2002.

64. Eross EG, Dodick DW. The effects of botulinum toxin type A on disability in episodic and chronic migraine. Paper presented at the American Headache Society 44th Annual Scientific Meeting, Seattle, WA; June 21–23, 2002.

65. Mathew NT, Kailasam J, Kaupp A, et al. "Disease modification" in chronic migraine with botulinum toxin type A: long-term experience. Paper presented at the American Headache Society 44th Annual Scientific Meeting, Seattle, WA; June 21–23, 2002.

66. Mauskop A. Long-term use of botulinum toxin type A (Botox®) in the treatment of episodic and chronic migraine headaches. Paper presented at the American Headache Society 44th Annual Scientific Meeting, Seattle, WA; June 21–23, 2002.

67. Klapper JA, Klapper A. Use of botulinum toxin in chronic daily headaches associated with migraine. *Headache Q* 1999;10: 141–143.

68. Klapper JA, Mathew NT, Klapper A, et al. Botulinum toxin type A (BTX-A) for the prophylaxis of chronic daily headache [abstract]. *Cephalalgia* 2000;20:292–293.

Chronic Daily Headache

Ninan T. Mathew

Chronic daily or near-daily headaches (CDH) are arbitrarily defined as headaches occurring more than 15 days per month or 180 days per year in the absence of an underlying structural or systemic disease.

CLASSIFICATION OF CHRONIC DAILY HEADACHE

Ample evidence indicates that patients with CDH are a heterogeneous group that can be subdivided into various categories. Approximately 20% of patients with CDH are primary (daily from the onset), whereas the majority, 80%, are transformed from intermittent headache. The International Headache Society classification (1) does not separately classify CDH but describes the various entities in the group. Table 5-1 shows an attempted broad classification of chronic daily headache (CDH).

CHRONIC DAILY HEADACHE IN THE HEADACHE CLINIC POPULATION

Approximately 35% to 40% of patients who seek treatment at the headache centers suffer from daily or near-daily headache (2). All those patients have headaches for more than 15 days a month or 180 days a year. The majority of patients with CDH seeking treatment in headache clinics have chronic migraine (CM) or transformed migraine (TM) (70%) (3). The headaches in these patients are more severe and more disabling as reported in the epidemiological study of frequent headaches (4). Pure chronic tension-type headache (CTTH) is relatively rare.

EPIDEMIOLOGY OF CHRONIC DAILY HEADACHES

Reported prevalence of CDH in the general population is 2.95% to 4.7% (4–7). Prevalence of CM and CTTH in the general population is equal, accounting for approximately one half of the CDH population. Scher et al. (4) found that CM is characterized by more severe pains and higher levels of disability than CTTH. This fact accounts for the higher percentage of patients with CM seen in headache centers. Epidemiology of CM is similar to that of episodic migraine because (a) gender ratio is 2.4:1 and (b) there is an inverse relation with low educational level.

Castillo et al. (5) reported that in Spain the prevalence of CDH in the general population is 4.7% of which 2.3% have CTTH and 2.4% CM. Medication overuse was found to be prevalent in 41% of CM patients and 18% of CTTH patients, indicating that TM patients have more severe pain requiring more medications. In France, Lanteri et al. (7) found the prevalence of CDH to be 2.95% of the population; two thirds of them had CM.

Table 5-1. Classification of chronic daily headache (CDH)

Chronic migraine (CM) or transformed migraine (TM) (2)
Chronic tension-type headache (CTTH)
New persistent daily headache (NPDH)
Hemicrania continua (HC)

Note: All of these categories can be associated with analgesic overuse.

CHRONIC MIGRAINE (CM) OR TRANSFORMED MIGRAINE (TM)

The term *transformed migraine* was first introduced in 1987 by Mathew et al. to describe a common, daily, or near-daily headache condition that constituted 77% of CDH patients seen at the Houston Headache Clinic (2). In two separate series Manzoni et al. reported that 71% and 75%, respectively, of their patients transformed their headaches into a chronic daily pattern from a distinct episodic pattern (8,9). Solomon et al. also recognized chronic daily headaches and mentioned that the majority of their 100 cases transformed from episodic migraine, even though actual percentages were not given (10).

Clinical Features of CM or TM

The second edition of the IHS Classification has adopted the term *CM* (1). In this chapter, the terms *CM* and *TM* are used interchangeably.

Typically the patient describes a history of distinct attacks of migraine with or without aura starting in the teens or early 20s, which eventually becomes more frequent. In addition, the patient develops interparoxysmal tension-type headache, which also becomes more frequent, eventually leading to a daily or near-daily headache. Women in this group may show definite exacerbations of their migraine perimenstrually. Many of the headaches retain certain characteristics of migraine, whereas others are indistinguishable from CTTH. Patients may suffer from a migraine one day and a tension-type headache the next day. Periods of prolonged, persistent, and continuous headache lasting for several weeks may occur in many. In a representative sample of 184 patients reported by Saper et al., mean number of headache days was 23 days per month, with 46% reporting daily headaches (11). Daily headache can be intermittent for a few hours per day or continuous. A single episode of a prolonged headache period, a relapsing remitting course, a relapsing progressive course, or a chronic progressive course can occur.

Manzoni et al. analyzed the evolutionary pattern of transformed migraine (8,9). The majority maintained migraine attacks in addition to developing tension-type headache daily or nearly daily. Others lost the temporal profile of migraine but developed continuous headache with many migrainous features. It has been suggested to subdivide transformed migraine into (a) migraine with interparoxysmal headache and (b) chronic migraine to accommodate these two presentations (12). In general, the transformed migraine group showed higher incidence

Table 5-2. Comparison of clinical characteristics of chronic migraine and chronic tension-type headache

Chronic migraine	Chronic tension-type headache
Headache >15 d/mo	Headache >15/mo
Headache >180 d/yr	Headache >180/yr
Previous history of distinct migraine attacks	No history of distinct migraine attacks
Increased incidence of headache in family	Positive family history less prominent
Retains migrainous characters to a significant degree, intermittently or continuously	Migrainous features absent or very insignificant
Increased neurological and gastrointestinal symptoms	Neurological and gastrointestinal symptoms minimal
Menstrual aggravation	No particular aggravation during menstruation
More relief during pregnancy	Less relief during pregnancy
Excessive intake of analgesics	Excessive intake of analgesics
Responds to antimigraine therapy	Response to antimigraine therapy may occur, but less striking
Behavioral and psychological factors prominent	Behavioral and psychological factors prominent
More disabling	Less disabling
Seeks medical help more often	Seeks medical help less often— more lapsed consultations

of family history of headache, more neurological and gastrointestinal (GI) symptoms, aggravation during menstruation, and relief during pregnancy, compared with other forms of chronic daily headaches, particularly CTTH. Table 5-2 compares the clinical characteristics of transformed migraine and CTTH.

Types of Transformation and Risk Factors for Chronic or Transformed Migraine

In approximately 70% of cases, the transformation from episodic headache to CDH is gradual, whereas it is sudden in about 30%. Factors aiding sudden transformation include trauma to the head and neck, flulike illness, aseptic meningitis, surgical interventions, myelography, lumbar puncture with initial low-pressure headache, epidural injections, and medical illnesses. In many cases the additional factors are not known.

Transformation from episodic migraine to CDH is an insidious process in many, taking years. Table 5-3 lists the factors for development of chronic migraine and chronic daily headache based on clinical observations (13,15) and epidemiological studies (4,14,16).

Table 5-3. Risk factors for chronic daily headache and chronic migraine

Head trauma (4)

Drug overuse
  Caffeine (14)
  Analgesics/caffeine/butalbital (13)

Ergotamine (15)

Opioids

Psychological comorbidities
  Depression
  Anxiety
  Bipolar illness
  Abnormal personality profile
  Sleep disorders

Stressful life events (16) (moving, changes in relationships, major problems with children, extremely stressful ongoing situations)

Analgesic Overuse as a Risk Factor in CDH

Analgesic overuse ranged from 50% to 82% in clinic-based samples of CDH (13,15,17–19), and community-based surveys showed analgesic overuse in 30% of CDH patients compared to 10% to 12% of patients with episodic headache (20).

Scher et al. conducted a case control study of CDH (206 CDH and 507 controls) looking into risk factors (14). They looked at current and previous exposure to excess analgesics and reported that over-the-counter (OTC) medications containing caffeine and caffeine in beverages may be a risk factor in developing CDH before the age of 40. They did not evaluate the role of butalbital/caffeine/analgesic combinations. Narcotics and NSAIDs were not found to be risk factors in this particular study, even though clinical experience is to the contrary. Aspirin was found to be protective.

It is not certain whether analgesic overuse is the cause of chronicity or whether it is the consequence. Arguments in favor of analgesic overuse being a consequence of frequent headaches rather than the cause claim that a significant percentage of CDH patients do not overuse analgesics. In countries like India, where analgesic overuse is rare, CDH exists (21) and withdrawal of analgesics alone does not eliminate headache in CDH. Whether analgesic overuse is the cause or consequence of CDH is still unsettled, but most headache experts would agree that analgesic overuse maintains and perpetuates headache.

Other Risk Factors

Scher et al. (4) reported other risk factors for CDH. Head injury was the most significant risk factor in their study. Relatively mild head injury is well known to initiate CDH in patients with a history of migraine; therefore it is important to get the history of episodic migraine before the head trauma.

Stressful life events such as moving, changes in relationships (breakup, widowhood, divorce, separation), major problems with children, and extremely stressful ongoing situations limited to the year of and year before CDH onset were reported to be significant risk factors by Stewart et al. based on epidemiological studies (16). This indicates a causal relationship between stressful life events and CDH. A greater frequency of attacks and obesity were also risk factors for progression from episodic to chronic daily headache. Whether weight loss would reduce the probability of progression is not known.

MEDICATION OVERUSE HEADACHE (MOH) (1) OR ANALGESIC REBOUND HEADACHE

Because medication overuse is a very important part of CDH, it is appropriate to examine this entity in some detail. Excessive and daily use of immediate-relief medications is seen in patients with CDH. Medication misuse headache has been referred to as "medication overuse (MOH)," "analgesic rebound headache," "ergotamine rebound headache," and "drug-induced headache." *Rebound headache* is often used to characterize the headache-perpetuating tendency when immediate-relief medications are used very frequently. The International Headache Society uses the term *medication overuse headache* (MOH).

There appears to be some confusion between the terms *recurrence* and *rebound*. Recurrence may be defined as the recurrence of the same headache that was significantly relieved by an abortive antimigraine agent. Recurrence should occur within the expected natural duration of that migraine attack. Recurrence of the same headache may occur when 5-HT1 agonists are used in acute migraine.

Rebound headache, in contrast, can be defined as perpetuation of head pain in chronic headache sufferers caused by frequent and excessive use of immediate-relief medication. It can also be defined as "a self-sustaining, rhythmic, headache-medication cycle characterized by daily or near daily headache and irresistible and predictable use of immediate relief medications as the only means of relieving headache attacks" (15).

Evidence for Rebound

The most convincing evidence for analgesic-ergotamine rebound is the fact that mere discontinuation of these medications results in significant improvement. There is ample data in the literature to support the existence of analgesic/ergotamine rebound headache (13,15,17–19,22–24). Silverman et al. (25) reported that moderate or severe headache occurred in 52% of patients on caffeine withdrawal based on a double-blind cessation of caffeine consumption. In a survey of physicians engaged in the treatment of headache, more than 40% of the respondents (174) indicated that analgesic rebound is present in at least 20% of their patients with headache (26).

Agents commonly associated with rebound in decreasing order include butalbital/caffeine/aspirin/acetaminophen combinations, caffeine-containing analgesic combinations, opioids, and ergotamine (23). Triptans have been reported to cause multiple recurrences and rebound (27,28), but the incidence is extremely low. Unlike patients with analgesic rebound, patients who overused triptans had a shorter and less severe withdrawal as well as a significantly lower relapse rate (28).

Clinical Features of Medication Overuse Headache (MOH), Analgesic Rebound Headache

A number of clinical characteristics help identify the occurrence of analgesic rebound headache in patients with primary headache disorders (23). The following are the clinical features of analgesic rebound:

1. The headaches are refractory, daily or near daily.
2. Headaches occur in a patient with primary headache disorder who uses immediate-relief medications very frequently, often in excessive quantities.
3. The headache itself varies in its severity, type, and location from time to time.
4. The slightest physical or intellectual effort will bring on the headaches. In other words, the threshold for head pain appears to be low.
5. Headaches are accompanied by asthenia, nausea, and other GI symptoms, restlessness, anxiety, irritability, memory problems, and difficulty in intellectual concentration and depression. Those consuming large quantities of ergot derivatives may exhibit cold extremities, tachycardia, paresthesias, diminished pulse, hypertension, lightheadedness, muscle pain of the extremities, weakness of the legs, and depression.
6. There is a drug-dependent rhythmicity of headaches. Predictable early morning (2 a.m. to 5 a.m.) headaches are frequent, particularly in patients who use large quantities of analgesic, sedative, caffeine, or ergotamine combinations. Butalbital, a short-acting barbiturate containing analgesics, suppresses REM sleep, which is followed by REM rebound and results in awaking with severe headache.
7. There is evidence of tolerance to analgesics over a period of time, patients needing increasing doses as time goes by.
8. Withdrawal symptoms are observed when the patients are taken off pain medications abruptly.
9. Spontaneous improvement of headache occurs on discontinuing the medications.
10. Concomitant prophylactic medications are relatively ineffective while the patients are consuming large excess amounts of immediate-relief medications.

Patterns of Medication Consumption in Patients with Medication Overuse Headache

Many patients consume analgesics in anticipation of headache. Fear of pain drives them to take medication even before the headache develops. There is a predictable and irresistible pattern of use in many patients. Multiple medications are used concomitantly, both prescription and nonprescription. Ferrari and Sternieri (29) analyzed the reasons for daily analgesic consumption in patients with chronic headache disorders. The reasons given by the patient were consumption under medical advice to take the analgesic at the moment of need (57%); because they cannot cope with pain (67%); apprehension about headache developing if drug is not taken (62%); recurrence of pain soon after previous consumption (30%); the notion there is no other cure (61%); because the analgesic makes headache more bearable and enables them to function at work (62%); to reduce tension and anxiety (41%); and to aid sleep (18%). It should be noted that many patients gave more than one of the reasons just cited for the daily analgesic consumption.

The behavioral aspect of the analgesic consumption is important. Relief of pain gives a negative reinforcement, and changes in mood produced by some of the agents containing barbiturates or stimulants such as caffeine may give a positive reinforcement for the behavior resulting in excessive use of immediate-relief medications. It is very rare for these patients to use the habit-forming doses of barbiturates, which is usually above 600 to 800 mg per day. Therefore addiction does not appear to be a problem in the majority of patients, even though there are exceptions of drug-seeking behavior.

Analgesic use does not usually interfere with the execution of normal social and/or occupational roles, as happens when the abuse substance is a narcotic or alcohol. On the contrary, the analgesic represents a kind of necessary crutch for his or her everyday functions.

Development of tolerance is evidenced by escalating consumption with no appropriate adverse consequences. Withdrawal symptoms upon discontinuation can be very prominent. These withdrawal symptoms include restlessness, sleeplessness, increased headache, diarrhea, and occasional seizures, especially in those who consume large amounts of butalbital-containing analgesics. Increase in headache pain with decrease in analgesic efficacy occurs over a period of time.

Consequence of Rebound

Clinical evidence from various centers around the world points to the fact that rebound phenomenon alters the natural history of migraine.

Is Medication Overuse or Analgesic Rebound an Addictive Behavior?

Analgesic rebound phenomenon is actually a paradoxical response. Those taking most medications experience most pain. The question then arises, is a high level of pain experience the cause of high analgesic consumption? Or is the overuse of analgesics due to certain psychological predispositions? That leads to this question: Is analgesic rebound headache due to addictive behavior?

There is no evidence of addictive personality in these patients (30). Sensation-seeking behaviors are not high in these patients with chronic headache (31).

Analgesic Rebound is Unique to Primary Headache Disorders

Relapses of migraine occur in migraineurs who have been placed on analgesics for other ailments (32). The association between analgesic overuse and headache has been studied in

Table 5-4.   Possible pathophysiological mechanisms of CDH and analgesic rebound

Serotonergic dysnociception (35–38)

Central sensitization (39–41)

Dysfunction of periaqueductal gray (PAG) (42,43)

Impaired opioid antinociception (44–47)

conditions other than primary headache disorders. Chronic overuse of analgesics does not cause increased headache in nonmigraineurs. For example, studying a group of pure arthritis patients who were consuming fairly large amounts of analgesics regularly for arthritis did not show increased incidence of headache (33). Of those patients taking regular analgesics for arthritis who had CDH, all gave a past history of migraine (34). CDH developed after regular analgesic use had been established in these patients. No patient without a past history of primary headache developed daily headache while taking regular analgesics (34). The conclusion from various clinical observations and studies is that analgesic rebound headache may be restricted to those who are already headache sufferers, particularly migraine.

Pathophysiology of CDH and Analgesic Rebound

Pathophysiology of CDH and analgesic rebound is poorly understood. Defective antinociceptive mechanisms may be responsible. Table 5-4 lists the various possible pathophysiological mechanisms.

There is experimental evidence that "opioid-induced pain" may occur as a result of activation of pain facilitatory mechanisms in the rostral ventral medulla (RVM), which involves increased activity of cholecystokinin (CCK) as up-regulation and increased expression of dynorphin. Enhanced release of excitatory neurotransmitters from primary afferens and increased expression of PGRP in dorsal route ganglia are additional factors involved in opioid-induced pain.

Comorbidity of Chronic Daily Headache

Behavioral and Psychiatric Comorbidity

A number of recent publications deal with the behavioral and psychiatric comorbidity of migraine (48–53). Those observations are highly relevant to chronic daily headache because the majority of severe chronic daily headaches are transformed migraine. Breslau et al. (48) found the estimated risk for major depression associated with prior migraine, adjusted for sex and education, was 3.2. The risk for migraine associated with prior depression was 3.1. The bidirectional influences, with each disorder increasing the risk of onset of the other, were shown in the study (50). A "shared etiology" between migraine and depression is implicated. A history of migraine is also associated with increased lifetime rates of anxiety disorders, illicit drug use disorders, nicotine dependence, and suicide attempts (48–50). Those with a history of migraine were more likely to report job absenteeism, assess their general health as fair or poor, and use mental health services (48–50). Breslau and Andreski (51) reported that migraine was associated with increased incidence of "neuroticism" defined as a general emotional overactivity, which may lead to neurotic disorders under stress. Merikangas et al. (52,53) also observed strong association between migraine and depression, bipolar illness, and anxiety and panic disorders. The epidemiological studies just cited confirm the association between migraine and primary psychiatric and behavioral disorders such as depression, anxiety, and neuroticism, which have been previously reported in the clinic-based population.

The psychiatric comorbidity in CDH was assessed by Sandrini et al. (54) in a series of 98 patients. DSM-III-R criteria was used to diagnose psychiatric conditions. Only 9.2% had no psychiatric diagnosis. Anxiety disorders were observed in 72.4%, mood disorders in 55.1%, combined anxiety and mood disorders in 46%, and somatoform disorders in 3.1%. Of those with mood disorders, one third suffered from major depression.

Neurological Comorbidity

The coexistence of migraine and idiopathic intracranial hypertension without papilledema may result in refractory chronic daily headache (55). A spinal tap to measure the cerebrospinal fluid (CSF) pressure is the only way to make a diagnosis of this condition. Headache characteristics of the two conditions may be very similar. In a refractory case of chronic daily headache with migrainous features, a spinal tap to rule out raised CSF pressure is in order (55). Another comorbid neurological condition associated with chronic daily headache is sleep apnea (56).

Quality of Life and Disability in CDH Patients

Health-related quality of life (HQL) using the short form (SF-36) questionnaire in patients with CDH showed significantly worse scores in physical functioning, role functioning (physical), bodily pain, general health perceptions, and mental health than patients with migraine headache (57). MIDAS Scale (58) showed very high disability scores in CDH patients (59).

MANAGEMENT OF CHRONIC DAILY HEADACHE

The two major factors that determine the prognosis of CDH are analgesic rebound and comorbidity. The first step in the management of CDH is to determine the presence or absence of rebound phenomenon. A person suffering from headache despite consuming analgesics and ergotamine on a daily basis could fall into the category of drug-induced headache or analgesic rebound headache. Concomitant use of prophylactic medications in this situation is usually ineffective.

The behavioral, psychological, and disability aspects of CDH need to be considered when treating patients with this form of headache. A multimodality approach is essential for satisfactory results, and a combination of pharmacological and behavioral interventions is necessary.

It is important to make as comprehensive a diagnosis as possible and attempt to recognize the subtype of CDH the patient is suffering from. Those with transformed migraine are significantly more responsive to treatment than those with CTTH. In all subtypes, the analgesic rebound has to be looked for.

These are the essential principles of management of CDH:

- Discontinuation of the offending medications—detoxification
- Attempts to break the cycle of continuous headache by pharmacotherapeutic agents
- Initiation of prophylactic pharmacotherapy
- Management of breakthrough headaches by specific agents such as triptans
- Recognition of comorbid psychiatric and behavioral issues with concomitant behavioral intervention, relaxation-based behavioral therapy such as biofeedback therapy, cognitive behavioral therapy, individual counseling, family therapy, physical exercise, and dietary instructions
- Adequate instructions about ill effects of medications with special focus on analgesics—education
- Continuity of care

The multimodality approach to treatment just outlined can be undertaken either with outpatients or inpatients.

Outpatient Treatment

Outpatient treatment is most suitable for highly motivated patients without serious comorbidities who are not very high consumers of opioids/butalbital/sedative-containing analgesics. Outpatient management will consist of (a) abrupt discontinuation for simple analgesics and triptans (for those with triptan rebound), (b) gradual taper of the butalbital/caffeine/opioid medications, (c) substituting such analgesics with nonsteroidal antiinflammatory agents (NSAIDs) (e.g., naproxen sodium 550 mg twice a day) or including COX_2 inhibitors during the withdrawal period, (d) introduction of appropriate prophylactic pharmacotherapy, (e) treating breakthrough headache with specific antimigraine drugs such as a triptan, and (f) combining all these with behavioral approaches and education.

Inpatient Treatment

Inpatient treatment is indicated in (a) those who fail outpatient treatment, (b) those who consume very large quantities of opioids/butalbital/tranquilizers containing analgesics, and (c) those with very significant psychological and behavioral comorbidities as well as medical comorbidities.

The essential differences in the inpatient approach are a more aggressive supervised withdrawal of offending medications, the use of agents to reduce the effect of abrupt withdrawal, intravenous administration of medication around the clock to break the cycle of headache, and initiating prophylaxis that often includes a rational combination of medications to treat comorbidities and adjusting the dosages. A hospital stay of 5 to 6 days is necessary in the majority of cases; it may extend to 10 or 15 days in more complicated cases.

Detoxification

Discontinuation of daily analgesics, narcotics, sedatives, caffeine, and ergotamine is the first step. A rare patient with triptan-induced rebound may also have to be taken off those medications, substituting a triptan with low recurrence rate such as naratriptan for infrequent use.

Opioid Withdrawal

Gradual withdrawal is the ideal approach. A formal schedule of withdrawal, decreasing the medication by one tablet per day every 3 days is recommended. The patient should be warned that the headache may get worse during the withdrawal period, 24 to 72 hours of stopping or decreasing the dosage of the medication. Other symptoms of withdrawal may occur, including anxiety, tremulousness, insomnia, and restlessness. Common symptoms of opioid withdrawal including codeine consist of nausea, vomiting, diarrhea, lacrimation, rhinorrhea, sweating, yawning, muscle aches, and craving for opioids.

Abrupt withdrawal of analgesics and narcotics is possible; however, it should be done under close supervision. Detoxification from opioids, particularly codeine, can be aided by using clonidine, which reduces the clinical symptoms of opioid withdrawal (60). Oral clonidine 0.1 mg two or three times a day is usually used. Another option is the transdermal clonidine patch (0.2 mg), which may be applied on the first day of withdrawal, to be changed after 1 week and discontinued after 2 weeks. Transdermal clonidine is more convenient for patients who may experience vomiting during the withdrawal period.

Butalbital Withdrawal

The most commonly prescribed and overused medication for the treatment of chronic headaches and one of the most common causes of analgesic rebound is butalbital/caffeine/aspirin/acetaminophen combinations with or without codeine. Butalbital is a short-acting barbiturate. Attempts at butalbital withdrawal using standard tapering methods require slow discontinuation over a number of days and are subject to patient noncompliance. If the patient does not report butalbital intake accurately or taper is too rapid, significant withdrawal symptoms can occur. Barbiturate withdrawal symptoms may include apprehension, muscle weakness, tremors, postural faintness, amnesia, twitches, seizures, and psychosis or delirium. Seizures usually occur on the second or third day of withdrawal but can occur up to the eighth day. In order to avoid seizure and other withdrawal reactions, a long-acting barbiturate such as phenobarbital may be substituted. Phenobarbital 30 mg three times daily for the first 2 days and 30 mg daily for the next 2 days is recommended during the withdrawal period (61). Phenobarbital loading protocol provides for more rapid and effective medication withdrawal, reduced opportunities for patient noncompliance, and medication "bargaining" behavior and superior safety.

Caffeine Withdrawal

Caffeine has been shown to cause rebound headache both in epidemiological surveys and double-blind controlled trials (14,25). Many OTC medications contain caffeine and are taken in large quantities by patients because they are nonprescription. The patient may not follow the instructions that come with the medications and end up taking as many as 10 to 20 caffeine-containing tablets a day. Dietary caffeine in the beverage adds to the total caffeine intake. These two sources of caffeine have to be discussed with each patient and appropriate steps taken to withdraw as quickly as possible. Note that some of the OTC medications have as high as 65 mg of caffeine in them (e.g., Excedrin Migraine).

Breaking the Cycle of Headache: Transitional Therapies

To further aid the withdrawal of opioids/butalbital/caffeine-containing agents and to help break the cycle of headache, any one of the following or an appropriate combination of these is recommended. Note: These agents are usually used for a few days to a week or two until the headache cycle is broken.

NSAIDs: naproxen (62), Tolfenamic acid (63), ketoprofen, diclofenac
Methylergonovine (64)
Sumatriptan subcutaneous (SC) injections (65)
Naratriptan oral
Oral corticosteroids (66,67)
Intravenous (IV) dihydroergotamine (68,69)
Continuous SC infusion of DHE (CS QI–DHE) (70)
IV prochlorperazine (71)
IV chlorpromazine (72)
IV droperidol (73)
Intramuscular (IM) droperidol (74)
IV diphenhydramine (75)
IV valproate sodium (76–79)
IV dexamethasone (80)

Evidence for the effectiveness of transitional therapy during the withdrawal period is best in Class II and in most instances Class III because there are no randomized placebo-controlled double-blind (RCDBT) trials.

NSAIDs, particularly naproxen sodium 500 mg twice daily, is useful in withdrawing patients from ergotamine (62). We use naproxen sodium or COX_2 inhibitors in patients being withdrawn from butalbital compounds. COX_2 inhibitors have the distinct advantage of fewer gastric side effects. NSAIDs should be taken after meals. Medications such as cimetidine, ranitidine, misoprostol, sucralfate, and omeprazole may be necessary to protect gastric and duodenal mucosa.

Using triptans as transitional therapy, Diener et al. (65) found that repeated SC injection of sumatriptan may be useful in breaking the cycle of TM. The maximum dose of SC sumatriptan per day is 12 mg. It may be given for 3 to 4 days. Because of the excellent tolerability of naratriptan, its prolonged effect and very low recurrence rate, many clinicians are using naratriptan (2.5 mg tablet twice daily) during the withdrawal period. There are no randomized controlled double-blind trials (RCDBT).

Corticosteroids may have a place in the transitional therapy even though RCDBT are lacking. Randomized open trial reports indicate that patients taking corticosteroids during withdrawal period experienced headache-free days earlier, milder withdrawal symptoms including nausea and headache, and needed less rescue medications (67). In the study, prednisolone was used in tapering doses for the 9 days of the study, with 100 mg daily for 3 days, 50 mg daily for 3 days, and 20 mg daily for 3 days. The author uses IV dexamethazone for 3 days during the withdrawal period (2 mg twice daily) in his inpatients. Prednisone as an initial treatment of analgesic-induced daily headache has been reported successful (81).

IV Dihydroergotamine

In most transformed migraine patients, the daily headache cycle can be broken by repetitive IV administration of dihydroergotamine (DHE) (68,69). A test dose of one third of a milliliter of DHE with 5 mg of metoclopramide or 10 mg of prochlorperazine may be used, followed by 0.5 mL of DHE with one of the antinausea medications every 6 hours for 48 to 72 hours. DHE may be given IV push or diluted in 50 ml of normal saline piggyback. Some patients may require the therapy for a few additional days. Approximately 70% to 80% of patients do respond to DHE. Nausea, diarrhea, leg cramps, and chest pain are seen as side effects in some patients. Nausea may occur in spite of metoclopramide or prochlorperazine. IV ondansetron (Zofran 4 mg) may be useful for nausea, even though ondansetron by itself has no headache-reducing efficacy in migraine (82). IV metoclopramide may cause akathisia and restlessness in some patients.

In-home IV administration of DHE by a visiting nurse is a cost-effective method of breaking the cycle of CDH (83). However, the nursing service should be reliable and prompt, with facilities to monitor and manage adverse events.

IM DHE is effective, as is SC, even though the degree of response is much less than with IV. Continuous in-home SC infusion (CSQI–DHE) using a programmable computerized infusion pump has been reported (70). Long-term local effect of SC DHE is not known. DHE is contraindicated in coronary and peripheral vascular disease. Triptans and DHE should not be combined.

Alternate IV Medications

In those who are unable to tolerate DHE or when it is contraindicated, alternative IV medications are possible. These include chlorpromazine (72) or prochlorperazine (71). In some patients, 12.5 mg of chlorpromazine given IV (piggyback) infused for 15 minutes every 6 hours for 2 days has been found effective. Orthostatic hypotension is a possible side effect, and precautions should be taken to prevent dizziness and syncope as a result of orthostatic hypotension.

Prochlorperazine at 5 to 10 mg IV is also effective and can be repeated. Extrapyramidal dystonic reactions are possible side effects that can be counteracted by benztropine mesylate (Cogentin).

Anecdotal reports also indicate the use of IV dexamethasone (80). Although there are no controlled studies to prove its clinical efficacy, those who have prolonged migraine seem to respond to such therapy. It can be combined with DHE or prochlorperazine.

Droperidol

Droperidol, an adjunct during general anesthesia, has been used to treat agitation, surgical pain, in combination with opioids, and nausea and vomiting. IV droperidol has been reported to be effective in acute migraine (73). A recent randomized placebo-controlled double-blind parallel group study in 22 centers showed that 2.75 mg droperidol IM resulted in a 2-hour headache response of over 80% (74). Two-hour pain-free response for 2.75 mg droperidol was 60% compared to 30% for the placebo. Higher doses were not more effective.

Adverse events included asthenia, anxiety, akathisia, and somnolence, which occurred in 15% to 30% of patients. Thirty percent of those were severe in intensity.

Thus there is evidence from one randomized double-blind placebo-controlled study that IM droperidol is effective in acute migraine even though side effects may prevent its routine use in many patients. Further studies are needed to confirm Class I evidence for efficacy. Because many of the agents are useful in acute migraine and effectively used for transitional treatment for CDH, IM droperidol may also be useful.

Miscellaneous Agents for IV Use

Anecdotal reports of the effectiveness of IV diphenhydramine (Benadryl) and magnesium sulphate expanded options for breaking the cycle of CDH. The recommended dose of diphenhydramine is 50 mg IV every 6 hours (75). Magnesium sulphate IV 1 g twice a day for 3 to 4 days may also help (84).

IV Valproate Sodium (Depacon)

Recently IV valproate sodium has been found useful for status migrainosus and can be given to break the cycle of CDH (76–79). Five hundred milligrams of valproate sodium diluted in 50 cc of IV saline given as fast drip or diluted in 20 mL N. saline as IV push are recommended. This can be repeated every 8 hours for 2 days. IV valproate is as effective as DHE but with fewer side effects such as nausea, leg cramps, and chest pain (85). In patients who cannot tolerate or have contraindications to DHE, IV valproate is an excellent option, especially because of its superior tolerability. It is a common practice to switch these patients to oral valproate (divalproex sodium) for prophylaxis once the headache is broken.

Infusion Center Treatments

Many treatments that used to be given only in an inpatient setting are now administered in outpatient infusion centers, after which patients are sent home. IV DHE and sodium valproate can be administered twice daily. Disadvantages of this treatment modality is that delayed side effects such as akathisia must be managed and patients should not drive home after receiving certain IV therapy. Cost effectiveness is the major advantage.

Tizanidine as Transitional Therapy

Tizanidine is a centrally acting alpha 2 adrenergic agonist. The effect of tizanidine is greatest on polysynaptic pathways, which, in turn, reduce facilitation of spinal motor neurons. It has very little direct effect on skeletal muscles. Even though it is chemically related to clonidine, tizanidine has significantly less effect on blood pressure.

There is Class II evidence that tizanidine is useful for CTTH (86), but those results have never been replicated. One open-label retrospective study report indicated that a combination of tizanidine 2 to 6 mg and naproxen sodium 550 mg twice daily was a useful strategy for transitional therapy during the detoxification phase of patients with analgesic rebound headache (87). This Class III evidence has to be improved by further controlled trials.

Prophylactic Pharmacotherapy

Patients with transformed migraine may respond to antimigraine prophylactic agents effectively, provided detoxification from analgesic has already been achieved. The clinician may choose a prophylactic agent or a combination of prophylactic agents depending on the clinical diagnosis and comorbid factors. Table 5-5 shows the commonly used prophylactic agents and their clinical usefulness.

Tizanidine Prophylaxis

One open-label study (88) and a double-blind placebo-controlled study (89) indicated tizanidine as an effective prophylactic agent for CDH. In the double-blind placebo-controlled study (89), Tizanidine was found to be significantly superior to placebo as follows: number of severe headache days per week, average headache intensity, peak headache intensity, and mean headache duration. Incidence of severe headache reduced by 55% compared to placebo in the tizanidine group, and the headache index reduced by 51%. No difference was seen between groups in the use of analgesic and abortive medications during the study. This study, even though it was double blind placebo controlled, is only Class II evidence because it has not been replicated and because the study had major deficiencies in that the patients were taking other preventive medications as well.

Tizanidine may have a role in prophylaxis of chronic daily headache; however, the high incidence of side effects such as somnolence in 47% of patients and dizziness in 24% of patients makes this medication a less than ideal agent for many patients.

Valproate Prophylaxis

In an open-label study on patients with CDH, divalproex sodium given daily reduced the frequency of migraine as well as total headache days (90). Tremor, weight gain, and loss of hair are some of the disturbing side effects.

Topiramate Prophylaxis

Because of its proven efficacy in episodic migraine, topiramate prophylaxis has an important place in the prophylactic therapy of chronic migraine. Universal lack of weight gain and weight loss in many patients is an added advantage. Topiramate can be combined with antidepressant effectively, and concomitant use of triptans is well tolerated.

Rational Copharmacy

There is a place for rational copharmacy in the prophylactic treatment of CDH. For example, one can combine a primary

Table 5-5.   Classes of drugs used in prophylaxis of CDH–TM

Class	FDA Approved for Migraine (Class I Evidence)	Other Agents in the Class	Most Appropriate Patients	Unsuitable Patients
Beta Adrenergic Blocking Agents	Propranolol Timolol	Nadolol Metoprolol Atenolol Pindolol	CDH with hypertension, stress, anxiety	CDH with asthma, congestive failure, brittle diabetes, hypotension
Tricyclic Antidepressants	None	Amitriptyline Nortriptyline Doxepin Imipramine Protriptyline	CDH with depression, sleep problems	CDH with obesity
Antiepileptic Drugs	Divalproex	Gabapentin Topiramate Levetiracetum Lamotrigine Tiagabin Zonisamide	CDH with bipolar disorder, epilepsy, essential tremor, neuropathy, obesity (Topiramate), ischemic heart disease, diabetes (Topiramate)	CDH with obesity (Valproate)
Calcium Channel Blocker	Verapamil Nicardipine Diltiazem		CDH with hypertension, angina, prolonged migraine aura, Raynaud's disease	

Serotonin Antagonists	Methysergide Cyproheptadine	CDH with intractable migraine symptoms, Cyproheptadine in CDH in children	CDH with ischemic heart disease, atherosclerotic disease
Alpha 2 Adrenergic Agonists	Tizanidine	CDH with insomnia	CDH with hepatic disorders, hypotension
SSRIs and Other Antidepressants	Fluoxetine Sertraline Paroxetine Fluvoxamine Nefazodone Venlafaxine	CDH with anxiety, depression, and OCDs	CDH with bipolar illness
Atypical Antipsychotics	Quetiapine	CDH with severe anxiety, insomnia, bipolar illness	
Botulinum Toxin	Type A Type B	Intractable CDH	CDH with Myasthenia or Myasthenic Syndrome, those on aminoglycosides
Miscellaneous Agents	Vitamin B2 Magnesium Oxide	CDH with prolonged migraine aura, familial forms of migraine with neurological symptoms	

antimigraine prophylactic agent, such as a beta-blocker, methysergide, or divalproex sodium, with agents that are effective for psychiatric comorbid conditions such as depression or anxiety. A combination of antidepressants or antianxiety agents with antimigraine prophylactic agents is a rational way of approaching the treatment of persistent CDH. Copharmacies are now accepted in most chronic disorders such as diabetes and hypertension. In fact, copharmacy is more relevant in the treatment of chronic daily headache because of significant comorbidities. Examples of combination therapy are beta-blockers plus tricyclic antidepressants in CDH patients with depression and insomnia, divalproex sodium plus SSRIs in patients with CDH, anxiety, and depression, and calcium channel blockers plus lithium in patients with migraine and bipolar illness.

Options in the Management of Severe Refractory CM/CDH

Various medications such as MAOI inhibitors, stimulants, long-acting opioids, botulinum toxin type A, daily triptans, particularly naratriptan, and daily DHE have been reported to be useful in very refractory cases (Class III evidence).

Long-acting Opioids

Long-acting opioids such as OxyContin, fentanyl patch, and methadone may have a place in selected intractable cases. However, long-term good control is obtained in only approximately 20% to 25% of cases (91). They are safe and do not cause weight gain. However, the drawbacks of long-term opioids are sedation, constipation, nausea, potential dose escalation of doses, and legal and regulatory issues for the physician. When abortive therapies such as triptans are contraindicated or when preventive pharmacotherapy is totally ineffective, long-acting opioids may be an option. Short-acting opioids should be avoided.

Atypical Antipsychotics

Patients with behavioral disorders such as borderline personality disorder and those with severe insomnia may benefit from relatively small doses of atypical antipsychotics such as quetiapine fumarate (Seroquel), risperidone (Risperdal), and ziprasidone (Geodon). Among these, ziprasidone has the least number of extrapyramidal effects. Most clinicians prefer quetiapine fumarate (Seroquel).

Botulinum Toxin in Chronic Headache

Botulinum toxin is a novel method of modification of chronic headache. Although the mechanism is not fully understood, it appears to act by a distinct antinociceptive action, possibly through an effect on muscle spindles or on the nociceptive pain pathways including C and A delta fibers, mechano and chemo receptors, or by effecting the release of substance P, CGRP, and glutamate (92). The muscle paralytic action may have no major role in pain relief.

A number of studies have been done in chronic tension-type headache and migraine (93–97). Silberstein and colleagues conducted a double-blind vehicle-controlled randomized trial in patients with IHS-defined migraine headache with or without aura (94). Subjects with a history of migraine diagnosis before age 50 with an average of two to eight moderate or severe migraines per month over the previous 3 months were eligible for enrollment. Patients were randomized to receive botulinum toxin type A, 25 units, or botulinum toxin type A, 75 units. The total dose was divided among various muscle groups in the frontal, temporal, and glabellar areas. The patients attended a baseline visit, an injection visit, and three monthly postinjection visits and kept a headache diary for the duration of the study. The frequency of moderate or severe migraine was recorded by the 122 patients who completed the study, which was the main outcome variable. There was a significant reduction in the number of moderate or severe migraine in the 25-unit group versus placebo at months 2 and 3 postinjection. Additionally, patients in the 25-unit group experienced a significantly greater reduction in migraine-associated vomiting versus placebo at month 3. The lack of significant effect of 75 units may be attributable to the lower frequency of migraine at baseline in that group. This study on migraine has not been duplicated. Further double-blind studies are in progress at the present time.

Brin and colleagues (95) conducted a double-blind placebo-controlled study of botulinum toxin type A in 56 patients with migraine. The authors found a significant reduction in the severity of pain and a trend toward reduction in headache frequency and duration. Retrospective analysis and open-label trials of various series have shown encouraging results in both chronic tension-type headache and migraine. No studies are available using botulinum type B.

The best indications for considering botulinum toxin therapy are primary disabling headaches including very frequent migraine, chronic daily headache (transformed migraine), chronic tension-type headache, medication overuse (drug-induced headache), patients with chronic jaw, neck, or muscle spasm associated with headache when acute medications like triptans are contraindicated, such as in patients with coronary artery disease, patients with compliance problems, and patients who are refractory to routine treatment.

Botulinum toxin is safe and well tolerated. Doses are over 30 times below the toxic doses, offering a large margin of safety. Adverse events are rare, mild, and reversible. All of the medications used to prevent migraine and transformed migraine are associated with adverse events, which can limit their utility. Thus botulinum toxin represents a new option for those who cannot tolerate or who do not respond to currently available preventive therapy.

Botulinum toxin has a long duration of action. It is readministered after beneficial effects wear off, which is usually 3 to 4 months. In patients who cannot or do not want to comply with a daily medication regime, botulinum toxin is a very viable option.

Thus evidence is beginning to accumulate regarding the efficacy of botulinum toxin in migraine. It must be tested in a large patient population to determine the optimum dose regimes and the best injection sites. It is not yet clear why some patients derive relief from botulinum toxin and others do not. Further trials should try to discern which patient characteristics are predictive of positive response to botulinum toxin. At the present time, there are two ways of using the injection: in preselected areas of the head and neck or in areas corresponding to the patient's maximum pain. On an average, 50 to 100 units of botulinum toxin type A divided into smaller units for each site of injection is recommended. In open trials, many patients seem to get relief, and they do not hesitate to get repeat treatment after approximately 3 months.

Concomitant Behavioral Therapy

Concomitant behavioral intervention, including biofeedback therapy, individual cognitive behavioral therapy, family therapy, physical exercise, and dietary instructions, is imperative for the successful management of patients with CDH. Details of these modes of treatment are beyond the scope of this chapter. Physical therapy (heat, massage, ultrasonography) to neck muscles may help partially. Selected application of trigger point injections may help as well.

Education

Adequate instruction about the nature of the patent's disorder and the ill effects of certain medications used in excessive and frequent quantities, particularly analgesics and narcotics, should be emphasized. The patients have to understand that this disorder is biological in nature, with neurochemical and physiological changes producing the headache. They should also appreciate the fact that behavioral factors, such as anxiety, depression, inability to relax, and stress, influence this biology a great deal, making headaches more frequent, more severe, and more difficult to manage. Every program that deals with CDH should have education as a part of the therapeutic program.

Continuity of Care

CDH is usually a prolonged problem occupying years of a person's life, and none of the preventive medications are 100% effective. Adverse effects prevent prolonged use of many medications. Patients develop tachyphylaxis to many medications. Therefore, continuity of care with frequency follow-up and adequate physician/patient communication is essential for the long term.

Psychiatric Referral

TM/CDH are not primary psychiatric disorders, although comorbidities are important. Referral to a psychiatrist should not be an end-of-the-road referral. If a psychiatrist is consulted, it should be in conjunction with the medical treatment. The physician who takes care of these patients should have full control of all aspects of treatment, and the psychiatric treatment should only be an adjunct in the overall management.

Referral to a Tertiary Care Headache Unit

A tertiary care headache center with facilities for inpatient and outpatient treatment is the most appropriate place for referral. Pain management clinics with emphasis on physical methods of treatment such as epidural blocks or heavy narcotics should be avoided.

Overall, from the experience of many centers treating chronic daily headache patients, it appears that approximately one third of patients show relapse of their daily headache and may have a tendency to go back to taking pain medications regularly unless they are supervised very carefully (98,99). In patients with this persistent, intractable chronic daily headache, the behavioral, psychological, and neuroendocrine features are strikingly different from the patients with CDH who show improvement (98). The Minnesota Multiphasic Personality Inventory (MMPI) was abnormal in 100% of intractable cases. High scores and hypochondriasis, depression, and hysteria (scores 1, 2, and 3) were consistent, and combinations of high scores of 6, 7, 8, and 9 were seen in 56% of those with intractable CDH. Among the parents of patients with intractable CDH, a high incidence of alcoholism was found. A high incidence of physical, emotional, and sexual abuse was also found in this group when compared to those who were treated successfully. The Zung Depression Scale and the Beck Depression Inventory were also higher in the intractable group when compared to the improved group.

Therefore, it appears that there is a group of patients with very persistent intractable chronic daily headache that is resistant to all currently available forms of treatment. It may signify some permanent abnormalities in the pain control systems of the brain.

REFERENCES

1. The International Classification of Headache Disorders, 2nd ed. *Cephalalgia* 2004;24(Suppl 1).
2. Mathew NT, Reuveni U, Perez F. Transformed or evolutive migraine. *Headache* 1987;27:102–106.
3. Sanin LC, Mathew NT, Bellmeyer LR, et al. International Headache Society (IHS) Headache Classification as applied to a headache clinic population. *Cephalalgia* 1994;14:443–446.
4. Scher A, Stewart W, Liberman J, et al. Prevalence of frequent headache in a population sample. *Headache* 1996;38(7): 497–596.
5. Castillo J, Munoz P, Guitera V, et al. Epidemiology of chronic daily headache in the general population. *Headache* 1999;39: 190–196.
6. Wang SJ, Fuh JL, Lu SR, et al. Chronic daily headache in Chinese elderly: prevalence, risk factors, and biannual follow-up. *Neurology* 2000;54(2):314–319.
7. Lanteri M, Minet J, Awiam G, et al. Prevalence and description of chronic daily headache in the general population in France in 2000. *Cephalalgia* 2001;21:468.
8. Manzoni GC, Micieli G, Granella F, et al. Daily chronic headache: classification and clinical features: observation on 250 patients. *Cephalalgia* 1987;7(Suppl 6):169–170.
9. Manzoni GC, Sandrini, Zanferrari C, et al. Clinical features of daily chronic headache and its different subtypes. *Cephalalgia* 1991;11(Suppl 11):292–293.
10. Solomon S, Lipton RB, Newman LC. Clinical features of chronic daily headache. *Headache* 1992;32:325–329.

11. Saper JR, Lake AE, Madden FF, et al. Comprehensive/tertiary care for headache: a 6-month outcome study. *Headache* 1999; 39(4):249–263.

12. Manzoni GC, Granella F, Sandrin G, et al. Classification of chronic daily headache by International Headache Society criteria: limits and new proposals. *Cephalalgia* 1995;15:37–43.

13. Mathew NT, Stubits E, Nigam MP. Transformation of episodic migraine into chronic daily headache: an analysis of factors. *Headache* 1982;22:66–68.

14. Scher AI, Lipton RB, Stewart WF. Is caffeine a risk factor for chronic daily headache? Results for the frequent headache epidemiology study (FRHE). *Cephalalgia* 2001;21:473.

15. Saper JR, Jones JM. Ergotamine dependency. *Clin Neuropharmacol* 1986;9:244.

16. Stewart WF, Scher AI, Lipton RB. Stressful life events and risk of chronic daily headache. Results from frequent headache epidemiology study (FRHE). *Cephalalgia* 2001;21:279.

17. Baldrati A, Bini L, D'Alessandro R, et al. Analysis of outcome predictors of migraine towards chronicity. *Cephalalgia* 1985;5(Suppl 2):195–199.

18. Giglio JA, Bruera OC, Leston JA. Hosp. Clinicas Bs.As. Hosp. R. Rossi La Plata. Argentina. *Cephalalgia* 1995;15(Suppl 14):165.

19. Srikiatkhachorn A, Phanthwychinda K. Prevalence and clinical features of chronic daily headache in a headache clinic. *Headache* 1997;37(5):277–280.

20. Gagnon CM, Lofland KR, Rokicki LA, et al. Chronic daily headache versus episodic headache in a large community based sample. *Headache* 1999;39:355.

21. Ravishanker K. Unusual Indian migraine trigger factors. *Cephalalgia* 2000;20:359.

22. Kudrow L. Paradoxical effects of frequent analgesic use. In: Critchley M, Friedman A, Gorini S, et al., eds. *Advances in neurology*, vol. 33. New York: Raven Press, 1982:335.

23. Mathew NT, Kurman R, Perez F. Drug induced refractory headache: clinical features and management. *Headache* 1990;30:634–638.

24. Rapoport AM, Weeks RE, Sheftell FD, et al. Analgesic rebound headache. Theoretical and practical implications. *Cephalalgia* 1985;5(Suppl 3):448.

25. Silverman K, Evans SM, Strain EC, et al. Withdrawal syndrome after the double blind cessation of caffeine consumption. *N Engl J Med* 1992;327:1109–1114.

26. Rapoport AM, Stang P, Gutterman DL, et al. Analgesic rebound headache in clinical practice—data from a physician survey. *Headache* 1996;36:14–19.

27. Limmroth V, Kazarawa Z, Fritsche G, et al. Headache after frequent use of serotonin agonists zolmitriptan and naratriptan. *Lancet* 1999; 353(9150):378.

28. Katsarava Z, Fritsche G, Finke M, et al. Clinical features of withdrawal headache and long term follow up after withdrawal from triptans in comparison to other antimigraine drugs. *Cephalalgia* 2001;21:278.

29. Ferrari A, Sternieri E. Chronic headache and analgesic abuse. In: DeMarinis M, Granella F, eds. *Ten years of headache research in Italy*. Rome: CIC Edizioni Internazionali, 1996:44–45.

30. Michultka DM, Blanchard EB, Appelbaum KA, et al. The refractory headache patient II high medication consumption (analgesic rebound) headache. *Behav Res Ther* 1989;27:411–420.
31. Wang W, Timsit-Berthier M, Schoenen J. Negative correlation between sensation seeking behavior and intensity dependence of auditory evoked potentials in migraine. *Cephalalgia* 1995; 15(Suppl 14):65.
32. Isler H. Migraine treatment as a cause of chronic migraine. In: Rose FC, ed. *Advances in migraine research and therapy.* New York: Raven Press, 1982:159.
33. Lance E, Parkes C, Wilkinson M. Does analgesic abuse cause headaches de novo? *Headache* 1988;28:61.
34. Bahra A, Walsh M, Menon S, et al. Does chronic daily headache arise de novo in association with regular analgesic use? *Cephalalgia* 2000;20:294.
35. Hering R, Glover V, Patichis K, et al. 5-HT in migraine patients with analgesic rebound headache. *Cephalalgia* 1993;13: 410–412.
36. Srikiatkhachorn A, Govitrapons P, Limthavon C. Up-regulation of 5-HT2 serotonin receptor; a possible mechanism of transformed migraine. *Headache* 1994;34:8–11.
37. Srikiatkhachorn A, Anthony M. Platelet 5-HT and 5-HT2 receptors in patients with analgesic induced headache. *Cephalalgia* 1995;15(Suppl 14):83.
38. Srikiatkhachorn A, Govitrapons P, Anthony M. Plasticity of serotonin symptoms and mechanisms of analgesic-abuse headache. *Cephalalgia* 2001;21:470–471.
39. Burstein R, Yarnitsky D, Gooraryeh I, et al. An association between migraine and cutaneous allodynia. *Ann Neurol* 2000;47:614–624.
40. Burstein R, Cutrer MF, Yarnitsky D. Development of cutaneous allodynia during a migraine attack—clinical evidence for the sequential recruitment of spinal and supraspinal neurons in migraine. *Brain* 2000;123:1703–1709.
41. Burstein R. Possible contribution of peripheral and central sensitization to chronic daily headache. *Cephalalgia* 2001;21:282.
42. Nagesh V, Welch M, Aurora SK, et al. Is there a brainstem generator of chronic daily headache? *J Headache Pain* 2000;2:67–71.
43. Welch KM, Nagesh V, Aurora S, et al. *Cephalalgia* 2001;21:281.
44. Sicuteri F. Opioid receptor impairment—underlying mechanism in "pain diseases"? *Cephalalgia* 1981;1:77–82.
45. Sicuteri F. Natural opioids in migraine. In: Critchley M, ed. *Advances in neurology.* New York: Raven Press, 1982:523–533.
46. Sicuteri F. Is acute tolerance to 5-hydroxytryptamine opioid dependent? Its absence in migraine sufferers. *Cephalalgia* 1983;3:187–190.
47. Fields HL, Heinricher MM. Brainstem modulation of nociceptor-driven withdrawal reflexes. *Ann NY Acad Sci* 1989;563:34–44.
48. Breslau N, Davis GC, Endreski P. Migraine, psychiatric disorders and suicide attempts: an epidemiological study of young adults. *Psychiatry Res* 1991;37(1):11–23.
49. Breslau N, Davis GC. Migraine, physical health and psychiatric disorder: a prospective epidemiologic study in young adults. *J Psychiatric Res* 1993;27(2):211–221.

50. Breslau N, Davis GC, Schultz LR. Migraine and major depression: a longitudinal study. *Headache* 1994;34(7):387–393.
51. Breslau N, Andreski P. Migraine, personality, and psychiatric comorbidity. *Headache* 1995;35:382–386.
52. Merikangas KR, Angst J, Isler H. Migraine and psychopathology: Results of the Zurich cohort study of young adults. *Arch Gen Psychiatry* 1990;47:849–853.
53. Merikangas KR, Angst J. Headache syndromes and psychiatric disorders: Association and familial transmission. *J Psychiatric Res* 1993;27(2):197–210.
54. Sandrini G, Verri AP, Barbieri E, et al. Psychiatric comorbidity in chronic daily headache. *Cephalalgia* 1995;15(Suppl 14):163.
55. Mathew NT, Ravishanker K, Sanin LC. Coexistence of migraine and idiopathic intracranial hypertension without papilledema. *Neurology* 1996;46:1226–1230.
56. Guilleminaut C, Dement WC. *Sleep apnea syndrome.* New York: LISS, 1978.
57. Monzon MJ, Lainez MJ. Quality of life in migraine and chronic daily headache patients. *Cephalalgia* 1998;18:638–643.
58. Stewart WF, Lipton RB, Kolodner K, et al. Reliability of the migraine disability assessment score in a population-based sample of headache sufferers. *Cephalalgia* 1999;19(2):107–114.
59. Mathew NT, Villarreal S, Kailasam J. Improvement in headache related disability in chronic daily: treatment outcome assessed by MIDAS. *Headache* 2000;40:420.
60. Jaffe JH. Drug dependence: opioids, non narcotics, nicotine (tobacco) and caffeine. In: Kaplan HI, Sadock BJ, eds. *Comprehensive textbook of psychiatry,* 5th ed. Philadelphia: W.B. Saunders, 1989: 642–686.
61. Sands GH. A protocol for butalbital, aspirin and caffeine (BAC) detoxification in headache patients. *Headache* 1990;30(8):491–496.
62. Mathew NT. Amelioration of ergotamine withdrawal symptoms with naproxen. *Headache* 1987;27:130–133.
63. Ala-Hurula V, Mylyla VV, Hokkanen E, et al. Tolfenamic acid and ergotamine abuse. *Headache* 1981;21:240–243.
64. Graff-Radford SB, Bittar CT. The use of methylergonovine (methergine) in the initial control of drug induced refractory headache. *Headache* 1993;(33):390–393.
65. Diener HC, Haab J, Peters C, et al. Subcutaneous sumatriptan in the treatment of headache during withdrawal from drug-induced headache. *Headache* 1991;31:205–209.
66. Bonuccelli U, Nuti A, Lucetti C, et al. Amitriptyline and dexamethasone combined treatment in drug-induced headache. *Cephalalgia* 1996;6:197–200.
67. Gobel H, Heinze A, Heinze-Kuhn K. Prednisolone alleviates and shortens withdrawal phase in drug induced headache. *Cephalalgia* 2001;21:481.
68. Raskin NH. Repetitive intravenous dihydroergotamine as therapy for intractable migraine. *Neurology* 1986;36:995–997.
69. Silberstein SD, Schulman EA, Hopkins MM. Repetitive intravenous DHE in the treatment of refractory headache. *Headache* 1990;30:334–339.
70. Stillman MJ, Zajac DE, Rybicki A. Pilot study of continuous subcutaneous infusion of DHE (CSQI–DHE) in the treatment of transformed migraine. *Cephalalgia* 2001;21:479.

71. Coppola M, Yealy DM, Leibold RA. Randomized, placebo-controlled evaluation of prochlorperazine versus metoclopramide for emergency department treatment of migraine headache. *Ann Emerg Med* 1995;26(5):541–546.
72. Lane PL, Ross R. Intravenous chlorpromazine-preliminary results in acute migraine. *Headache* 1985;25(6):302–304.
73. Wang SJ, Silberstein SD, Young WB. Droperidol treatment of status migrainosus and refractory migraine. *Headache* 1997; 37(6):377–382.
74. Silberstein S, Young WB, Mendizabal JE, et al. Efficacy of intramuscular droperidol for migraine treatment—a dosage response study. *Cephalalgia* 2001;21:271–272.
75. Swidan SZ, Hamel RL, Saper JR, et al. The efficacy of intravenously administered diphenhydramine versus dihydroergotamine, ketorolac, chlorpromazine, and droperidol in the treatment of refractory daily chronic headache. *Neurology* 1999;(Suppl 2):A255.
76. Mathew NT, Kailasam J, Meadors L, et al. Intravenous valproate sodium (Depacon) aborts migraine rapidly, a preliminary report. *Headache* 2000;40:720–723.
77. Krusz JC. Intravenous valproate sodium in the treatment of intractable migraine in the headache clinic. *Cephalalgia* 2001;21:433.
78. Edwards K, Norton J, Behnke J, et al. Comparison of intravenous valproate vs. intramuscular dihydroergotamine and metoclopramide for acute treatment of migraine headache. *Cephalalgia* 2001;21:433.
79. Karpitsky VV, Schwartz TH, Gunett CA, et al. Intravenous valproate in the treatment of chronic daily headache. *Cephalalgia* 2001;21:479.
80. Saadah HA. Abortive migraine therapy in the office with dexamethasone and prochlorperazine. *Headache* 1994;34(6): 366–370.
81. Krymchantowski AV, Barbosa JS. Prednisone as an initial treatment of analgesic induced daily headache. *Cephalalgia* 2000;20: 70–113.
82. Ferrari MD. 5-HT receptor antagonists and migraine therapy. *J Neurol* 1991;238:S53–S56.
83. Norris LL, Serowoky M, Aurora SK, et al. Outpatient intravenous dihydroergotamine is effective in chronic daily headache. *Cephalalgia* 2001;21:477–478.
84. Mauskop A, Altura B, Cracco R. Intravenous magnesium sulphate rapidly alleviates headache of various types. *Headache* 1996;36:154–160.
85. Mathew NT, Kailasam J. Repetitive intravenous administration of valproate sodium in intractable migraine: comparison with intravenous dihydroergotamine (DHE). *Neurology* 2000;54:A22(abst).
86. Fogelholm R, Murros K. Tizanidine in chronic tension-type headache. A placebo controlled double blind crossover study. *Headache* 1992;32:509–513.
87. Smith TR. Low dose tizanidine combined with long-acting NSAIDs for detoxification from analgesic rebound headache: a retrospective review. *Cephalalgia* 2000;20:381.
88. Saper JR, Winner PK, Lake AE. An open label dose titration study of the efficacy and tolerability of tizanidine hydrochloride

tablets in the prophylaxis of chronic daily headache. *Headache* 2001;41:357–368.

89. Lake AE. Chronic headache. New advances in treatment strategies. Presented at the World Congress of Neurology, London, 2001.

90. Mathew NT, Ali S. Valproate in the treatment of persistent chronic daily headache. An open label study. *Headache* 1991;31:71–76.

91. Saper JR, Lake III AE, Hamel RL, et al.. Long-termed scheduled opioid treatment for intractable headache: 3-year outcome report. *Cephalalgia* 2000;20:380(abst).

92. Akoi KR. Pharmacology and immunology of botulinum toxin serotypes. *J Neurol Sci* 2001;248(Suppl 3-10).

93. Binder WJ, Brin MF, Blitzer A, et al. Botulinum toxin type A (Botox) for the treatment of migraine headaches: an open-label study. *Otolaryngol Head Neck Surg* 2000;123:669–676.

94. Silberstein S, Mathew N, Saper J, et al. Botulinum toxin type A as a migraine preventive treatment. *Headache* 2000;40:445–450.

95. Brin MF, Swope DM, O'Brien C, et al. Botox for migraine: double-blind, placebo-controlled, region-specific evaluation. *Cephalalgia* 2000;20:421–422.

96. Mauskop A, Basdeo R. Botulinum toxin A is an effective prophylactic therapy for migraines. *Cephalalgia* 2000;20:422.

97. Relja M. Treatment of tension-type headache with botulinum toxin: 1-year follow-up. *Cephalagia* 2000;20:336.

98. Mathew NT, Kurman R, Perez F. Intractable chronic daily headache. A persistent neurobiobehavioral disorder. *Cephalalgia* 1989;9(Suppl 10):180–181.

99. Pini L, Bigarelli M, Vitale G, et al. Headaches associated with chronic use of analgesics: A therapeutic approach. *Headache* 1996;36:433–439.

Tension-type Headache and Miscellaneous Primary Headache Disorders

Ninan T. Mathew

TENSION-TYPE HEADACHE

Tension-type headache is the most common type of primary headache disorder; its lifetime prevalence in the general population ranges in different studies from 30% to 78%. At the same time, it is the least studied of primary headache disorders. Recent research has indicated a neurobiological basis at least for the more severe subtypes of tension-type headaches. The IHS classification of tension-type headache is given in Table 6-1 (1).

Tension-type headaches are divided into episodic and chronic. The episodic variety is further subdivided into infrequent and frequent subtypes. The infrequent tension-type headache occurs less than once a month and does not have any significant impact on the individual. Thus it does not deserve much attention from the medical profession. However, patients with frequent episodic tension-type headache can encounter considerable disability that sometimes warrants expensive drugs and prophylactic medications. Chronic tension-type headache is, of course, always associated with disability and high personal and socioeconomic costs.

All three subtypes of tension-type headache are divided into those associated with pericranial tenderness and those without pericranial tenderness. Manual palpation, preferably as a pressure control palpation, is recommended to assess muscle tenderness. It should be noted that patients with migraine can exhibit soreness and tenderness of the pericranial and neck muscles, making the distinction between tension-type headache and migraine more difficult.

The mechanism of the pathophysiology of tension-type headache is poorly understood. It is thought that episodic tension-type headaches may be due to peripheral pain mechanisms, whereas in chronic tension-type headache, central nociceptive mechanisms may play an important role. Central sensitization of the nociceptive system may be an underlying reason for the chronic tension-type headache.

Note that patients with chronic migraine are prone to exhibit headaches that may meet the criteria of a chronic tension-type headache from time to time. This causes diagnostic confusion in chronic daily headache with a mixed picture of migraine and tension-type headache. The treatment approach does not change from that of chronic migraine without interictal tension-type headache.

The clinical characteristics of tension-type headache as defined by IHS are (a) bilateral location, (b) pressing or tightening (nonpulsating) quality, (c) mild or moderate intensity, and

Table 6-1. Tension-type headache (TTH) (1)

2.1 Infrequent episodic tension-type headache (ETTH)
  2.1.1 Infrequent episodic tension-type headache associated with pericranial tenderness
  2.1.2 Infrequent episodic tension-type headache not associated with pericranial tenderness
2.2 Frequent episodic tension-type headache
  2.2.1 Frequent episodic tension-type headache associated with pericranial tenderness
  2.2.2 Frequent episodic tension-type headache not associated with pericranial tenderness
2.3 Chronic tension-type headache (CTTH)
  2.3.1 Chronic tension-type headache associated with pericranial tenderness
  2.3.2 Chronic tension-type headache not associated with pericranial tenderness
2.4 Probable tension-type headache
  2.4.1 Probable infrequent episodic tension-type headache
  2.4.2 Probable frequent episodic tension-type headache
  2.4.3 Probable chronic tension-type headache

(d) not aggravated by routine physical activity such as walking or climbing stairs. There is no associated nausea or vomiting (anorexia may occur) and no more than one symptom of photophobia or phonophobia.

To diagnose the frequent episodic tension-type headache variety, at least 10 episodes occurring on one or more, but less than 15 days per month for at least 3 months should occur, whereas in the infrequent variety, the frequency is less than one per month. Chronic tension-type headache is attributed to tension-type headache occurring more than 15 days or more per month on an average of more than 3 months. Chronic tension-type headache may evolve from episodic tension-type headache over time. It should be noted that like chronic migraine, chronic tension-type headache can also be associated with medication overuse.

TENSION-TYPE HEADACHE IN MIGRAINEURS

A great deal of evidence now suggests that tension-type headache in migraineurs and chronic tension-type of headache may be different from episodic tension-type headache. Tension-type headache in migraineurs are frequent, severe, and of longer duration than in nonmigraineurs (2). They are associated with more photophobia, phonophobia, and nausea than tension-type headache in nonmigraineurs (3). Only migraineurs have episodic tension-type headache precipitated by alcohol, aged cheese, chocolate, and physical activity (4). Tension-type headache in migraineurs respond to agents such as sumatriptan (5,6). Sumatriptan has significant effect on chronic tension-type headache (7), but it has no clinically relevant effect in the treatment of episodic tension-type headache (8).

The preceding observations plus epidemiological data on chronic tension-type headache make a strong argument to consider tension-type headache in migraineurs and chronic tension-type headache, with many features in common with migraine without aura, as different from episodic tension-type headache.

MANAGEMENT OF TENSION-TYPE HEADACHE

Episodic tension-type headache (ETTH) is typically treated with aspirin and/or acetaminophen often combined with caffeine or alternatively with nonsteroidal antiinflammatory drugs (NSAIDs) such as ibuprofen, naproxen sodium, or ketoprofen. Adequate doses of nonsteroidals are necessary. The most effective dose is 600 to 800 mg of ibuprofen, 500 to 750 mg of naproxen sodium, or 75 mg of ketoprofen. Combination analgesics containing caffeine, if used frequently, may result in medication overuse headache. Therefore, the author discourages patients from taking caffeine-containing medications even though they are effective for individual attacks. Moderate intensity ETTH may respond to a combination of acetaminophen, isometheptene, and dichloralphenazone (Midrin). Combination analgesics containing butalbital should be avoided because of the high potential for medication overuse headache. Patients with frequent ETTH may benefit from prophylactic medications using tricyclic antidepressants such as amitriptyline or nortriptyline. If a high degree of depression and anxiety is associated with frequent episodic tension-type headache, addition of an SSRI may be beneficial.

Nonmedication approaches that may benefit some patients include progressive relaxation training, biofeedback, hypnosis, acupuncture, and physical therapy modalities. The management of the chronic tension-type headache, often associated with analgesic overuse and comorbidities, is described in Chapter 5.

NEW DAILY PERSISTENT HEADACHE (NDPH)

NDPH is a condition in which the headaches are of fairly sudden onset, which becomes daily and unremitting without a previous history of episodic headaches of any kind (9–11). The pain is typically bilateral, pressing or tightening in quality, and of mild to moderate intensity. There may be photophobia, sonophobia, and mild nausea.

The IHS diagnostic criteria (1) include (a) headache for more than 3 months fulfilling criteria b to d; (b) headache is daily and unremitting from the onset or from less than 3 days from the onset, (c) at least two of the following pain characteristics should be present: bilateral location, pressing/tightening (nonpulsating) quality, mild or moderate intensity, not aggravated by routine physical activity such as walking or climbing stairs; (d) both of the following: no more than one of photophobia, phonophobia, or mild nausea and neither moderate nor severe nausea or vomiting; (e) not attributed to another disorder.

Characteristically, the headache may be unremitting from the moment of onset and build very rapidly to a continuous unremitting course. Such onset or rapid development must be clearly recalled. It is usually clearly recalled by the patient and described unambiguously.

Secondary headache such as low-pressure cerebrospinal fluid (CSF) volume headache, raised CSF pressure headache, post-traumatic headache, and headache attributed to infection (particularly viral) should be ruled out by appropriate investigations.

NPDH may take either of two subforms: a self-limiting subform, which typically resolves without therapy within several months, and a refractory subform, which is resistant to aggressive treatment programs. This variety of headaches needs further research to understand the nature of the illness. At the present time, it is treated as a chronic daily headache. If there is overuse of medication involved, the patients have to be detoxified. Preventive medications used for the treatment of chronic tension-type headache or chronic migraine may be effective in some patients.

PRIMARY STABBING HEADACHE

The previously used term for primary stabbing headache was ice-pick pains, jabs and jolts, ophthalmodynia periodica (1). Primary stabbing headache is a transient localized stab of pain in the head that occurs spontaneously in the absence of organic degree of underlying structures or of the cranial nerves (12). The head pains, occurring as a single stab or a series of stabs, are exclusively or predominantly felt in the distribution of the first division of the trigeminal nerve (orbit, temple, and parietal area) (12). The stabs last up to a few seconds and recur with irregular frequency ranging from one to many per day. There are no accompanying symptoms. It is not attributed to any other disorder. The majority of the stabs last 3 seconds or less. In rare cases, stabs occur repeatedly over days, and there has been one description of a status lasting 1 week. Stabs may move from one area to another in either the same or the opposite hemicrania. When they are strictly localized to one area, structural changes at this site and in the distribution of the affected cranial nerve must be excluded.

Stabbing pains are more commonly experienced by people subject to migraine (about 40%) or cluster headache (about 30%), in which cases they are felt in the sites habitually affected by these headaches. These patients need a thorough physical examination as well as imaging to exclude any underlying organic condition.

Treatment

Reassurance is key to the successful management of this condition. Patients with migraine who may have episodes of primary stabbing headache should also be reassured. It is very important to let patients know that sudden stabs of this kind do not mean there is an aneurysm in the brain. Many patients have been reported to respond to indomethacin, and it is definitely worthwhile as a primary drug in this condition. As a preventive, there is no purpose in using triptans in this disorder.

HYPNIC HEADACHE

Hypnic headaches are also referred to as alarm clock headache (13). This is mostly a disorder of the elderly. Patients who have hypnic headache get attacks of dull headache that always awaken them from sleep (14–16). The headache develops only during sleep and awakens the patient and does not occur during the waking hours. At least two of the following characteristics are seen: (a) occurs more than 15 times per month, and (b) it lasts 15 or more minutes after waking and usually starts occurring after the age of 50.

Autonomic symptoms such as associated nausea, photophobia, or phonophobia may occur but not more than one of them. Like any other primary headache disorder, intracranial disorders must be excluded. Distinction from one of the trigeminal autonomic cephalalgias is necessary for effective management. The pain of hypnic headache is usually mild or moderate, but severe pain is reported by approximately 20% of patients. Pain is bilateral in about two thirds of cases. Headaches usually last from 15 to 180 minutes, but longer duration has been described.

Treatment

Hypnic headache responds to lithium and also to caffeine. There is no evidence that these headaches respond to triptans. Lithium is given in a prophylactic fashion. The author starts lithium with 150 mg twice daily and increases to 300 mg twice daily. One hundred milligrams of caffeine before going to sleep may be an effective preventive agent. However, some patients may find it difficult to go to sleep after taking caffeine.

REFERENCES

1. The International Classification of Headache Disorders, 2nd Ed. *Cephalalgia* 2004;[Suppl 1].
2. Rasmussen BK, Jensen R, Schroll M, et al. Interrelations between migraine and tension-type headache in general population. *Arch Neurol* 1992;49:914–918.
3. Iverson HK, Langemark M, Andersson PG, et al. Clinical characteristics of migraine and episodic tension-type headache in relation to old and new diagnostic criteria. *Headache* 1990; 30:514–519.
4. Ulrich V, Russell MB, Jensen R, et al. A comparison of tension-type headache in migraineurs and in non-migraineurs: a population-based study. *Pain* 1996;67:501-506.
5. Cady RK, Gutterman D, Saiers JA, et al. Responsiveness of non-IHS migraine and tension-type headache to sumatriptan. *Cephalalgia* 1997;17:588–590.
6. Lipton RB, Cady RK, O'Quinn S, et al. Effects of sumatriptan on the full spectrum of headaches in individuals with disabling IHS migraine. *Cephalalgia* 1999;19:370.
7. Brennum J, Kjeldsen M, Olesen J. The $5HT_1$-like agonist sumatriptan has a significant effect in chronic tension-type headache. *Cephalalgia* 1992;12:375–379.
8. Brennum J, Brinck T, Schriver L, et al. Sumatriptan has no clinically relevant effect in the treatment of episodic tension-type headache. *Eur J Neurol* 1996;3:23–28.
9. Evans RW, Rozen TD. Etiology and treatment of new daily persistent headache. *Headache* 2001;4:380–382.
10. Goadsby PJ, Boes C. New daily persistent headache. *J Neurol Neurosurg Psychiatry* 2002;72[Suppl 2]:ii6–ii9.
11. Silberstein SD, Lipton RB, Solomon S, et al. Classification of daily and near daily headaches: proposed revisions to the IHS-criteria. *Headache* 1994;34:1–7.

12. Pareja JA, Ruiz J, de Isla C, et al. Idiopathic stabbing headache (jabs and jolts syndrome). *Cephalalgia* 1996;16:93–96.
13. Dodick DW, Mosek AC, Campbell IK. The hypnic ('alarm clock') headache syndrome. *Cephalalgia* 1998;18:152–156.
14. Ghiotto N, Sances G, DiLorenzo G, et al. Report of eight new cases of hypnic headache and a mini-review of the literature. *Funct Neurol* 2002;17:211–219.
15. Newman LC, Lipton RB, Solomon S. The hypnic headache syndrome: a benign headache disorder of the elderly. *Neurology* 1990;40:1904–1905.
16. Raskin NH. The hypnic headache syndrome. *Headache* 1988; 28:534–536.

Cluster Headache and Other Trigeminal Autonomic Cephalalgias

Ninan T. Mathew

Trigeminal autonomic cephalalgias share clinical features of headache and prominent cranial parasympathetic autonomic features. Experimental and human functional imaging suggests that these syndromes activate a normal human trigeminal parasympathetic reflex with clinical signs of cranial sympathetic dysfunction being secondary.

Cluster headache (CH), one of the most severe forms of head pain, is a typical example of a periodic disease and distinct from other forms of headache. The term *cluster headache* recognizes periodicity as a major clinical feature of the disorder (1,2).

CLASSIFICATION AND CLINICAL TERMS

The International Headache Society (IHS) recognizes various forms of trigeminal autonomic cephalalgias (3). Table 7-1 shows the classification of cluster headache and other autonomic cephalalgias.

CLUSTER HEADACHE

The terms used in describing cluster headache include *attack,* meaning individual attacks of cluster headache pain; *cluster period,* periods during which patients have repeated attacks; *remission,* a period of freedom from attacks; and *minibouts,* periods of attacks lasting less than 7 days.

Description

Cluster headache consists of attacks of severe, strictly unilateral pain, which is orbital, supraorbital, temporal, or in any combination of these sites lasting 15 to 180 minutes and occurring from once every other day to eight times a day. The attacks are associated with one or more of the following, all of which are ipsilateral: conjunctival injection, lacrimation, nasal congestion, rhinorrhea, forehead and facial sweating, miosis, ptosis, and eyelid edema. Most patients are restless or agitated during an attack.

Diagnostic Criteria (Table 7-2)

During a particular cluster period, some of the attacks may be very severe, and others may be less severe. The duration of the attack also may vary. Some are short and some are longer. The attacks may be less frequent at certain times during the cluster period, particularly at the beginning and toward the end.

Episodic cluster headache is characterized by cluster periods of 7 days to 1 year with periods of remission of more than 14 days up to months or years and occasional minibouts. Chronic

Table 7-2. IHS Diagnostic Criteria for Cluster Headache (3)

At least 5 attacks fulfilling criteria B–D

Severe or very severe unilateral orbital, supraorbital, and/or temporal pain lasting 15–180 minutes if untreated

Headache is accompanied by at least one of the following:
1. ipsilateral conjunctival injection and/or lacrimation
2. ipsilateral nasal congestion and/or rhinorrhea
3. ipsilateral eyelid edema
4. ipsilateral forehead and facial sweating
5. ipsilateral miosis and/or ptosis
6. a sense of restlessness or agitation

D. Attacks have a frequency from one every other day to 8 per day

E. Not attributed to another disorder

cluster headache is characterized by absence of remission for 1 year or short remission of less than 14 days, increased frequency of attacks, and relative resistance to pharmacotherapy.

Clinical Manifestations

CH, predominantly a disease of men (the male-to-female ratio is approximately 9:1), has an approximate prevalence of 0.1% to 0.4% in the general population (4). It usually begins between the ages of 20 and 40, although there are well-documented cases outside that range. The unique head pain profile, periodicity, and autonomic features distinguish cluster headache from other headache disorders.

The Headache Pain Profile

The headache pain profile consists of rapid onset of headache reaching a peak in intensity in 10 to 15 minutes, lasting generally from 30 to 45 minutes. As indicated in the IHS diagnostic criteria, the range of pain duration could be 15 minutes to 180 minutes. The pain may remain severe for an hour or more, and then after a period of fluctuating peaks of pain, it rapidly subsides leaving the sufferer exhausted. The headache is almost always unilateral, the most common site of pain being orbital, retroorbital, temporal, supraorbital, and infraorbital in the order of decreasing frequency. Rarer cases occur outside the trigeminal territory (5). A few to several attacks usually occur with a frequency of range of one a week to eight or more per day.

In any cluster period, pain remains on the same side and may affect the same side year after year. Occasionally, pain may be contralateral in a subsequent cluster period; even most rarely it alternates from side to side, headache to headache. Pain is of terrible intensity and usually described as boring or tearing, like a "hot poker in the eye" or as if "the eye is being pushed out." This is distinctly different from the dull, throbbing pain of migraine.

Periodicity

There is a clocklike regularity in the timing of attacks (6), a phenomenon thought to be due to a dysfunction of the hypothalamic biological clock mechanism. Acute attacks involve activation of posterior hypothalamic gray matter as detected in recent imaging studies (7). Onset shortly after falling asleep is common and, at least in some subjects, it corresponds to the onset of rapid eye movement (REM) sleep (8). Nocturnal attacks also occur during non-REM periods (8). Sleep apnea and resultant oxygen desaturation could act as a trigger for cluster headache attacks (9). At times, three or four attacks per night rapidly leads to sleep deprivation, which in turn can result in frequent daytime naps, often with further painful attacks. Circum annual periodicity also occurs.

Autonomic Symptoms

Parasympathetic overactivity resulting in ipsilateral lacrimation, injection of the conjunctiva, and nasal stuffiness or rhinorrhea is regular. Partial sympathetic paresis resulting in ptosis and miosis also occurs. Facial flushing or pallor, scalp and facial tenderness, tenderness of the ipsilateral carotid artery, and bradycardia are other common associated symptoms. Some of these features also occur in patients with CPH or other conditions such as dissection of the carotid artery, but the temporal profile for cluster headache is virtually specific.

Behavior during Attacks

During a cluster headache attack, patients have a sense of restlessness or agitation. Some patients pace the floor or sit in a position that gives them maximum relief (10). Patients find it difficult to lie down because it aggravates pain, distinct from migraine during which the patient retreats into a dark, quiet room. The CH patients may behave in irrational and bizarre ways, moaning, crying, or screaming, and they may threaten suicide. Some patients find relief by physical exercise such as jogging in place. They may press on the eye or temples with the hand or with an ice pack or a hot washcloth. Many prefer to be alone or go outside even in colder weather. After attacks, the patient may be exhausted. Fear of further attacks with the onset of sleep may lead to prolonged attempts to remain awake. This futile behavior results in the rapid onset of REM activity when sleep eventually overcomes the patient, and a further attack often occurs within minutes of falling asleep.

Provocation of Attacks

Alcohol frequently triggers an attack while the patient is in an active cluster phase. In patients with periods of remission, alcohol rarely precipitates an attack during a pain-free period. Most subjects give up the use of alcohol as soon as they realize a cluster headache has begun. Some patients who are receiving prophylactic treatment can consume alcohol without developing an attack. Some can imbibe without any effect on the attacks regardless of the phase of the disorder, and a very small percentage actually use excess quantities of alcohol to try to get to sleep without provoking an attack. Unlike migraine, cluster headache may be precipitated by any type of alcoholic beverage: beer, spirits, and wine have the same effect. Whether alcohol acts simply as a vasodilator is uncertain.

Other vasodilators such as nitroglycerin tablets (11) and histamine also induce attacks of cluster headache in susceptible patients. A transient, mild hypoxemia occurs following the administration of nitroglycerin (12). Kudrow and Kudrow reported that cluster headache in patients in remission and nonheadache control had no headache following nitroglycerin despite transient oxygen desaturation (13). In the active cluster group, low-grade oxygen desaturation persisted, never returning to baseline, and resulted in cluster attacks. Altitude hypoxemia and sleep apnea–induced hypoxemia can also induce cluster headache attacks during the cluster period. Kudrow and Kudrow offered the hypothesis, based on observations, that the carotid body chemoreceptors are involved in cluster headache pathogenesis (14).

Food items and food additives do not appear to be triggers for cluster headache attacks. Frequency of smoking is greatly increased among cluster headache patients, and some achieve remission after abstinence.

For patients in the episodic phase, the factors that determine the beginning and end of a cluster period or period of remission are unknown. Stress, depression, and psychological factors seem to have less importance in the pathogenesis of cluster headache than other headache types. Behavior of some patients during the attack that resembles a manic episode, periodicity of the cluster headache, and the beneficial effects of lithium in some patients suggests some resemblance to bipolar disorder.

Course

Both the episodic form and the chronic form of cluster headache continue to occur for years. In the episodic form, remissions may last many years, but the subject remains at risk for recurrence until old age. In a large series of patients followed by Krabbe1 (15), only a small minority appear to have lost the propensity to attacks with age. Chronic form may revert to episodic form (16).

Pathophysiology of Cluster Headache

Although a unifying pathophysiological explanation of cluster headache is not yet available, any attempt to understand this syndrome must take into account the three cardinal features of the disorder: pain, autonomic features, and periodicity. Some observations on the neurobiology of cluster headache have recently been made. To recognize the significance, a basic understanding of the neurovascular anatomy is essential. Cephalic pain is relayed to the central nervous system through nociceptive ophthalmic branches of the trigeminal nerve, which innervates pain-sensitive intracranial structures such as dura matter and the dural blood vessels. Substance P and calcitonin gene-related peptide (CGRP) are trigeminal vascular neuropeptides released in both animals and humans when trigeminal nerves, trigeminal fibers, or ganglion are activated. CGRP, the most potent vasodilator in the human body and in animal models, when released, leads to production of neurogenic inflammation and dilation of dural blood vessels. Activation of the trigeminal vascular system in cluster headache has been corroborated by evidence demonstrating markedly elevated blood levels of CGRP in the external jugular vein (EJV) of patients during cluster attack (17).

A number of observations have indicated vasodilation of the ophthalmic artery during cluster headache attack. These include tonometry, corneal indentation, pulse amplitude studies, and thermography showing focal hyperthermia. Doppler studies showing decreased velocities in the ophthalmic artery, conventional angiography showing dilation of the ophthalmic artery (18), and recent magnetic resonance angiographic studies confirm the same (19). Vasodilation has been shown to follow the onset of pain and is not the initial event (20). Thus pain and vasodilation are due to activation of the trigeminal vascular system.

The autonomic features of cluster headache indicate activation of the cranial parasympathetic fibers. These fibers originate from first-order neurons within the superior salivatory nucleus, which has functional brain stem connections to the trigeminal nucleus caudalis. These fibers travel with the seventh cranial nerve and synapse in the pterygopalatine ganglia. Postganglionic fibers provide vasomotor and secretomotor innervation to the cranial blood vessels and the lacrimal and nasal mucosal glands, respectively. Activation of this pathway has been similarly supported by the finding of dramatically elevated blood levels of vasoactive intestinal polypeptide (VIP) in the EJV of sufferers during an attack (17). Involvement of the parasympathetic system in cluster headache is thought to be due to a collateral activation of the parasympathetic pathways from trigeminal nucleus caudalis.

The presence of a postganglionic Horner's syndrome during attacks of cluster headache indicates involvement of the carotid sympathetic plexus. The cavernous carotid artery is likely the location because it is the level where parasympathetic, sympathetic, and trigeminal nerve fibers converge (21). Indeed, evidence from a variety of imaging sources has demonstrated the presence of arterial dilation and venous outflow obstruction in the region of cavernous sinus in patients with cluster headache. Periodicity of the syndrome will have to be explained by changes that happen in the areas of the brain that control biological clock mechanisms, namely, the hypothalamus.

Hypothalamic Dysfunction in Cluster Headache

One study of nine patients with chronic cluster headache used PET imaging during acute nitroglycerin-induced cluster headache attacks and found marked activation in the hypothalamic gray, an area specific for cluster headache (7). This activation pattern has not been observed in migraine or experimental ophthalmic division head pain. Furthermore, hypothalamic activation was not seen in the control group of cluster headache patients given nitroglycerin to induce an attack while they were in remission. This finding implies that the hypothalamus is involved in the pain process in a permissive and triggering manner, rather than simply as a response to first-division nociception. Furthermore, given that this area is involved in circadian rhythms and sleep wake cycles, this data established an involvement of the hypothalamic gray in the genesis of an acute cluster headache attack (7). Another study that also supports the idea of involvement of hypothalamic area in cluster headache pathogenesis provides for the tantalizing evidence that primary headache disorders may be associated with abnormal brain structure as well as function (22). Voxel-based morphometric MR imaging, an objective and automated method of analyzing changes in brain structure, was used to study the brain structure of patients with cluster headache. A significant structural difference was found in the hypothalamic gray compared with controls (22). This structural anomaly correlated with the area of activation demonstrated in the PET scan studies (22).

The remarkable circadian, circannual, and seasonal rhythmicity of cluster headache suggests periodic disturbance and hypothalamic activity. Over a period of 20 years, studies have found abnormal pituitary hormone levels during cluster periods, indicating altered secretory hypothalamic rhythms in these patients (23). Most of these rhythms return to normal during periods of cluster headache remission. Hormonal abnormalities in cluster headaches are associated with disorder of hypothalamic function.

Circadian and circannual rhythmicity including the sleep wake cycle is under the control of the supracharismatic nucleus (SCN), located in the periventricular group of hypothalamic neurons. SCN also regulates secretion of melatonin by the pineal gland. Dysfunction of hypothalamic nucleus may explain the rhythmic periodicity of cluster headache. Peak incidence of cluster headache occurs around changing of the clock for daylight savings and standard time, predilection of attacks to occur during sleep, and alteration in secretory circadian hormone rhythms, including melatonin, which have been reported to be effective in treating cluster headache in some patients.

To summarize the current knowledge of cluster headache pathophysiology, we can envision a model whereby there is dural activation of trigeminal vascular and cranial parasympathetic systems from central or peripherally acting triggers at a permissive time, known as the "cluster period," which is determined by a dysfunctional hypothalamic pacemaker. Whether or not hypothalamic activity participates in this process is unclear. Anatomical substrate is clearly present because the hypothalamus has well-recognized functional connections to salivatory and other parasympathetic nucleus, as well as preganglionic sympathetic neurons within the brain stem and spinal cord. Activation of these pathways may lead to painful vascular changes within the cavernous sinus, secondary involvement of sympathetic plexus overlying the cavernous carotid artery, and stimulation of secretory function of the lacrimal and other mucosal glands.

EXAMINATION

The only abnormal physical sign that may be seen between attacks of CH, either permanently or for a few hours, is an ipsilateral partial Horner's syndrome with a minor degree of upper lid ptosis and miosis. Pharmacological testing of the pupillary response suggests the Horner's syndrome is a third-order neuron disorder (24).

During an attack, an ipsilateral Horner's syndrome, conjunctival injection, tearing, and nasal obstruction are common. Flushing and ipsilateral facial sweating are relatively rare. An occasional patient will complain of swelling of the temple, cheek, palate, or gums ipsilateral to the pain. In most instances, swelling cannot be detected by an examiner, although occasionally there is apparent edema and soft tissue swelling in the region described by the sufferer.

Results of neurogenic imaging studies, including computed tomography (CT) and magnetic resonance imaging (MRI) scans of the head and neck, are normal, and cerebral angiography, performed between attacks, is unremarkable. Arteriography or magnetic resonance angiography (MRA) during the attack has been performed only a few times (18,19). In the best documented cases, the carotid artery appeared to be in spasm or to be irregularly compressed in the region of the siphon, with dilated ophthalmic artery (18,19).

DIAGNOSIS

The diagnosis of CH, which is primarily clinical, is based on the history of the attacks, a careful description of the pain, the temporal profile, the trigger factors, and the associated autonomic manifestations. The rapid escalation of the pain, the predominance of nocturnal attacks, and the limited duration of each headache are important details of the history. Despite the rarity of associated structural abnormalities, it is appropriate to obtain a neuroimage, preferably a MRI of the brain or a contrast-enhanced CT.

Differential Diagnosis

CH is distinguished from migraine by the male predominance, strict unilaterality of pain, short-lived attacks (45 minutes to 1 hour), multiple attacks per day, associated autonomic features, restlessness and inability to lie down during the attack, and the periodicity (clustering) of attacks. Migraines tend to occur

Table 7-3.   Comparison of cluster headache and migraine

Clinical Feature	Cluster Headache	Migraine
Gender ratio (M:F)	90:10	25:75
Unilateral pain	−100%	−68%
Duration	15–180 min	4–72 hrs
Associated with		
Nausea	+	+++
Photophobia, phonophobia	+	+++
Exacerbation by movement	−	+++
Family history	+	+++
Neurological aura	−	+
Autonomic features, such as lacrimation, rhinorrhea, and ptosis	+++	±

primarily in women. Attacks may be associated with prodrome or aura and last a number of hours to days. Nausea, vomiting, and photophobia are prominent features in migraine; they are absent in CH (Table 7-3).

Symptomatic Cluster Headache

Symptomatic CHs (25) are CH-like attacks that occur as a result of an underlying intracranial lesion. Parasellar meningioma, adenoma of the pituitary, calcified lesion in the region of the third ventricle, anterior carotid artery aneurysm, epidermoid tumor of the clivus expanding into the suprasellar cistern, vertebral artery aneurysms, nasopharyngeal carcinoma, ipsilateral large hemispheric arteriovenous malformation, and upper cervical meningioma have been reported to produce symptomatic CH, which should be suspected when clinical features are atypical. Atypical features include the following:

1. Absence of typical periodicity seen in episodic CH. In other words, the headaches behave more like chronic CH.
2. A certain degree of background headache that does not subside between attacks.
3. Inadequate or unsatisfactory response to treatments that are effective in idiopathic CH, such as oxygen inhalation or ergotamine.
4. Presence of neurological signs other than miosis and ptosis.

A careful neurological examination is essential. Diminished corneal reflex and other signs of involvement of the fifth nerve and signs of involvement of other cranial nerves have to be looked for. Most cases of symptomatic CH reported have had some parasellar abnormality, especially around the distal portions of the carotid artery in the cavernous sinus area, where nociceptive fibers of the trigeminal nerve and sympathetic and parasympathetic nerves come together. Clusterlike headaches have been reported following head and facial trauma involving the trigeminal nerve territory (26,27).

Differentiating from Trigeminal Neuralgia

Trigeminal neuralgia is a short-lived lancinating pain confined to the second and third divisions of the trigeminal nerve. The most common areas of pain are perioral, around the angle of the mouth, or periorbital, in the distribution of the second division of the trigeminal nerve. Presence of trigger zones of the face, stimulation of which brings on severe attacks, is characteristic of trigeminal neuralgia. The patient prefers not to touch the face, unlike the patient with CH, who may press on the areas to obtain some relief. Trigeminal neuralgia is more common above 50 years of age. Each attack lasts for only a few seconds.

MANAGEMENT OF CLUSTER HEADACHE

Treatment of Acute Attacks of Cluster Headache

Acute attacks are of sudden onset and short duration. Therefore agents that give immediate relief are essential. Only agents that reach the site of action rapidly are effective in acute CH. Analgesics and oral ergotamine, which are effective in migraine, tend not to be useful in CH because their rate of onset is slow relative to severe and short-lasting CH pain. The most effective agents are oxygen inhalation (28) and subcutaneous sumatriptan (29,30). Nasal sumatriptan (31), nasal zolmitriptan (32), and oral zolmitriptan (33) are also used.

Oxygen

The recommended dose for oxygen inhalation by face mask is 7 liters per minute for 10 minutes at the onset of headache. Approximately 60% to 70% of patients respond to oxygen, the effect being evident in approximately 5 minutes (28). Oxygen may delay an attack rather than abort it completely in some patients. Oxygen has a significant cerebral vasoconstrictive property and reduces calcitonin gene-related peptide (CGRP) release during CH attacks (17).

Sumatriptan

In a double-blind placebo-combined study, it was shown that 15 minutes after treatment, 74% of active subcutaneous (SC) sumatriptan and 26% of placebo-treated patients had reported relief (29). With SC sumatriptan the headache relief is very rapid, commencing within 5 minutes. The recommended dose is 6 mg SC. Increasing the dose from 6 mg to 12 mg did not result in either more responders or quicker effect (34). Long-term repeated use of sumatriptan for acute attacks of CH has been investigated (35). In the first 3 months of a 24-month European multicenter open study (35) to assess the safety and efficacy of SC sumatriptan (6 mg) in the long-term acute treatment of CH, 138 patients each treated a maximum of two attacks daily with a single 6 mg injection. (The effect of oral sumatriptan is slower than that of SC injection; hence oral administration is not the ideal route for CH attacks.) A total of 6,353 attacks were treated.

Adverse events, reported in 28% of sumatriptan-treated attacks, were qualitatively similar to those seen in long-term trails for migraine. Their incidence did not increase with frequent use of sumatriptan. There were no clinically significant treatment effects on vital signs, electrocardiographic recordings, or laboratory parameters.

Headache relief (a reduction from very severe, severe, or moderate pain to mild or no pain) at 15 minutes was obtained for a median of 96% of attacks treated. There was no indication of tachyphylaxis or increased frequency of attacks with long-term treatment. This study demonstrated that, in long-term use, 6 mg of SC sumatriptan is a well-tolerated and effective acute treatment for CH.

Preemptive treatment with oral sumatriptan in a regimen of 100 mg three times daily does not affect either the timing or frequency of headache (36). Sumatriptan is contraindicated in patients with ischemic heart disease or uncontrolled hypertension. Both oxygen and sumatriptan reduce CGRP in the external jugular vein during a CH attack, whereas opioids do not (17).

In a double-blind placebo-controlled randomized trial, patients with episodic or chronic cluster headache treated one attack with 20 mg sumatriptan nasal spray and then treated a second attack, at least 24 hours later, with matching placebo (31). Headache scores were rated on a 5-point scale (very severe, severe, moderate, mild, or none) at 5, 10, 15, 20, and 30 minutes. Overall, five centers enrolled 118 patients who treated 154 cluster attacks: 77 with sumatriptan and 77 with placebo.

At 30 minutes following treatment, 57% of attacks treated with sumatriptan and 26% treated with placebo achieved a headache response (P = 0.002). Thirty-minute pain-free rates were 47% for sumatriptan and 18% for placebo (P = 0.003). Sumatriptan was also more efficacious than placebo in achieving meaningful relief and relief of associated symptoms. There were no serious adverse events reported for either treatment group.

In 26 patients, four consecutive attacks were treated alternately with nasal spray and SC injection (37). Treatment was given within 5 minutes of onset of pain, and the time interval for the start and completeness of pain relief, provided these occurred within 15 minutes of administration, were recorded by the patient. After completion of the study, the patients were also asked to indicate which treatment they preferred, based on efficacy, side effects, and handling of the preparation. Forty-nine of the 52 treatments with injection resulted in complete relief of pain within 15 minutes, with a mean of 9.6 minutes. The remaining three attacks were reduced by a mean of 86.7% at 15 minutes. Only 7 of the 52 treatments with nasal spray in the nostril ipsilateral to pain resulted in complete relief within this time period, with a mean of 13.0 minutes. In 18 of these treatments, pain was reduced by a mean of 42.2% at 15 minutes, whereas no effect on pain was obtained at this time in the remaining 27 treatments. The effect was almost identical when the nasal spray was administered in the nostril on the nonpainful side. As an overall judgment, only 2 of the 26 patients preferred nasal spray to injection. Conclusion of the study indicates that sumatriptan nasal spray 20 mg per dose is less effective than SC injection in relieving pain in the great majority of cluster headache sufferers.

Zolmitriptan Nasal Spray

Rapidity of onset of action, convenience of use, and lack of unpleasant taste make zolmitriptan nasal spray an attractive agent for acute cluster headache attacks. In a single-blind study of 5 mg zolmitriptan nasal spray, 60 out of 76 (78%) cluster headache attacks became pain free within 15 minutes, and 35 (46%) within 10 minutes (32). None of the attacks treated with placebo had response until 25 minutes. Large-scale double-blind placebo-controlled trials are in progress. Fast onset of action, the portability (unlike oxygen), and convenience of use (unlike SC sumatriptan) makes nasal zolmitriptan a very significant agent in the management of acute cluster attacks.

Zolmitriptan Tablets

In a randomized, placebo-controlled, three-period crossover study, adult patients with an established diagnosis of CH were given three oral doses (placebo, 5 mg zolmitriptan, and 10 mg zolmitriptan) for the acute treatment of three CHs (33). Headache was rated on a 5-point verbal scale of nil, mild, moderate, severe, and very severe, and patients were asked to treat attacks of moderate or greater severity. Headache response was an improvement of two or more points on this scale.

Zolmitriptan is the first orally administered triptan to demonstrate efficacy in the acute treatment of episodic cluster headache. Zolmitriptan (10 mg and 5 mg) provided relief from CH at 30 minutes following treatment in patients with episodic CH and was well tolerated.

The intention-to-treat population consisted of 124 patients who took trial medication. The majority (73%) had episodic CH; the rest (27%) had chronic CH. Of the 124, 102 treated three attacks, 13 treated two attacks, 8 treated one attack, and 1 was lost to follow-up. Considering both episodic and chronic CH, response rates were 30% for placebo (PLB), 33% for zolmitriptan 5 mg (Z-5), and 41% for zolmitriptan 10 mg (P = 0.11; Z-10). A similar but insignificant dose response was seen for the subgroup of patients with episodic CH; 29% (PLB, n = 83), 40% (P = 0.11; Z-5, n = 83), and 47% (P = 0.102; Z-10, n = 79). There was no evidence for a headache response in chronic CH patients. For episodic patients, mild or no pain 30 minutes after treatment was observed in a higher proportion of patients treated with zolmitriptan compared with placebo, 42% (PLB), 57% (Z-5; P = 0.01), and 60% (Z-10; P = 0.01). Response rates for mild/no pain at 30 minutes in patients with chronic CH were not significantly better than placebo. To wait for 30 minutes for a pain-free response is not acceptable for the majority of patients.

Dihydroergotamine

Dihydroergotamine (DHE), available in injectable and nasal form in the United States, is effective in the relief of acute attacks of CH. Intravenous (IV) injection gives rapid relief in less than 10 minutes, whereas intramuscular (IM) injection and nasal DHE takes longer.

Ergotamine

Ergotamine, available only in tablet or suppository form, is not particularly useful in acute management because it takes longer to be effective and the attack may subside spontaneously before the medicine has a chance to work. However, some patients may respond fairly quickly to the suppository form of ergotamine. In general, use of oral or suppository ergotamine is not highly effective in the management of acute attacks of CH because of the delayed action.

Topical Local Anesthetics

Locally applied lidocaine nasal drops have been reported effective (38). The use of 4% lidocaine nasal drops is recommended. Patients are told to lie supine with the head tilted backward toward the floor at 30 degrees and turned to the side of the headache. A medicine dropper may be used, and the dose (1 ml of 4% lidocaine) may be repeated once, 15 minutes after the initial dose. The beneficial effect is purely from local anesthetic action that interferes with the nociceptive circuits involving the nasal mucosa and the sphenopalatine ganglion and, in turn, decreases the afferent activity in the trigeminal system. Lidocaine nasal spray or peg pushing may also be tried. Many physicians, however, do not find lidocaine a reliable agent.

Analgesics and Narcotics

Analgesics and narcotics have little value in the treatment of acute attacks of CH. Because the pain is of short duration and self-limited, administration of oral medication is futile most of the time because these medications reach the bloodstream in adequate levels only after the headache is almost terminated. Repeated use may result in habit formation. In most patients, narcotics are not necessary. In patients with coronary artery disease, in whom $5HT_{1B/1D}$ agonists are contraindicated, butorphanol nasal spray (Stadol) may be used to relieve pain.

Prophylactic Pharmacotherapy of Cluster Headache

Prophylactic pharmacotherapy is the mainstay in the management of CH. Medications are used daily during the cluster period for the episodic variety and continuously for the chronic variety (39). The most effective agents include ergotamine, verapamil, lithium carbonate, corticosteroids, methysergide, and valproate. Indomethacin is specific for paroxysmal hemicrania. Beta-adrenergic blocking agents and tricyclic antidepressants are of no particular value.

Principles of prophylactic pharmacotherapy include starting medications early in the cluster period using medications daily until the patient is free of headache for at least 2 weeks, tapering the medications gradually rather than abruptly withdrawing them toward the end of the treatment period, and restarting them at the beginning of the next cluster period. The side effects of the medications have to be explained to the patient in every case. A few attacks occur despite preventive medications, and, in those situations, abortive agents such as oxygen or sumatriptan can be used.

The criteria for selection of a particular medication for prophylactic treatment depend on previous response to prophylactic medications, adverse reactions to medications, presence of contraindications for the use of a particular medication, type of CH (episodic vs. chronic vs. CPH, age of the patient, frequency of attacks, timing of attack (nocturnal vs. diurnal), and expected length of cluster period. Combinations of two or more medications may be necessary for proper control in some patients.

If a patient is seen in the midst of a series of CHs and indicates that previous clusters have lasted a few weeks or a few months, it is likely he or she is still in the episodic phase of the disease. For such an individual, prophylactic therapy will probably be needed for only a limited time, and this permits the use of regimens that would not be suitable for long-term or continuous use.

Corticosteroids

Although there is little understanding of the beneficial mode of action, a short course of corticosteroids is one of the most effective means of providing quick protection against frequent attacks of CH. Several regimens have proven effective; each was an empirical choice, and other dosages might be equally effective. Provided there are no known medical contraindications, a tapering course of oral prednisone can be given as follows: prednisone (60 mg) as a single morning dose for 3 days, followed by a 10 mg reduction every third day, then tapering the dose to zero over 18 days. The prednisone is given each morning to reduce interference with sleep; despite this, many subjects feel stimulated while on the higher doses.

For some patients, the corticosteroid taper is sufficient to give protection from the attacks, and by the time the course is over, the current cluster period has ended. It often happens that the headaches return as the dose is lowered. To prevent a return of the attacks when the corticosteroids are withdrawn, we initiate prophylactic therapy with oral ergotamine or verapamil, along with corticosteroid. (This allows time for verapamil and ergotamine to become effective when the effects of corticosteroid wane.) In some patients, repeat of the corticosteroid taper may be required because the CH attacks return with full vigor. Repeat courses of corticosteroids should be avoided, whenever possible. Repeat courses might induce serious steroid side effects such as weight gain, fluid retention, gastric irritation, hyperglycemia, or a more permanent side effect such as osteonecrosis. For these patients, an alternative form of prophylaxis is indicated.

Corticosteroids are also useful in chronic CH; however, when the medication is tapered, the headache tends to return. If steroids are going to be effective, they are usually effective after the first couple of doses, and certainly by the third day as a general guideline.

The mechanism of action of steroids in CH is speculative. Suppression of the inflammatory reaction, possibly in the cavernous sinus area (venous vasculitis), is a possible explanation. It is also possible that corticosteroids exert some control on serotonergic neurotransmission in the central nervous system

(CNS). The side effects of steroids prevent long-term use. Necrosis of the joints and bones is of particular concern. In general, use of corticosteroids should be limited to short periods of time as an attempt to break the cycle of headache in the episodic variety and for extreme flare-ups in the chronic variety. Long-term use should be avoided.

Ergotamine

One milligram of ergotamine tartrate twice a day given prophylactically is very useful. There is no evidence that ergotamine causes rebound phenomenon in CH, as it does in migraine. Ergotamine is particularly useful in controlling nocturnal attacks when taken at bedtime. Ergotamine is contraindicated in peripheral and cardiovascular disease.

Verapamil

Verapamil is the prophylactic drug of choice in both episodic and chronic CH; doses typically range between 120 and 480 mg daily in divided doses, but doses up to 1,200 mg daily have been used in chronic CH (40). Constipation and water retention are the usual side effects. Verapamil can be combined with ergotamine, and this combination is the treatment of choice in episodic CH prophylaxis. Prior to initiating the calcium blocker, it is appropriate to perform an ECG to rule out any cryptic conduction defect. Hypotension, peripheral edema, and severe constipation are potential side effects.

Methysergide

Methysergide is useful as a prophylactic agent. It is best indicated in younger patients with CH. In older patients with potential atherosclerotic heart disease, this agent has to be used with care. Methysergide has a number of side effects, including muscle cramps and muscle pain, water retention, and fibrotic reactions (retroperitoneal, pleural, pulmonary, and cardia valvular). Because the duration of episodic CH is usually less than 4 months, the use of methysergide is quite acceptable for that period of time. However, in chronic CH, methysergide must be used with caution, with provision for drug holidays between treatment periods. Six months of treatment with 2-month drug holidays is essential if the patient is to have repeated treatments with methysergide. Investigations, including periodic chest roentgenogram, echocardiogram, and intravenous pyelogram (IVP), are recommended to check for the development of any fibrotic reactions.

Intravenous Dihydroergotamine (DHE)

If different combinations of corticosteroid, ergotamine, verapamil, and methysergide do not result in a remission of the cluster period, a 3- to 4-day course of IV DHE (0.5 ml every 6 hours) is helpful in breaking the cycle (41).

Lithium Carbonate

Lithium carbonate is used mostly in the prophylactic treatment of chronic CH, even though it is helpful in the episodic variety (42,43). Lithium is a mood-stabilizing agent. The mechanism of the beneficial action of lithium in CH is not fully understood. Lithium stabilizes and enhances serotonergic neurotransmission within the CNS. The usual dose of lithium is 600 to 900 mg per day in divided doses. Lithium levels should be obtained within the first week and periodically thereafter. The serum level required for therapeutic response is usually 0.4 to 0.8 mEq per liter, which is less than the standard recommended dose in cases of bipolar psychosis. Patients who respond to lithium experience dramatic relief in the first week. Chronic CH patients appear to be more responsive than those with episodic patterns. Approximately 20% of chronic CH may become episodic on lithium treatment, and many patients may require an additional agent such as ergotamine or verapamil with lithium (44). As months go by, there is a tendency for the effect of lithium to wane, and some patients have become resistant to lithium after months of treatment (44). Lithium dose does not appear to prevent alcohol-induced CH.

The side effects of lithium need to be carefully monitored. Neurotoxic effects such as tremor, lethargy, slurred speech, blurred vision, confusion, nystagmus, ataxia, extrapyramidal signs, and seizures may occur if toxic levels are reached. Concomitant use of sodium-depleting diuretics should be avoided because sodium depletion will result in high lithium levels and neurotoxicity. Long-term effects such as hypothyroidism and renal complications must be monitored in chronic CH patients who use lithium for a long time. Polymorphonuclear leukocytosis is a common reaction to lithium often mistaken for occult infection.

Sodium Valproate

Sodium valproate, 600 to 2,000 mg per day in divided doses, has been reported to be an effective agent in reducing the frequency of CH attacks (45). Valproate is fairly well tolerated. Lethargy, tremor, weight gain, and hair loss are some of the common side effects. The valproate level has to be maintained between 50 and 100 µg/ml, and periodic estimations of blood count and liver enzymes are essential. Valproate should not be used in patients with hepatic disorders. IV sodium valproate, which has recently been shown to be effective in migraine, may be worthwhile to use in CH (46).

Topiramate

Topiramate may be effective for CH. Two prospective open-label studies found topiramate effective at terminating or reducing attacks of both the episodic and chronic forms with a mean dose of 100 mg and a range of 25 mg to 200 mg (46a, 46b). The medication may be started at 25 mg once a day and then titrated upward by 25 mg once every 3 to 7 days by another 25 mg depending on the response to as high as 200 mg. However, another prospective open-label study did not find topiramate effective (46c).

Topical Capsaicin

It has been suggested that treatment of CH patients with topical capsaicin may desensitize sensory neurons by depleting the nerve terminals of substance P. In a double-blind placebo-controlled study using intranasal capsaicin (0.025% cream) applied via a cotton-tipped applicator 0.5 inch up the nostril, ipsilateral to the side of the headache twice daily for 7 days, patients who received the active drug had significantly less frequent and less severe attacks (47). Application of capsaicin in the eye should be avoided. Local burning sensations in the nasal mucosa were an unpleasant side effect. Further experience is needed before this mode of therapy is recommended for routine use.

Civamide

Intranasal civamide, a derivative of capsaicin, has been reported to have modest effect in preventing CH attacks, in placebo-controlled trial (48). Civamide is less irritating to the mucosa than capsaicin.

Transdermal Clonidine

Some clinical as well as pharmacological indications seem to suggest that a reduction of the noradrenergic tone occurs in CH, during both the active and remission periods. But sharp fluctuations of the sympathetic system may trigger the attacks. Clonidine, an alpha-2-adrenergic presynaptic agonist, regulates the sympathetic tone in the central nervous system. Therefore, a continuous administration of low-dose clonidine could be beneficial in the active phase of CH by antagonizing the variations in noradrenergic tone. After a run-in week, transdermal clonidine (5 to 7.5 mg) was administered for 1 week to 13 patients suffering from CH, either episodic (eight cases) or chronic (five cases) (49). During clonidine treatment, the mean weekly frequency of attacks dropped from 17.7 ± 7.0 to 8.7 ± 6.6 (P = 0.0005); the pain intensity of attacks measured on the visual analogue scale, from 98.0 ± 7.2 to 41.1 ± 36.1 mm (P = 0.001); and the duration, from 59.3 ± 21.9 to 34.3 ± 24.6 min (P = 0.02). This open pilot study strongly suggests that transdermal clonidine may be an effective drug in the preventive treatment of CH. Its efficacy may be due to its central sympathoinhibition, which reduces or prevents the occurrence of fluctuations of noradrenaline release that may induce the attacks (49).

In another study, a 2-week course of transdermal clonidine (5 mg the first week, 7.5 mg the second week), preceded by a 5-day run-in period, was administered to 16 patients with episodic CH in an active cluster period. In five patients, the painful attacks disappeared after the seventh day of treatment (50). For the group as a whole, no significant variations in headache frequency, pain intensity, or attack duration were observed between the run-in period and the first and second weeks of treatment (ANOVA) (50). Further studies are necessary to clarify the effectiveness of transdermal clonidine in the prophylaxis of episodic CH.

Indomethacin

Indomethacin has not been shown to be significantly effective in cluster headache. However, indomethacin is particularly useful in the treatment of CPH. Benefit usually appears within 48 hours. Indomethacin is a powerful prostaglandin inhibitor and reduces cerebral blood flow. Other indomethacin-responsive headache syndromes include hemicrania continua, benign exertional headache, benign cough headache, idiopathic stabbing headache, and headache associated with sexual activity (51).

Prioritization of Prophylactic Therapy

For episodic CH, ergotamine 1 mg twice a day is the first choice followed by verapamil 360 mg to 480 mg a day. In more resistant cases a combination of ergotamine and verapamil is recommended. Methysergide 2 mg three to four times a day is an effective alternative, especially in younger patients. Methysergide should not be combined with ergotamine. Corticosteroids may be used for short periods of time to break the cycle of headache or to treat severe exacerbations.

For chronic CH, the preference is a combination of verapamil and lithium. In more resistant cases of chronic CH, triple therapy using ergotamine, verapamil, and lithium or using methysergide, verapamil, and lithium may be considered. There is very little experience with valproate for CH; therefore it is considered a low priority. Careful monitoring of blood levels of lithium and valproate are essential.

Nerve Blocks and Injections

Occipital nerve steroid injections of 120 mg of methylprednisolone with lidocaine into the greater occipital nerve ipsilateral to the site of attack have been reported to have resulted in remissions lasting from 5 to 73 days (52). This procedure is a reasonably effective temporary measure to give the patient freedom from pain for a short period of time. Decrease in the afferent input to the trigeminal vascular system via C2 and the spinal tract and nucleus of the trigeminal nerve may be the mechanism by which occipital nerve injections help CH control. Blockade of the sphenopalatine ganglion using cocaine or lidocaine is a useful temporary measure to give freedom from attacks for a few days; however, the reoccurrence rate is high.

Surgical Treatment of Chronic Intractable
Cluster Headache

The following are indications for surgery in chronic CH: total resistance to medical treatment, strictly unilateral case, and stable psychological and personality profiles, including low addiction proneness. Over the last decades, a number of procedures have been tried for surgical treatment of CH (Table 7-4).

Of all the procedures listed in Table 7-4, those directed toward the trigeminal nerve, particularly percutaneous radiofrequency trigeminal rhizotomy, have been the most effective. A number of related articles have appeared in the literature (53–58). The radiofrequency trigeminal rhizotomy utilizes the thermocoagulation of the pain-carrying fibers of the trigeminal nerve. It is a stereotactic procedure.

Results

Experience in many centers indicates that approximately 70% to 75% of patients obtain beneficial effects from radiofrequency trigeminal rhizotomy. In the majority, the CH attacks stop. In a

Table 7-4. Surgical procedures for cluster headache

Procedures directed towards sensory trigeminal nerve
Alcohol injection into supraorbital and intraorbital nerves
Alcohol injection into Gasserian ganglion
Avulsion of infraorbital, supraorbital, and supratrochlear nerves
Retrogasserian glycerol injection
Radiofrequency trigeminal gangliorhizolysis
Gamma knife trigeminal rhizotomy
Microvascular decompression of trigeminal root (Jannetta)
Trigeminal sensory root sections

Procedures directed toward autonomic pathways
Section of greater superficial petrosal nerve
Section of nervus intermedius
Section or cocainization of sphenopalatine ganglion

Procedures directed toward the "cluster headache generator"
Deep brain stimulation of the posterior hypothalamus
Radiofrequency trigeminal rhizotomy

smaller percentage, there is a substantial improvement, with occasional mild episodes. The results are not fully satisfactory, and failure of the procedure can occur in approximately 15% of patients.

Those who show excellent and good results continue to improve for a number of years. Long-term follow-up for more than 20 years has indicated continuing good results. Recurrence of pain is seen in approximately 20% of patients who had excellent or very good results initially. Patients who have recurrence can undergo repeat surgery, which may take place on the opposite side. It is our experience that patients who have had a history of an occasional headache on the opposite side may develop recurrence on the opposite side. Therefore, we recommend selecting patients with a history of strictly unilateral headache.

Complications

A number of relatively minor complications can occur, especially in the immediate postoperative period. These include transient diplopia, stabbing pain in the distribution of the trigeminal nerve, difficulty in chewing on the side of the lesion, and jaw deviation. These complications are usually transient, and complete recovery is the rule. A more troublesome complication is anesthesia dolorosa. The incidence of anesthesia dolorosa is very low. In our series of 98 patients on long-term follow-up, only 2 had moderately severe symptoms of anesthesia dolorosa. Because of corneal analgesia produced by the radiofrequency lesion, patients must be instructed to take proper care of their eyes after surgery. Untreated corneal infections can easily result in corneal opacification because of lack of corneal sensation.

Some Observations on the Radiofrequency Procedure

In the last 17 years, some of our observations of 106 patients who have undergone radiofrequency lesions are as follows:

1. Complete analgesia is necessary for adequate beneficial effects. In contrast, in trigeminal neuralgia, partial analgesia is all that is necessary.
2. If the pain is confined to the orbital, retroorbital, infraorbital, or supraorbital area, a lesion involving V1 and V2 divisions of the trigeminal nerve is adequate. If the pain is also in the temple and the area of the ear, a lesion of the third division is necessary because the auricular branch of the mandibular nerve supplies the temple and the ear.

Gamma knife procedure directed to the trigeminal root and ganglia is gaining acceptance in a few centers (59). It is too early to recommend gamma knife procedures for chronic cluster headache until published reports in large series are available.

DEEP BRAIN STIMULATION

A recent report of deep brain stimulation of the homolateral posterior inferior hypothalamus, as a beneficial treatment in cluster headache prophylaxis, is promising (60). Of course it would need expert teams who are well versed with the procedure.

Cluster-Tic Syndrome

Cluster headache with coexistent trigeminal neuralgia can occur in some patients. They have to be treated concomitantly in order to make patients headache free.

PAROXYSMAL HEMICRANIAS

The paroxysmal hemicranias (PH) are a group of rare benign headache disorders that clinically resemble cluster headache but fail to remit with standard anticluster therapy (Table 7-5).

Table 7-5. IHS diagnostic criteria for paroxysmal hemicrania

At least 20 attacks fulfilling criteria B–D

Attacks of severe unilateral, orbital, supraorbital temporal pain lasting 2–30 minutes

Headache is accompanied by at least one of the following:
  Ipsilateral conjunctival injection and/or lacrimation
  Ipsilateral nasal congestion and/or rhinorrhea
  Ipsilateral eyelid edema
  Ipsilateral forehead and facial sweating
  Ipsilateral miosis and/or ptosis

Attacks are at frequency above 5 per day for more than half the time, although periods with lower frequency may occur.

Attacks are prevented completely by therapeutic doses of indomethacin

Not attributed to another disorder

Attacks of PH have similar characteristics of pain and associated symptoms and signs to those of cluster headache, but they are short lasting, more frequent, occur more commonly in women, and exhibit an absolute responsiveness to indomethacin. Chronic paroxysmal hemicrania (CPH) (61,62) with an unremitting course was the first entity described in this group; later, an episodic variety (with remissions) was reported, and the term *episodic paroxysmal hemicrania (EPH)* was given (63). CPH can evolve from EPH.

Sometimes, the responsiveness to indomethacin may be incomplete because of poor dosing. In general, a dose of 150 mg or more orally or rectally may be required initially with a lower maintenance dose later.

One of the major differences between cluster headache and paroxysmal hemicrania is the lack of male predominance. In fact, the female-to-male ratio is 3:1. Onset is usually in adulthood, although childhood cases have been reported. Table 7-6 summarizes the differential diagnosis of short-lasting headaches.

A family history of CPH or EPH is not at all common. In 21% of reported cases, there was a documented family history of migraine. Only one patient reported a positive family history for CH (64).

The pain is strictly unilateral and without side shift in the vast majority of patients. The maximum pain is experienced in the ocular, temporal, maxillary, and frontal regions: nuchal, occipital, and retroorbital pain has less often been described. The pain may occasionally radiate into the ipsilateral shoulder and arm. The pain is described as a throbbing, boring, pulsatile, or stabbing sensation that ranges in severity from moderate to excruciating. In 28 previous reports, mild discomfort was noted interictally at the usual sites of pain (64). During headaches, sufferers usually prefer to sit quietly or lie in bed in the fetal position; rarely, however, some sufferers assume the pacing activity usually seen in CH.

In CPH, attacks recur from 1 to 40 times daily. However, there is a marked variability in attack frequency; the frequency of mild attacks ranges from 2 to 14 daily, and severe attacks recur 6 to 40 times daily. Most patients report 15 or more attacks per day. Headaches usually last between 2 and 25 minutes each (range, 2 to 120 minutes).

In EPH, the daily attack frequency ranges from 2 to 30, with attacks lasting 3 to 30 minutes each. The headache phase lasts from 2 weeks to 4.5 months, whereas remission periods range from 1 to 36 months.

Both EPH and CPH are characterized by excruciatingly severe throbbing or piercing headaches localized in the temple and orbital regions and accompanied by the ipsilateral autonomic features typical of CH. Both EPH and CPH have clinically similar features: multiple short-duration daily headaches, nocturnal attacks, precipitation by alcoholic beverages, and absolute response to treatment with indomethacin.

EPH differs from CPH by temporal profile. EPH is characterized by discrete attack and remission phases, whereas CPH occurs chronically without remissions. EPH is therefore frequently mistaken for episodic CH (ECH) because both EPH and ECH occur as active periods consisting of brief excruciating

Table 7-6. Differential diagnosis of paroxysmal hemicranias

Feature	Cluster headache	Chronic paroxysmal hemicrania	Episodic paroxysmal hemicrania	SUNCT	Idiopathic stabbing headache	Trigeminal neuralgia
Gender (M:F)	9:1	1:3	1:1	8:1	F>M	F>M
Pain type	Boring	Throbbing/boring	Throbbing	Stabbing	Stabbing	Stabbing
Severity	Very severe	Very severe	Very severe	More severe	Severe	Very severe
Location	Orbital Temporal	Orbital Temporal	Orbital Temporal	Orbital Temporal	Any part	V2/V3
Attack duration	15–180 min	2–45 min	1–30 min	5–250 s	<1 a	<1 a
Attack frequency	1–8/day	1–40/day	3–30/day	1/day to 30/h	Few to many/day	Few to many/day
Autonomic features	+++	++	++	+++	–	–
Alcohol PPT	+	+	+	+	–	–
Indomethacin	±	+++	+++	–	+	–

Modified from: Silberstein SD, Lipton RB, Goadsby PJ. *Headache in clinical practice.* Oxford: Isis, Medical Media, 1998:132, with permission. Abbreviations: F, female; M, male; V1, ophthalmic; V2, maxiliary; V3, mandibular divisions of the trigeminal innervation; +, precipitates headaches; ±, effect not consistent; –, no effect on headache.

headaches recurring numerous times daily with associated ipsi-lateral autonomic disturbances, separated by pain-free remis-sions. Both EPH and CPH may occur nocturnally, and both may be triggered by alcohol. EPH is differentiated from ECH by the increased frequency and shorter duration of individual headaches, and by its absolute response to indomethacin thera-py. CPH must be differentiated from chronic CH.

Diagnostic Workup

It is important to examine the patient carefully just like in any other headache disorder and rule out any organic condition. Every patient with possible paroxysmal hemicrania must have diagnostic neuroimaging to exclude an underlying secondary cause. Structural mimics of CPH have included a parasellar pituitary adenoma, maxillary cyst, occipital infarction, ganglio-cytoma growing from the sella turcica, ophthalmic herpes zoster infection, arteriovenous malformation, cavernous sinus menin-gioma, frontal lobe tumor, and Pancoast's tumor. Magnetic reso-nance imaging is suggested as the neuroimaging procedure of choice because of its higher sensitivity than computerized tomography for visualizing tumors and vascular malformations.

Treatment

CPH by definition responds totally to indomethacin. The usual initial dose should be 50 mg twice daily; those who respond par-tially should have the benefit of receiving 150 or 200 mg of indomethacin. Most patients will respond to 150 mg daily and response can be dramatic with quick dissipation of headache symptoms. A beneficial effect normally will be seen within 48 hours after the correct dose is administered. Rarely, an occasion-al patient may need dosage as high as 300 mg daily. The lack of responsiveness to indomethacin should make one suspect a CPH-like presentation secondary to an underlying lesion.

The gastrointestinal (GI) side effects are a major problem on prolonged use. The GI side effects normally can be controlled with a histamine type II receptor antagonist, proton pump inhibitors, or prostaglandin. Misoprostol doses of 100 to 200 mg four times a day is very successful in preventing nonsteroidal-induced gastric ulcers. The length of treatment with indomethacin varies. Many patients with CPH may need pro-longed use of indomethacin. Those with EPH will need it only for the short periods. Some patients may be able to stop indomethacin without headache recurrence. Some patients may have to stop the indomethacin because of side effects. If indomethacin is no longer a viable treatment option for CPH, COX_2 inhibitors have provided relief in some patients. The author has successfully used celecoxib in a patient who could not tolerate indomethacin (65).

Short-lasting Unilateral Neuralgiform Pain with Conjunctival Injection and Tearing (SUNCT Syndrome)

Short-lasting unilateral neuralgiform pain with conjunctival injection and tearing (SUNCT) is a curious benign short-lasting headache with autonomic features (66). SUNCT is distinguished from paroxysmal hemicranias and cluster headache by the ultrashort attack duration (average 61 seconds) and high frequency of attacks (average 28.3).

Most attacks occur during the day, with a bimodal distribution (there is morning and afternoon/evening peak) (67). Nocturnal attacks are rare. Pain is confined to the first division of the trigeminal nerve. A statuslike pattern has been reported in SUNCT syndromes (68). SUNCT syndrome is characterized by less severe pain but marked autonomic activation during the attacks. The most important autonomic feature is tearing and conjunctival injection. Some patients may have nasal symptoms as well. Treatment of this condition is difficult.

Treatment

SUNCT syndrome does not respond to indomethacin and in general is resistant to many therapeutic agents. Recent reports have indicated that lamotrigine (69), topiramate (70), and gabapentin (71) may have a role in the treatment of SUNCT syndrome. Most of the other agents used for primary headache disorders have no effect.

Like the paroxysmal hemicranias, there have been several secondary SUNCT syndromes reported, which include organic lesions, particularly posterior fossa abnormalities such as cerebellopontine angle arteriovenous malformation, cavernous angioma of the pons, brain stem infarction, basilar impression, craniostenosis, and HIV infection.

Because the attacks are extremely short lived, there is absolutely no point in trying to treat the individual episodes. The only logical approach is to attempt to use an agent, which may have some effect in reducing the frequency of the episodes.

Hemicrania Continua

Hemicrania continua (HC) is another rare unilateral continuous headache disorder that responds to indomethacin (72). Remitting and unremitting forms have been described (73).

HC remains a rare disorder with less than 120 reported cases found in the literature. Recent clinical experience suggests that the disorder may be more common than previously recognized. HC is one of the causes of refractory, unilateral, chronic daily headaches. This disorder demonstrates a marked female preponderance, with a female-to-male ratio of 1.9:1. Age of onset of the disorder ranges from 11 to 58 years (mean, 44 years). Response to indomethacin is diagnostic. Table 7-7 lists indomethacin responsive headache disorders.

Patients with hemicrania continua tend to have an ongoing continuous low-grade headache with exacerbations of the pain. During the exacerbations, there may be a number of migrainous features such as throbbing pain, nausea, sometimes vomiting, photophobia, and sonophobia. The exacerbations of hemicrania continua may sometimes be indistinguishable from migraine. The differential diagnosis in this situation would be a side-locked migraine. Response to indomethacin differentiates the two conditions. Side-locked migraine would respond to triptans during the exacerbations.

In addition to the continuous hemicrania pain, during the exacerbations there are autonomic symptoms as seen in cluster

Table 7-7. Indomethacin responsive headache syndromes

A. Absolute Responsiveness
  1. Paroxysmal hemicranias
  2. Chronic paroxysmal hemicrania (CPH)
  3. Episodic paroxysmal hemicrania (EPH)
  4. Hemicrania continua
B. Relative or Partial Responsiveness
  1. Primary stabbing headache or idiopathic stabbing headache
  2. Benign cough headache
  3. Benign exertional headache

headaches; however, the degree of autonomic symptoms may not be that striking. Because of the presence of autonomic symptoms, hemicrania continua is also classified as a trigeminal autonomic cephalalgia.

REFERENCES

1. Ekbom KA. Ergotamine tartrate orally in Horten's "Histaminic Cephalgia" (also called Harris's "Ciliary Neuralgia"). *Acta Psychiatr Scand* 1947;46:106–113.
2. Kunkle EC, Pfeiffer JB Jr, Wilhoit WM, et al. Recurrent brief headache in cluster pattern. *Trans Am Neurol Assoc* 1952; 77:240–243.
3. The International Classification of Headache Disorders. *Cephalalgia* 2004;24[Suppl 1].
4. Manzoni GC, Prusinski A. Cluster headache: introduction. In Olesen J, Tfelt-Hansen P, Welch KMA, eds. *The headaches.* New York: Raven Press, 1993:543–545.
5. Sanin LC, Mathew NT, Ali S. Extratrigeminal cluster headache. *Headache* 1993;33:369–371.
6. Ekbom K. Pattern of cluster headache with a note on the relation to angina pectoris and peptic ulcer. *Acta Neurol Scand* 1970;45:225–237.
7. May A, Bahara A, Buchel C, et al. Hypothalamic activation in cluster headache. *Lancet* 1998;352:275–278.
8. Kudrow L, McGinty DJ, Philips ER, et al. Sleep apnea in cluster headache. *Cephalalgia* 1984;4:33–38.
9. Mathew NT, Glaze D, Frost JR. Sleep apnea and other sleep abnormalities in primary headache disorders. In Clifford Rose F, ed. *Migraine clinical and research advances.* London: Karger, 1985:40–49.
10. Kudrow L. *Cluster headache. Mechanisms and management.* Oxford: Oxford University Press, 1980.
11. Ekbom K. Nitroglycerin as a provocative agent in cluster headache. *Arch Neurol* 1968;19:487–493.
12. Hales CA, Westphal D. Hypoxemia following the administration of sublingual nitroglycerin. *Am J Med* 1978;65:911–917.
13. Kudrow L, Kudrow DB. Association of sustained oxyhemoglobin desaturation and arrest of cluster headache attacks. *Headache* 1990;30:474–480.

14. Kudrow L, Kudrow DB. The role of chemoreceptor activity and oxyhemoglobin desaturation in cluster headache. *Headache* 1993; 33:483–484.
15. Krabbe A. The prognosis of cluster headache: a long-term observation of 226 cluster headache patients. *Cephalalgia* 1991; 11[Suppl 11]:250–251.
16. Manzoni GC, Terzano MG, Bono G, et al. Cluster headache: clinical findings in 180 patients. *Cephalalgia* 1983;3:21–30.
17. Goadsby PJ, Edvinsson L. Human in vivo evidence of trigemino-vascular activation in cluster headache: neuropeptide changes and effects of acute attacks therapies. *Brain* 1994;117:427–434.
18. Ekbom K, Greitz T. Carotid angiography in cluster headaches. *Acta Radiol Diagn* 1970;10:177–183.
19. Waldenlind E, Ekbom K, Torhall J. MR angiography during spontaneous attacks of cluster headache. A case report. *Headache* 1993;33:291–295.
20. Drummond PD, Lance JW. Thermographic changes in cluster headache. *Neurology* 1984;34:1292–1295.
21. Moskowitz MA. Cluster headache: evidence for a pathophysiologic focus in the superior pericarotid cavernous sinus plexus. *Headache* 1988;28:584–586.
22. May A, Ashburner J, Buchel C, et al. Correlation between structural and functional changes in brain in an idiopathic headache syndrome. *NAT Medicine* 1999;5:836–838.
23. Leone M, Bussone G. A review of hormonal findings in cluster headache: evidence for hypothalamic involvement. *Cephalalgia* 1993;13:309–317.
24. Watson C, Vijayan N. Evaluation of oculocephalic sympathetic function in vascular headache syndromes. Part 1. Methods of evaluation. *Headache* 1982;22:192–199.
25. Mathew NT. Symptomatic cluster. *Neurology* 1993;43:1270.
26. Reik L. Cluster headache after head injury. *Headache* 1987;27: 509–511.
27. Mathew NT, Rueveni U. Cluster-like headache following head trauma. *Headache* 1988;28:297.
28. Kudrow L. Response of cluster headache attacks to oxygen inhalation. *Headache* 1981;21:1–4.
29. The Sumatriptan Cluster Headache Study Group. Treatment of acute cluster headache with sumatriptan. *N Engl J Med* 1991;325:322–326.
30. Ekbom K, Cole JA. Subcutaneous sumatriptan in the acute treatment of cluster headache attacks. *Can J Neurol Sci* 1993;20 [Suppl 4]:F61.
31. Van Vliet JA, Bahra A, Martin V, et al. Intranasal sumatriptan in cluster headache: randomized placebo-controlled double blind study. *Neurology* 2003;60:630–633.
32. Mathew NT, Kailasam J, Seifert T, et al. Zolmitriptan (Zomig) nasal spray in cluster headache attacks: a single blind observation, a preliminary report. *Headache* 2004;44:483.
33. Goadsby PJ, Gawel M, Hardebo J, et al. Oral zolmitriptan is effective in the acute treatment of episodic cluster headache. *Neurology* 1999;52[Suppl 2]:A257.
34. Ekbom K, Monstad I, Prusinski A, et al. Subcutaneous sumatriptan in the acute treatment of cluster headache. A dose comparison study. *Acta Neurol Scand* 1993;88:63–69.

35. Ekbom K, Krabbe A, Micelli G, et al. Cluster headache attacks treated for up to three months with subcutaneous sumatriptan. *Cephalalgia* 1995;15:230–236.

36. Monstad I. Preemptive oral treatment with sumatriptan during a cluster period. *Cephalalgia* 1993;13[Suppl 13]:35.

37. Hardebo JE, Dahlof C. Sumatriptan nasal spray (20 mg/dose) in the acute treatment of cluster headache. *Cephalalgia* 1998; 18(7):487–489.

38. Kitelle JP, Grouse DS, Seyburn ME. Cluster headache: local anesthetic abortive agents. *Arch Neurol* 1985;42:496–499.

39. Raskin NH. *Headache.* New York: Churchill Livingstone, 1988.

40. Gabal U, Spierings EL. Prophylactic treatment of cluster headache with verapamil. *Headache* 1989;29:167–168.

41. Muther PJ, Silberstein SD, Schulman EA, et al. The treatment of cluster headache with repetitive intravenous dihydroergotamine. *Headache* 1991:31;25–32.

42. Mathew NT. Clinical subtypes of cluster headache and response to lithium therapy. *Headache* 1978;18:26–30.

43. Manzoni GC, Bono G, Lanfrenchi M, et al. Lithium carbonate in cluster headache: assessment of its short term and long term therapeutic efficacy. *Cephalalgia* 1983;3:109–114.

44. Ekbom K. Lithium for cluster headache: a review of the literature and preliminary results of long-term treatment. *Headache* 1981;21:132–139.

45. Hering R, Kuritzsky A. Sodium valproate in the treatment of cluster headache: an open trial. *Cephalalgia* 1989;9:195–198.

46. Mathew NT, Kailasam J, Meadors L, et al. Intravenous sodium valproate (Depacon) aborts migraine rapidly: a preliminary report. *Headache* 2000;40:720–723.

46a. Wheeler SD, Carrazana EJ. Topiramate-treated cluster headache. *Neurology* 1999;53(1):234–236.

46b. Lainez MJ, Pascual J, Pascual AM, et al. Topiramate in the prophylactic treatment of cluster headache. *Headache* 2003; 43(7):784–789.

46c. Leone M, Dodick D, Rigamonti A, et al. Topiramate in cluster headache prophylaxis: an open trial. *Cephalalgia* 2003; 23(10):1001–1002.

47. Marks DR, Rapoport A, Padia D, et al. A double-blind placebo-controlled trial of internasal capsaicin for cluster headache. *Cephalalgia* 1993;13:114–116.

48. Saper JR, Klapper RJ, Mathew NT, et al. Intranasal civamide for the treatment of episodic cluster headaches. *Arch Neurol* 2002;59:990–994.

49. D'Andrea G, Perini F, Granella F, et al. Efficacy of transdermal clonidine in short-term treatment of cluster headache: a pilot study. *Cephalalgia* 1995;15:430–433.

50. Leone M, Attanasio A, Grazzi L, et al. Transdermal clonidine in the prophylaxis of episodic cluster headache: an open study. *Headache* 1997;37:559–560.

51. Mathew NT. Indomethacin responsive headache syndrome. *Headache* 1980;21:147–150.

52. Anthony M. Arrest of attacks of cluster headache by local steroid injection of the occipital nerve. In Clifford Rose F, ed. *Migraine: clinical and research advances.* London: Karger, 1985:169–173.

53. Maxwell RE. Surgical control of chronic migrainous neuralgia by trigeminal gangliorhizolysis. *J Neurosurg* 1982;57:459–466.

54. Onoforio BM, Campbell JK. Surgical treatment of chronic cluster headache. *Mayo Clin Proc* 1986;61:537–544.

55. Sweet WH, Wepsie JG. Controlled thermocoagulation of trigeminal ganglion and rootlets for differential destruction of pain fibers. Part 1. Trigeminal neuralgia. *J Neurosurg* 1974;40: 143–156.

56. Mathew NT, Hurt W. Percutaneous radiofrequency trigeminal gangliorhizolysis in intractable cluster headache. *Headache* 1988;28:328–331.

57. Taha JM, Tew JM. Long-term results of radiofrequency rhizotomy in the treatment of cluster headache. *Headache* 1995; 35:193–196.

58. Waltz TA, Dalessio DJ, Ott KH, et al. Trigeminal cistern glycerol injections for facial pain. *Headache* 1985;25:354–357.

59. Ford RG, Fort DT, Swaid S, et al. Gamma knife treatment of refractory cluster headache. *Headache* 1998;38:3–9.

60. Leone M, Franzini A, Bussone G. Stereotactic stimulation of posterior hypothalamus gray matter in a patient with intractable cluster headache (letter). *N Engl J Med* 2001;345: 1428–1429.

61. Sjaastad O, Dale I. Evidence for a new (?) treatable headache entity. *Headache* 1974;14:105–108.

62. Sjaastad O, Dale I. A new (?) clinical headache entity "chronic paroxysmal hemicrania" 2. *Acta Neurol Scand* 1976;54:140–159.

63. Kudrow L, Esperanz AP, Vijaya NN. Episodic paroxysmal hemicrania? *Cephalalgia* 1987;7:197–201.

64. Antonaci F, Sjaastad O. Chronic paroxysmal hemicrania (CPH): a review of the clinical manifestations. *Headache* 1989;29:648–656.

65. Mathew NT, Kailasam J, Fischer A. Responsiveness to celecoxib in chronic paroxysmal hemicrania. *Neurology* 2000;55:316.

66. Sjaastad O, Saunt EC, Salvese NR, et al. Short-lasting, unilateral neuralgiform headache attacks with conjunctival injection, tearing, sweating, and rhinorrhea. *Cephalalgia* 1989;9: 147–156.

67. Pareja JA, Shen JM, Kruszewski P, et al. SUNCT syndrome: duration, frequency, and temporal distribution of attacks. *Headache* 1996;36:161–165.

68. Pareja JS, Caballero V, Sjaastad O. SUNCT syndrome: status-like pattern. *Headache* 1996;36:622–624.

69. D'Andrea G, Granella F, Ghiotto N, et al. Lamotrigine in the treatment of SUNCT syndrome. *Neurology* 2001, 57:1723–1725.

70. Rossi P, Cesarino F, Faroni J, et al. SUNCT syndrome successfully treated with topiramate: case reports. *Cephalalgia* 2003, 23:998–1000.

71. Porta-Etessam J, Martinez-Salio A, Berbel A, et al. Gabapentin (Neurontin) in the treatment of SUNCT syndrome. *Cephalalgia* 2002;22:249.

72. Sjaastad O, Spierings ELH. "Hemicrania continua": another headache absolutely responsive to indomethacin. *Cephalalgia* 1984;4:65–70.

73. Newman LC, Lipton RB, Solomon S. Hemicrania continua: ten new cases and a review of the literature. *Neurology* 1994;44:2111–2114.

First or Worst Headaches

Randolph W. Evans

First or worst refers to a new type of headache that may be the first episode of a primary headache, such as migraine or cluster, or the worst headache, which could be due to a primary or secondary headache disorder. About 1% of patients presenting to the emergency department have headache of acute onset as their chief complaint. About 20% of patients presenting to the emergency department with the "worst headache of my life" have a subarachnoid hemorrhage (1)

There are numerous possible causes of the acute severe new-onset headache (Table 8-1). The following may cause a sudden-onset headache but more often have a subacute onset: meningitis, encephalitis, sinusitis, periorbital cellulitis, cerebral vein thrombosis, optic neuritis, migraine, ischemic cerebrovascular disease, and cerebral vasculitis. An acute severe headache associated with neck rigidity raises concern about subarachnoid hemorrhage, meningitis, and systemic infections. Although many first or worst headaches are due to migraine, remember that migraine is a diagnosis of exclusion. Many secondary headaches mimic migraine. This chapter reviews headaches due to subarachnoid hemorrhage and thunderclap headache. Other types and causes of first or worst headaches are described in other chapters.

SUBARACHNOID HEMORRHAGE

Epidemiology

There are about 32,500 cases of nontraumatic subarachnoid hemorrhage (SAH) per year in the United States. About 80% are due to ruptured intracranial aneurysms (with a yearly incidence of about 10 in 100,000, resulting in 18,000 deaths) and 5% due to rupture of an intracranial arteriovenous malformation (AVM). In about 15% of cases, an arteriogram does not reveal the cause of the bleeding. In about 50% of these arteriogram-negative cases, the computed tomography (CT) scan demonstrates blood confined to the cisterns around the midbrain. Perimesencephalic hemorrhage usually indicates a ruptured prepontine or interpeduncular cistern dilated vein or venous malformation, although about 5% of the time a basilar artery aneurysm may be responsible. Other causes of SAH with a negative arteriogram include occult aneurysm, vertebral or carotid artery dissection, dural arteriovenous malformation, spinal arteriovenous malformation, mycotic aneurysm, pituitary hemorrhage, sickle-cell anemia, coagulation disorders, drug abuse (methamphetamine and cocaine use), primary or metastatic intracranial or cervical tumors, infections (e.g., herpes encephalitis), and vasculitis (Table 8-2) (2).

The prevalence of intracranial saccular aneurysms is about 2%, with 93% of aneurysms ≤10 mm. Ten to 15 million people in

Table 8-1. Differential diagnosis of the acute severe new-onset headache ("first or worst")

Primary headache disorders
    Migraine
    Cluster
    Primary exertional headache
    Primary orgasmic headache

Posttraumatic

Associated with vascular disorders
    Acute ischemic cerebrovascular disease
    Subdural and epidural hematomas
    Parenchymal hemorrhage
    Unruptured saccular aneurysm
    Subarachnoid hemorrhage
    Systemic lupus erythematosis
    Temporal arteritis
    Internal carotid and vertebral artery dissection
    Cerebral venous thrombosis
    Acute hypertension
        Pressor response
        Pheochromocytoma
        Preeclampsia

Associated with nonvascular intracranial disorders
    Intermittent hydrocephalus
    Benign intracranial hypertension
    Post-lumbar puncture
    Spontaneous intracranial hypotension
    Related to intrathecal injections
    Intracranial neoplasm
    Pituitary apoplexy

Acute intoxications

Associated with noncephalic infection
    Acute febrile illness
    Acute pyelonephritis

Cephalic infection
    Meningoencephalitis
    Acute sinusitis

Acute mountain sickness

Disorders of eyes
    Acute optic neuritis
    Acute glaucoma

Cervicogenic
    Greater occipital neuralgia
    Cervical myositis

Trigeminal neuralgia

Table 8-2. Causes of nontraumatic subarachnoid hemorrhage

80% intracranial saccular aneurysm

5% intracranial arteriovenous malformation

15% negative arteriogram

  50% benign perimesencephalic hemorrhage

  50% other causes

    Occult aneurysm

    Mycotic aneurysm

    Vertebral or carotid artery dissection

    Dural arteriovenous malformation

    Spinal arteriovenous malformation

    Sickle-cell anemia

    Coagulation disorders

    Drug abuse (especially cocaine)

    Primary or metastatic intracranial tumors

    Primary or metastatic cervical tumors

    Central nervous system (CNS) infection

    CNS vasculitides

the United States have or will have intracranial aneurysms. The mean age of rupture of aneurysms is around 50 years, with an increasing frequency of rupture until at least the eighth decade. Before 50 years of age, ruptured aneurysms are more common in men; after 50 years of age they are more frequent in women. In children and young adults, aneurysmal SAH is uncommon (less than 10% in 30 years of age or younger and less than 2% of those under 18 years of age) and SAH is more likely due to ruptured AVMs.

About 85% of aneurysms are located in the anterior circulation, most commonly at the junction of the internal carotid artery and the posterior communicating artery, the junction of the anterior cerebral artery and the anterior communicating artery, or the trifurcation of the middle cerebral artery (Fig. 8-1) (3). Posterior circulation aneurysms are most frequently located at the bifurcation of the basilar artery or the junction of a vertebral artery and the ipsilateral posterior inferior cerebellar artery. About 20% to 30% of patients have multiple aneurysms (especially in mirror locations), usually two or three.

Risk factors for rupture include size and location of the aneurysm, a history of prior SAH from a separate aneurysm (11 times higher risk), cigarette smoking (up to 11 times higher), hypertension, a moderate to high level of alcohol consumption, cocaine use, lean body weight, pregnancy (up to 20% of ruptures occur during pregnancy and during the early postpartum period), and a positive family history of aneurysms (Table 8-3) (4,5).

Familial disorders are associated with an increased risk of intracranial aneurysms. Seven percent to 20% of those with a

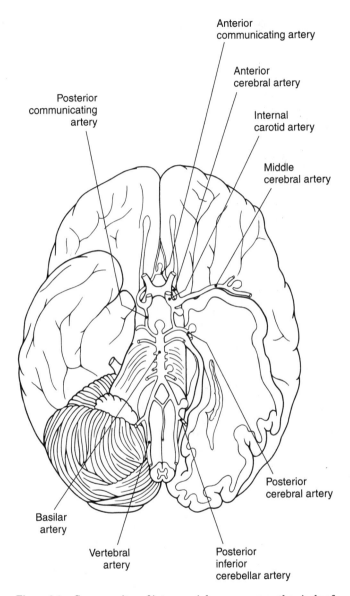

Figure 8-1. Common sites of intracranial aneurysms on the circle of Willis at the base of the brain.

Table 8-3.   Risk factors for rupture of intracranial saccular aneurysms

Older age

Size and location of the aneurysm

History of prior subarachnoid hemorrhage from a separate aneurysm

Cigarette smoking

Hypertension

Cocaine use

Lean body mass

Moderate to high level of alcohol consumption

Pregnancy

Positive family history of intracranial aneurysms

ruptured aneurysm have a first- or second-degree relative with an intracranial aneurysm (6). The risk of rupture of first-degree relatives (highest in siblings) of those with aneurysmal SAH is four times greater than in the general population. Other hereditable connective tissue disorders associated with an increased risk of aneurysms include polycystic kidney disease (10% have intracranial aneurysms), Ehlers-Danlos syndrome type IV, neurofibromatosis type I, and Marfan's syndrome.

Aneurysmal rupture occurs with the following activities: one third occur during sleep, one third during routine daily activities, and one third during strenuous activities such as bending, lifting, defecation, or sexual intercourse. Most episodes of rupture occur in the morning (9 A.M.) and evening (9 P.M.); the fewest occur during the night (3 A.M.). The rate of rupture is lowest in the summer and increases within 3 days of a substantial climatic change and within 24 hours of a large change in barometric pressure.

In a large prospective study, 5-year cumulative rupture rates for patients who did not have a history of subarachnoid hemorrhage with aneurysms located in internal carotid artery, anterior communicating or anterior cerebral artery, or middle cerebral artery were 0%, 2.6%, 14.5%, and 40% for aneurysms less than 7 mm, 7–12 mm, 13–24 mm, and 25 mm or greater, respectively, compared with rates of 2.5%, 14.5%, 18.4%, and 50%, respectively, for the same size categories involving posterior circulation and posterior communicating artery aneurysms (19).

Headache from SAH

Headache occurs in about 90% of people with SAH (7). The classic headache due to SAH is acute, severe, continuous, and generalized and often associated with nausea, vomiting, meningismus, focal neurological symptoms, and loss of consciousness. This explosive headache is typically described as the "worst headache of my life." Twelve percent report a feeling of a "burst." In a series of 42 patients with aneurysmal SAH, the onset of headache was as follows: almost instantaneous, 50%; 2 to 60 seconds, 24%; and

1 to 5 minutes, 19% (8). The headaches, which can occur in any location, may start in one location ipsilateral to the site of the ruptured aneurysm and then generalize or persist unilaterally. The headache typically reaches maximum intensity rapidly and then decreases in intensity over hours to days. The headache almost always has a minimum duration of 1 hour. However, 8% of those with SAH describe a mild, gradually increasing headache.

Clinical Presentation of SAH

Headache and findings on examination are variable. Perhaps 50% of patients with SAHs present with none or minimal headache and slight nuchal rigidity or moderate to severe headache with no neurological deficit or a cranial nerve palsy. Occasionally, patients can present with a stiff neck and no headache. Meningeal irritation may also cause back pain and radicular symptoms in the extremities. A supple neck does not exclude SAH. A stiff neck is present in the following percentages at various times after aneurysm rupture: 74%, day of rupture; 85%, second day; 83%, third day; and 75%, fourth day. During the first 24 hours of aneurysmal SAH, 40% of patients are alert, 67% have normal speech, and 69% have a normal motor examination (9). About 50% of patients have a presentation similar to meningitis with headache, stiff neck, nausea and vomiting, photophobia, and low-grade fever. Table 8-4 summarizes the presentation of SAH.

Table 8-4. Presentations of subarachnoid hemorrhage

Headache present in 90%

Classic headache: sudden, severe, and continuous, often with nausea, vomiting, meningismus, focal neurological findings, and loss of consciousness

Explosive headache: "worst headache of my life"

Feeling of a "burst" in 12%

Mild, gradually increasing headache in 8%, sudden severe in 92%

Can occur in any location, unilateral or bilateral

33% present with headache only

75% present with headache, nausea, and vomiting

66% sudden severe headache with loss of consciousness or focal deficits

50% present with none or minimal headache and slight nuchal rigidity or moderate to severe headache with no neurological deficit or a cranial nerve palsy

Stiff neck present in 75% during first 24 hours and on fourth day after subarachnoid hemorrhage

During first 24 hours: 40% alert, 67% have normal speech, and 69% have a normal motor examination

50% have presentation similar to meningitis: headache, stiff neck, nausea and vomiting, photophobia, and low-grade fever

Transient loss of consciousness in up to 33%

Sentinel Headache or Warning Leak

A sentinel headache (a retrospective diagnosis) or warning leak occurs in about 50% of patients before a major rupture of a saccular aneurysm. However, the concept of a warning leak headache has been challenged as due to recall bias (10). Accurate diagnosis of the headache can be lifesaving because major SAH has a morbidity and mortality of 50% to 70% and occurs in 30% to 50% of patients in the days or weeks after the sentinel headache. About 50% of the major SAHs occur within 1 week of the sentinel headache.

Sentinel headaches can be in any location and unilateral or bilateral. They typically have a sudden onset and are usually present for 1 or 2 days but can last from only several minutes to several hours or persist for 2 weeks. Associated symptoms or signs occur in about 70% of cases, including the following: nausea and vomiting in about 30% of cases; neck pain or stiffness in about 30%; visual disturbances such as blurred or double vision in about 15%; motor or sensory abnormalities in about 20%; and drowsiness, dizziness, or transient loss of consciousness, each of which occurs in about 20% of cases (11). In more than 50% of cases, the headache may be followed by nuchal rigidity and pain and/or nausea and vomiting, and/or transient loss of consciousness.

Perhaps 50% of those with sentinel headaches do not seek medical attention. When these patients see doctors, they are commonly misdiagnosed at the peril of themselves and their doctors (who are subject to malpractice suits). Common misdiagnoses include migraine, hypertension, sinusitis, and flu. *Beware of new-onset "migraine."* The diagnosis of sentinel headache and SAH should be considered in every patient with sudden, severe, and unusual headache or face pain. Features of sentinel headache are summarized in Table 8-5.

From time to time, patients present with a history of what may have been a sentinel headache some weeks or months earlier

Table 8-5.   Features of sentinel headache

Any location, unilateral or bilateral

Occurs before major subarachnoid hemorrhage in 50%

Usually sudden onset

Duration usually 1 to 2 days but can last several minutes to several hours to 2 weeks

Associated symptoms or signs in 70%

    30% nausea and vomiting

    30% neck pain or stiffness

    15% blurred or double vision

    20% motor or sensory abnormalities

    20% drowsiness

    20% dizziness

    20% transient loss of consciousness

    50% of these patients see a doctor and are frequently misdiagnosed where either they did not seek medical attention or they saw a physician but had no evaluation or an incomplete acute evaluation (e.g., a normal CT scan but no lumbar puncture). The possible life-threatening significance of the headache should be explained and then an appropriate investigation obtained (see following section on cerebral angiography).

CT and Magnetic Resonance Imaging Scans in SAH

A CT scan of the brain is the initial imaging study of choice to detect SAH. During the first 24 hours, aneurysmal SAH is present on 95% of scans but decreases to 50% by the end of the first week (Table 8-6) (12,13). In the absence of an intracranial hematoma, the pattern of hemorrhage helps suggest the location of the ruptured saccular aneurysm (Table 8-7). From more than 3 to 14 days after the hemorrhage, magnetic resonance imaging (MRI) (using the fluid-attenuated inversion recovery [FLAIR] sequence) is more sensitive than CT scan in the identification and delineation of SAH.

Lumbar Puncture and SAH

In cases of suspected SAH, a CT or MRI scan of the brain should be performed first because lumbar puncture can result in clinical deterioration and death after SAH. *A lumbar puncture should be performed on all patients with a new-onset headache suspicious for SAH who have normal CT or MRI scans.*

Red blood cells (RBCs) are present in virtually all cases of SAH and variably clear from about 6 to 30 days. When the

Table 8-6. Approximate probability of detecting aneurysmal hemorrhage on CT scan after the initial event

Time	Probability (%)
First 24 hours	95
Day 3	74
1 week	50
2 weeks	30
3 weeks	Almost 0

Table 8-7. Aneurysm sites suggested by the location of subarachnoid hemorrhage

Site of aneurysm	Predominant location of SAH
Anterior communicating artery	Interhemispheric fissure and/or septum pellucidum
Middle cerebral artery	Sylvian fissure cistern
Posterior communicating artery	Suprasellar cistern
Infratentorial arteries	Posterior fossa cistern
Unknown origin	Diffuse, symmetric cisterns

cerebrospinal fluid (CSF) obtained from the first lumbar puncture is bloody, the only certain way to distinguish SAH from a traumatic tap is the presence of a xanthochromia. (*Xanthochromia* literally means "yellow color" but generally refers to a colored supernatant.) Although a decrease in RBC from the first to the third test tube can be seen after a traumatic tap, a decrease may not be present or a similar decrease may be seen after a previous bleed. The presence of crenated RBC is not a reliable sign of SAH.

The breakdown of RBC in the CSF releases oxyhemoglobin from 2 to 12 hours after the SAH. Oxyhemoglobin is degraded by macrophages and other cells in the leptomeninges to bilirubin by the third to fourth day. Oxyhemoglobin and bilirubin are responsible for xanthochromia after SAH. The CSF supernatant is pink or pink-orange due to oxyhemoglobin, yellow due to bilirubin, and an intermediate color if both are present. Methemoglobin, a reduction product of hemoglobin, is found in encapsulated subdural hematomas and in old-loculated intracerebral hemorrhages. Because of the variability of the time for oxyhemoglobin release, some authorities recommend delaying the lumbar puncture for 12 hours after the ictus to avoid confusing a traumatic tap with a SAH.

Absorption spectrophotometry is more sensitive for the detection of xanthochromia than the naked eye (14), although most laboratories use visual inspection. Because oxyhemoglobin can form in vitro due to a traumatic tap, false positives can occur. Table 8-8 provides the probability of detecting xanthochromia by spectrophotometry at various times after SAH (15). There are other causes of xanthochromia, including the following: CSF protein more than 150 mg/dl; jaundice, usually with a total plasma bilirubin of 10 to 15 mg/dl; dietary hypercarotenemia; oral intake of rifampin; malignant melanomatosis; and an earlier traumatic lumbar puncture (Table 8-9).

Cerebral Arteriography, Magnetic Resonance Angiography, and Spiral CT Angiography (16)

If the CT or MRI scan and/or lumbar puncture demonstrate a SAH, a four-vessel digital subtraction cerebral arteriogram should be performed to try to identify the source of the bleed and to exclude multiple aneurysms that can occur in 20% to 30% of cases. In up to 16% of cases, the initial arteriogram may fail to identify the aneurysm, especially of the anterior communicating

Table 8-8. The probability of detecting xanthochromia with spectrophotometry in the cerebrospinal fluid at various times after a subarachnoid hemorrhage

12 hours	100%
1 week	100%
2 weeks	100%
3 weeks	over 70%
4 weeks	over 40%

Table 8-9. Causes of cerebrospinal fluid xanthochromia

Subarachnoid hemorrhage
  Breakdown of red blood cells produces xanthochromia
  Oxyhemoglobin is released after 2–12 hours: pink or pink-orange color
  Bilirubin is produced by the third or fourth day: yellow color
CSF protein >150 mg/dl
Total plasma bilirubin of 10–15 mg/dl
Dietary hypercarotenemia
Malignant melanomatosis
Oral intake of rifampin
Earlier traumatic lumbar puncture

artery. Potential reasons for the false-negative study include vasospasm, thrombosis of the aneurysm, observer error, and technical factors such as inadequate oblique views. Indications for a repeat arteriogram after about 2 weeks include the following: findings of vasospasm; an aneurysmal pattern of blood on the initial CT scan; and thin or thick subarachnoid blood, particularly with a great deal of blood in the basal frontal interhemispheric fissure, when a CT scan is performed within 4 days after the SAH.

Magnetic resonance (MR) angiography can detect about 90% of saccular aneurysms with a size of more than or equal to 5 mm (17). False-positive studies can occur, and confirmation with cerebral arteriography is necessary. MR angiography is very useful as a screening procedure. The treatment of incidental aneurysms, particularly those less than 10 cm in diameter with no prior history of aneurysmal rupture, depends on a number of factors and is controversial (18,19). Spiral (helical) CT angiography can detect perhaps 93% of intracranial saccular aneurysms. Spiral CT can be very useful instead of or as an alternative to MR angiography for patients with contraindications to MRI such as pacemakers, intracranial ferromagnetic clips, and severe claustrophobia. However, in addition to contrast allergy, there is additional risk of intravenous contrast in patients with renal insufficiency, dehydration, and diabetes. In practice, MR and CT angiography are both limited, of course, by the quality of the images and the ability of the interpreting physician.

THUNDERCLAP HEADACHES

A sudden severe headache with maximal onset within 1 minute without evidence of SAH is termed a *thunderclap headache*. A small percentage of these patients will have unruptured aneurysms, benign angiopathy of the CNS, CNS angiitis, intracerebral hemorrhage, cerebral venous thrombosis, carotid artery or vertebral artery dissections, pituitary apoplexy, occipital neuralgia, spontaneous intracranial hypotension, hypertensive encephalopathy, a colloid cyst of the third ventricle, acute sinusitis (particularly with barotrauma), spontaneous retroclival hematomas, and possibly Erve virus (Table 8-10). Most cases

Table 8-10.   Causes of thunderclap headache

Primary causes
  Migraine
  Primary thunderclap headache
  Primary orgasmic headache
Secondary causes
  Unruptured intracranial saccular aneurysm
  Benign angiopathy of the CNS
  CNS angiitis
  Intracerebral hemorrhage
  Cerebral venous thrombosis
  Carotid artery or vertebral artery dissection
  Pituitary apoplexy
  Occipital neuralgia
  Spontaneous intracranial hypotension
  Hypertensive encephalopathy
  Colloid cyst of the third ventricle
  Acute sinusitis
  Spontaneous retroclival hematoma
  Erve virus

are due to primary disorders (primary—benign or idiopathic—thunderclap headache, migraine, and orgasmic headache), which is a diagnosis of exclusion.

Further investigations should be considered when the initial scan and CSF examinations are normal. A normal CT scan does not mean the absence of pathology because the various secondary causes of thunderclap headache can be easily missed. An MRI scan including MR angiography can detect unruptured aneurysms, cerebral venous sinus thrombosis (a MR venogram may also be indicated), carotid or vertebral artery dissections, and pituitary hemorrhage. A spiral CT angiogram is another noninvasive alternative for detection of aneurysms. However, as noted, aneurysms can be missed on MR and CT angiograms. Postulated aneurysmal mechanisms of thunderclap headache include aneurysmal expansion, thrombosis, and intramural hemorrhage.

Primary (idiopathic) thunderclap headache, which is sudden and reaches maximum intensity within 30 seconds, usually lasts up to several hours, although a lingering less severe headache may persist for weeks (20). Episodes of thunderclap headache may occur repeatedly over a 7- to 14-day period. In up to one third of patients, the headache may recur over subsequent months to years. The headache may be precipitated by exercise, weight lifting, or sexual intercourse in up to 33% of patients. Other triggers include Valsalva, bathing in warm water, diving into cold water, brushing the teeth with cold water, walking into cold wind, coughing, and the postpartum period.

Primary thunderclap headache is variably associated with hypertension, posterior leukoencephalopathy, and angiographic evidence of reversible diffuse segmental vasospasm. In some cases with reversible vasospasm, CSF pleocytosis and protein elevation may be present. However, vasospasm is uncommon. Rarely, transient neurological deficits or cerebral infarction may occur. Nimodipine might be an effective treatment for patients with vasospasm and symptoms of cerebral ischemia.

REFERENCES

1. Morgenstern LB, Luna-Gonzales H, Huber JC, et al. Worst headache and subarachnoid hemorrhage: prospective, modern computed tomography and spinal fluid analysis. *Ann Emerg Med* 1998;32:297–304.
2. Khajavi K, Chyatte D. Subarachnoid hemorrhage. In: Gilman S, ed. *MedLink neurology*. San Diego, MedLink Corp. Available at www.medlink.com, 2004.
3. Schievink WI. Intracranial aneurysms. *N Engl J Med* 1997;336: 28–40.
4. Becker K. Epidemiology and clinical presentation of aneurysmal subarachnoid hemorrhage. *Neurosurg Clin N Am* 1998;9:435–444.
5. Juvela S. Natural history of unruptured intracranial aneurysms: risks for aneurysm formation, growth, and rupture. *Acta Neurochir Suppl* 2002;82:27–30.
6. Evans RW, Gorelick PB, Rothbart D. Should you screen for an aneurysm in a migraineur whose mother died from a ruptured intracranial saccular aneurysm? *Headache* 2001;41(2):204–205.
7. Weir B. Headaches from aneurysms. *Cephalalgia* 1994;14:79–87.
8. Linn FHH, Rinkel GJE, Algra A, et al. Headache characteristics in subarachnoid haemorrhage and benign thunderclap headache. *J Neurol Neurosurg Psychiatry* 1998;65:791–793.
9. Kassell NF, Torner JC, Haley EC, et al. The international cooperative study on the timing of aneurysm surgery. Part 1. Overall management results. *J Neurosurg* 1990;73:18–36.
10. Linn FH, Rinkel GJ, Algra A, et al.. The notion of "warning leaks" in subarachnoid haemorrhage: are such patients in fact admitted with a rebleed? *J Neurol Neurosurg Psychiatry* 2000; 68(3):332–336.
11. Hauerberg J, Anderssen BB, Eskesen V, et al. Importance of the recognition of a warning leak as a sign of a ruptured intracranial aneurysm. *Acta Neurol Scand* 1991; 83:61–64.
12. Adams HP, Kassell NF, Torner JC, et al. CT and clinical correlations in recent aneurysmal subarachnoid hemorrhage: a preliminary report of the cooperative aneurysm study. *Neurology* 1983; 33:981–988.
13. Van Gijn J, Van Dongen KG. The time course of aneurysmal hemorrhage on computed tomograms. *Neuroradiology* 1982;23: 153–156.
14. Cruickshank AM. ACP best practice no. 166: CSF spectrophotometry in the diagnosis of subarachnoid haemorrhage. *J Clin Pathol* 2001;54(11):827–830.
15. Vermeulen M, Hasan D, Blijenberg BG, et al. Xanthochromia after subarachnoid haemorrhage needs no revisitation. *J Neurol Neurosurg Psychiatry* 1989;52:826–828.

16. Baxter AB, Cohen WA, Maravilla KR. Imaging of intracranial aneurysms and subarachnoid hemorrhage. *Neurosurg Clin N Am* 1998;9:445–462.

17. Medina LS, D'Souza B, Vasconcellos E. Adults and children with headache: evidence-based diagnostic evaluation. *Neuroimaging Clin N Am* 2003;13(2):225–235.

18. Caplan LR. Should intracranial aneurysms be treated before they rupture? *N Engl J Med* 1998;339:1774–1775.

19. Wiebers DO, Whisnant JP, Huston J III, et al. Unruptured intracranial aneurysms: natural history, clinical outcome, and risks of surgical and endovascular treatment. *Lancet* 2003;12: 362:103–110.

20. Dodick DW. Thunderclap headache. *J Neurol Neurosurg Psychiatry* 2002;72(1):6–11.

Posttraumatic Headaches

Randolph W. Evans

Headaches commonly occur following head and neck injuries. This chapter reviews mild head injury and the postconcussion syndrome and whiplash injuries that are two of the most controversial topics in medicine. The types of headaches due to other neck injuries are similar to those following whiplash injuries.

MILD HEAD INJURY AND THE POSTCONCUSSION SYNDROME

Epidemiology

Mild head injury accounts for 75% or more of all brain injuries. Mild closed head injury is typically defined by the following criteria: a duration of loss of consciousness of 30 minutes or less or being dazed without loss of consciousness; an initial Glasgow Coma Scale score of 13 to 15 without subsequent deterioration; and absence of focal neurological deficits without evidence of depressed skull fractures, intracranial hematomas, or other neurosurgical pathology. The annual incidence of mild head injury in the United States is about 140 in 100,000. The causes of head injuries are as follows: motor vehicle accidents, 45%; falls, 30%; occupational accidents, 10%; recreational accidents, 10%; and assaults, 5% (Table 9-1). Motor vehicle accidents are more common in the young, and falls are more common in the elderly. Men are more frequently injured than women by a factor of 2 to 1. About one-half of all patients with mild head injury are between the ages of 15 and 34. Over 50% of patients with mild head injury will develop the postconcussion syndrome. About 20% to 40% of people with mild head injuries in the United States do not seek treatment.

Clinical Manifestations

Concussion is a trauma-induced alteration in mental status that may or may not involve loss of consciousness. The postconcussion syndrome follows usually mild head injury and comprises one or more of a large constellation of symptoms and signs, including the following categories: headaches, cranial nerve symptoms and signs, psychological and somatic complaints, cognitive impairment, and rare sequelae (Table 9-2) (1). The most common complaints are headaches, dizziness, fatigue, irritability, anxiety, insomnia, loss of concentration and memory, and noise sensitivity. Loss of consciousness does not have to occur for the postconcussion syndrome to develop.

Headache Types

Headaches are variably estimated as occurring in 30% to 90% of those who are symptomatic following mild head injury. Paradoxically, headache prevalence and lifetime duration are

Motor vehicle accidents	45%
Falls	30%
Occupational injuries	10%
Recreational accidents	10%
Assaults	5%

Table 9-2.   Sequelae of mild head injury

Headache types and causes
  Tension type
    Cranial myofascial injury
  Secondary to neck injury (cervicogenic)
    Myofascial injury
    Intervertebral discs
    Cervical spondylosis
    C2-3 facet joint (third occipital headache)
  Greater and lesser occipital neuralgia
  Secondary to temporomandibular joint injury
  Migraine
    Without and with aura
    Footballer's migraine
  Mixed
  Medication rebound
  Cluster
  Supraorbital and infraorbital neuralgia
  Due to scalp lacerations or local trauma
  Low-CSF-pressure headache
  Dysautonomic cephalalgia
  Orgasmic cephalalgia
  Carotid or vertebral artery dissection
  Subdural or epidural hematomas
  Hemorrhagic cortical contusions
  Hemicrania continua
Cranial nerve symptoms and signs
  Dizziness
  Vertigo
  Tinnitus
  Hearing loss
  Blurred vision
  Diplopia
  Convergence insufficiency
  Light and noise sensitivity
  Diminished taste and smell
Psychological and somatic complaints
  Irritability
  Anxiety
  Depression
  Personality change

Table 9-2. *Continued*

Fatigue
Sleep disturbance
Decreased libido
Decreased appetite
Posttraumatic stress disorder

Cognitive impairment
Memory dysfunction
Impaired concentration and attention
Slowing of reaction time
Slowing of information-processing speed

Uncommon and rare sequelae
Subdural and epidural hematomas
Cerebral venous thrombosis
Second impact syndrome
Seizures
Nonepileptic seizures (pseudoseizures)
Transient global amnesia
Tremor
Dystonia

greater in those with mild head injury than in those with more severe trauma. Posttraumatic headaches are more common in people with a history of headache.

Interestingly, patients who sustain iatrogenic trauma when undergoing a craniotomy for brain tumor (other than acoustic neuroma) or intractable epilepsy often have a self-limited combination of tension type and site of injury headache, if any headache at all (2). However, 3 months following removal of a vestibular schwannoma via the retrosigmoid approach, 34% of patients still complain of severe headaches.

According to the International Headache Society second edition criteria, the onset of the headache should be less than 7 days after the injury (3). The less than 7-day onset is arbitrary, particularly because the etiology of posttraumatic migraine is not understood. For example, posttraumatic epilepsy may have a latency of months or years. Similarly, it would not be surprising if there was a latency of weeks or months for posttraumatic migraine to develop (4). Conversely, because migraine is a rather common disorder, the longer the latency between the trauma and onset, the more likely the trauma may not have been causative. Consider the hypothetical case of a 27-year-old man who develops new-onset migraine 2 months after a mild head injury in a motor vehicle accident. The incidence of migraine in males under the age of 30 is 0.25% per year or, in this case, 0.042% per 2 months. Was the new-onset migraine due to the mild head injury or coincidence? Three months seems a more reasonable latency for onset than does 7 days (5).

Many patients have more than one type of headache or have headaches with tension and migraine features. Neck injuries commonly accompany head trauma and can produce headaches. Headaches from neck trauma are discussed in the next section on whiplash injuries.

Tension Type

Eighty-five percent of posttraumatic headaches are of the tension type. The headaches can occur in a variety of distributions, including generalized, nuchal-occipital, bifrontal, bitemporal, caplike, or headband. The headache, which may be constant or intermittent with variable duration, is usually described as a feeling of pressure, tightness, or dull aching. The headache may be present on a daily basis. Temporomandibular joint injury can be caused either by direct trauma or jarring associated with the head injury. Patients may complain of jaw pain and hemicranial or ipsilateral frontotemporal aching or pressure headaches.

Occipital Neuralgia

The term *occipital neuralgia* is in some ways a misnomer because the pain is not necessarily from the occipital nerve and does not usually have a neuralgic quality. Greater occipital neuralgia is a common type of posttraumatic headache but frequently is seen without injury as well. The aching, pressure, stabbing, or throbbing pain may be in a nuchal-occipital and/or parietal, temporal, frontal, or periorbital or retroorbital distribution. Occasionally, a true neuralgia may be present with paroxysmal, shooting pain. The headache may last for minutes to hours to days and can be unilateral or bilateral. Lesser occipital neuralgia can similarly occur, with pain generally referred more laterally over the head.

The headache may be due to an entrapment of the greater occipital nerve in the aponeurosis of the superior trapezius or semispinalis capitis muscle, or it can be referred without nerve compression from trigger points in these or other suboccipital muscles. Digital pressure over the greater occipital nerve at the midsuperior nuchal line (halfway between the posterior mastoid and the occipital protuberance) reproduces the headache (Fig. 9-1). However, pain referred from the C2-3 facet joint or other upper cervical spine pathology and posterior fossa pathology may produce a similar headache. A head injury can also injure the C2-3 facet joint and cause a third occipital headache (see later under whiplash injuries).

Migraine

Recurring attacks of migraine (4) with and without aura can result from mild head injury. Impact can also cause acute migraine episodes often in adolescents with a family history of migraine. This was originally termed *footballer's migraine* to describe young men playing soccer who had multiple migraine with aura attacks triggered only by impact (6). Similar attacks can be triggered by mild head injury in any sport. The most famous example involved the running back of the Denver Broncos and was witnessed by hundreds of millions of people around the world during the 1998 Super Bowl. Terrell Davis, who had preexisting migraine, developed a migraine with aura after a ding on the head at the end of the first quarter. After successfully using dihydroergotamine (DHE) nasal spray, he was able to return for the third quarter, scored the winning touchdown, set a Super Bowl rushing record, and was voted most valuable player.

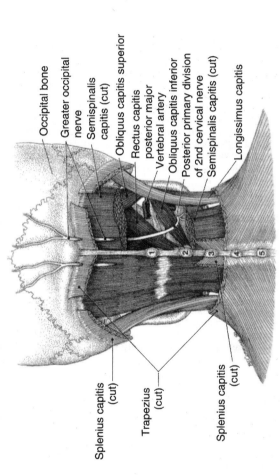

Figure 9-1. Course of the second cervical nerve, which becomes the greater occipital nerve and then penetrates the semispinalis capitis and trapezius muscles to continue beneath the scalp. Entrapment can occur where the nerve passes through the semispinalis muscle. Note the vertebral artery in the suboccipital triangle, which is bounded by the rectus capitis posterior major and the obliqui capitis superior and inferior muscles. (From Travell JG, Simons DG. *Myofascial pain and dysfunction: the trigger point manual.* Baltimore: Williams & Wilkins, 1983:313, with permission.)

Occipital bone
Greater occipital nerve
Semispinalis capitis (cut)
Obliquus capitis superior
Rectus capitis posterior major
Vertebral artery
Obliquus capitis inferior
Posterior primary division of 2nd cervical nerve
Semispinalis capitis (cut)
Longissimus capitis

Splenius capitis (cut)

Trapezius (cut)

Splenius capitis (cut)

Following minor head trauma, children, adolescents, and young adults can develop a variety of transient neurological sequelae that are not always associated with headache and may be due to vasospasm. Four clinical types can cause hemiparesis; somnolence, irritability, and vomiting; transient blindness, often precipitated by occipital impacts; and brain stem signs (7)

Cluster Headaches

Rarely are cluster headaches due to mild head injuries.

Supraorbital and Infraorbital Neuralgia

Injury of the supraorbital branch of the first trigeminal division as it passes through the supraorbital foramen just inferior to the medial eyebrow can cause supraorbital neuralgia. Similarly, infraorbital neuralgia can result from trauma to the inferior orbit. Shooting, tingling, aching, or burning pain along with decreased or altered sensation and sometimes decreased sweating in the appropriate nerve distribution may be present. The pain can be paroxysmal or fairly constant. A dull aching or throbbing pain may also occur around the area of injury.

Scalp Lacerations and Local Trauma

Dysesthesias over scalp lacerations occur frequently. In the presence or absence of a laceration, an aching, soreness, tingling, or shooting pain over the site of the original trauma can develop. The symptoms may persist for weeks or months but rarely for more than 1 year.

Subdural Hematomas

Tearing of the parasagittal bridging veins (which drain blood from the surface of the hemisphere into the dural venous sinuses) leads to hematoma formation within the subdural space. Even minor injuries without loss of consciousness such as bumps on the head or riding a roller coaster can result in this tearing. Falls and assaults are more likely to cause subdurals than motor vehicle accidents.

Subdural hematomas are usually located over the hemispheres, although other locations such as between the occipital lobe and tentorium cerebelli or between the temporal lobe and base of the skull can occur. A subdural hematoma becomes subacute between 2 and 14 days after the injury when there is a mixture of clotted and fluid blood, and it becomes chronic when the hematoma is filled with fluid more than 14 days after the injury. Rebleeding can occur in the chronic phase. Most patients with chronic subdural hematomas are in late middle age or are elderly. Subdural hematomas can be present with a normal neurological examination.

The headaches associated with subdurals are nonspecific and range from mild to severe and paroxysmal to constant. Unilateral headaches are usually due to ipsilateral subdural hematomas. Headaches associated with chronic subdural hematomas have at least one of the following features present in 75% of cases: sudden onset; severe pain; exacerbation with coughing, straining, or exercise; and vomiting and/or nausea.

Epidural Hematomas

Bleeding into the epidural space from a direct blow to the head produces an epidural hematoma. The source of the bleeding is variable and can be arterial, venous, or both. In the supratentorial compartment, bleeding can result from the following origins: middle meningeal artery (50%), middle meningeal veins (33%), dural venous sinus (10%), and other sources, including hemorrhage from a fracture line (7%). Most epidural hematomas in the posterior fossa are due to dural venous sinus bleeding. The locations of epidurals are as follows: temporal region—usually under a fractured squamous temporal bone (70%), frontal convexity (15%), parietooccipital (10%), parasagittal or posterior fossa (5%). Ninety-five percent of epidurals are unilateral.

Epidural hematomas usually occur between the ages of 10 and 40 and much less frequently in those under 2 or over 60. Motor vehicle accidents or falls are the most common causes. Trivial trauma without loss of consciousness can be a cause.

Forty percent of patients with an epidural hematoma present with a Glasgow Coma Score of 14 or 15. Less than one-third of patients have the classic "lucid interval" (initially unconscious, then recovery, and then unconscious again).

Up to 30% of epidural hematomas are of the chronic type. The patient is often a child or young adult who sustains what appears to be a trivial injury often without loss of consciousness. A persistent headache then develops, often associated with nausea, vomiting, and memory impairment, which might seem consistent with a postconcussion syndrome. After the passage of days to weeks, focal findings develop. The headaches of acute and chronic epidural may be unilateral or bilateral and can be nonspecific.

Low-Cerebrospinal-Fluid-Pressure Headache

Trauma can cause a cerebrospinal fluid (CSF) leak through a dural root sleeve tear or a cribiform plat fracture and result in a low-CSF-pressure headache with the same features as a post–lumbar puncture headache.

Dysautonomic Cephalalgia

This is a rare headache due to injury of the anterior triangle of the neck or carotid sheath. Acute local pain and tenderness in anterior triangle can be followed weeks or months later by severe unilateral frontotemporal headache, ipsilateral increased sweating of the face, dilation of the ipsilateral pupil, blurred vision, ipsilateral photophobia, and nausea. The headache can occur a few times per month and last hours to days.

Other Types

New-onset orgasmic cephalalgia can follow mild head trauma within 3 to 4 weeks. The headaches associated with carotid and vertebral artery dissections are discussed in Chapter 13. Hemorrhagic cortical contusions can cause a headache due to subarachnoid hemorrhage. Rarely, hemicrania continua can result from mild head injury (8).

Cranial Nerve Symptoms and Signs

Various cranial nerve symptoms and signs can occur following mild head injury. Within 1 week of injury, about 50% of patients report dizziness. Central and peripheral pathologies include labyrinthine concussion, perilymph fistula, and benign positional vertigo. Fourteen percent of patients report blurred vision, usually due to convergence insufficiency. Optic nerve contusions can result in decreased visual acuity and hue discrimination. Diplopia due to cranial nerve III, IV, and VI palsies can result. Light and noise sensitivity are reported by about 10% of patients.

Psychological and Somatic Complaints

Within 3 months of injury, up to 84% of patients have posttraumatic psychological symptoms. The prevalence of depression is at least 34%. Posttraumatic stress disorder may be present in about 25% of patients 6 months after the injury. Fatigue is a common complaint, reported by 29% of patients at 4 weeks and by 23% of patients 6 months after the trauma. Sleep disturbance is also frequent.

Cognitive Impairment

Four weeks following mild head injury, about 20% of patients complain of loss of memory and about 20% complain of difficulty with concentration. Neuropsychological testing can document deficits in information-processing speed, attention, reaction time, and memory for new information.

Rare Sequelae

A variety of other problems can occur uncommonly or rarely. Subdural and epidural hematomas each occur following up to 1% of mild head injuries. Subdural and epidural hematomas can occur after an initially normal computed tomography (CT) scan, but this is rare. Cerebral venous thrombosis is rarely caused by mild head injury.

Diffuse cerebral swelling is a rare complication of mild head injury; it usually occurs in children and adolescents and results in death or a persistent vegetative state. When diffuse cerebral swelling occurs after a second concussion when an athlete is still symptomatic from an earlier concussion, the term *second-impact syndrome* is used. Although the second-impact syndrome is a rare complication and somewhat controversial, expert opinion based guidelines have been suggested for return to play after concussion (9).

Occasionally, mild head injuries result in a posttraumatic seizure disorder. Nonepileptic seizures or pseudoseizures usually follow mild rather than more severe degrees of head injury and typically present during the first year after the injury.

Rarely, mild head injury triggers transient global amnesia, which in children may actually be due to confusional migraine. An essential-type tremor can also result from mild head injury. Finally, multiple episodes of mild head injury can result in Parkinson's syndrome (e.g., Muhammad Ali).

Biological Basis (10)

Mild head injury may result in cortical contusions due to coup and contrecoup injuries and diffuse axonal injury resulting from sheer and tensile strain damage. Subdural and epidural hematomas occasionally result. Release of excitatory neurotransmitters—including acetylcholine, glutamate, and aspartate—may be a neurochemical substrate for mild head injury. Neuroimaging studies—including magnetic resonance imaging (MRI), functional MRI, single photon emission computerized tomography (SPECT), and positron emission tomography (PET)—can show structural and functional deficits. Neuropsychological testing can reveal cognitive deficits.

There can be a different basis for each complaint. The cause of posttraumatic migraine is unknown but could be due to neurochemical abnormalities. Local extracerebral injury can lead to other symptoms such as benign positional nystagmus (caused by the shifting of position of free debris within the semicircular canals that is traumatically dislodged from the otolith organs) and occipital neuralgia.

The basis for persistent postconcussion syndrome is controversial. Most physicians believe there is a neuropathological substrate. However, others differ and suggest nonorganic causes, especially in cases involving litigation dealing with such matters as secondary pain, malingering, and conversion disorder. Psychological factors and such common symptoms as headaches, dizziness, and memory complaints that would have been present anyway are misattributed to the mild head injury. Each patient needs to be individually evaluated to try and determine the best explanation for persistent problems.

Diagnostic Evaluation

The judicious use of testing needs to be individualized for each patient. CT and MRI scans may be appropriate to evaluate many cases of mild head injury, particularly to exclude subdural and epidural hematomas. MRI is more sensitive than CT scanning for the detection of brain contusions and diffuse axonal injury. Occasionally, MRI detects isodense subdural and vertex epidural hematomas that may not be evident on CT scan.

Neuropsychological testing may be appropriate for patients with prominent cognitive and psychological complaints. However, there are numerous problems with test sensitivity, specificity, reliability, and confounding subject characteristics (11). The physician should be wary: Patients are often misdiagnosed as brain injured. The psychologist also needs to be familiar with findings in malingering and exaggerated memory deficits.

Evaluation by an ear, nose, and throat physician, including an audiogram and electronystagmogram, may be warranted for those with persisting vertigo or complaints of hearing loss. Patients with visual complaints may benefit from ophthalmological examination. Electroencephalographic studies are generally not indicated unless there is a suspicion of a seizure disorder.

Management

Treatment should be individualized after the patient's particular problems are diagnosed. Tension and migraine headaches can be treated with the usual symptomatic and preventive medications. The physician should be concerned about the potential for medication rebound headaches with the frequent use of over-the-counter medications such as acetaminophen, aspirin, and combination products containing caffeine and prescription drugs that also contain narcotics, butalbital, and benzodiazepines. Habituation is also a concern with narcotics, butalbital, and benzodiazepines. Posttraumatic chronic daily headache may respond to an intravenous DHE regimen. Botulinum toxin injections may also be beneficial for posttraumatic headaches.

Occipital neuralgia may improve with local anesthetic nerve blocks, which can be effective alone or combined with an injectable corticosteroid (e.g., 3 ml of 1% xylocaine or 2.5 ml of 1% xylocaine and 3 mg of betamethasone). Before injection, the physician should aspirate to avoid inadvertent injection into the occipital or vertebral artery. Nonsteroidal antiinflammatory drugs (NSAIDs) and muscle relaxants may also be of benefit. If there is a true occipital neuralgia with paroxysmal lancinating pain, baclofen, carbamazepine, tiazanidine, and gabapentin may help. Physical therapy and transcutaneous electrical nerve stimulation (TENS) may help some headaches.

For patients with cognitive dysfunction after mild head injury, the efficacy of cognitive retraining has not yet been well-established by prospective studies. Those with prominent psychological symptoms may benefit from supportive psychotherapy and the use of antidepressant and antianxiety medications. Tricyclic antidepressants such as amitriptyline and nortriptyline may be particularly useful in patients with posttraumatic headaches, depression, and sleep disturbances.

One of the most important roles for the physician is education of the patient and family members, other physicians, and, when appropriate, employers, attorneys, and representatives of insurance companies. There is widespread ignorance about the potential effects of mild head injury due to what Evans has termed the "Hollywood head injury myth" (12). Most people's knowledge of the sequelae of mild head injuries is largely the result of movie magic. Some of the funniest scenes in slapstick comedies and cartoons depict the character sustaining single or multiple head injuries, looking dazed, and then recovering immediately. In cowboy, action and detective, and boxing and martial arts films, seemingly serious head trauma is often inflicted by blows from guns and heavy objects, motor vehicle accidents, falls, fists, and kicks, all without lasting consequences. Our experience is minimal compared with the thousands of simulated head injuries seen in the movies and on television.

The physician can provide education by summarizing the literature and can use vivid examples from sports. The public is very familiar with dementia pugilistica, or punch-drunk syndrome of cumulative head injury in boxers. The examples of Joe Louis and Muhammad Ali are well known. Many have witnessed powerful punches resulting in dazed, disoriented boxers or knockouts. In other sports, there is also growing awareness of the effects of cumulative concussions in professional football (e.g., quarterbacks Steve Young, Troy Aikman, and Stan Humphries) and hockey (e.g., Pat Lafontaine and Mike Richter).

Prognosis

Risk Factors

The persistence and severity of symptoms and neuropsychological deficits are not predicted by a loss of consciousness of less than 1 hour as compared with a patient being just dazed. Lesions present on MRI scanning, usually in the frontal and temporal lobes, have prognostic value for deficits of frontal lobe functioning and memory. Significant predictors for return to work by 3 months after mild head injury include older age; higher level of education, employment, and socioeconomic status; and greater income. High-IQ patients recover faster than low-IQ patients. Age over 40 years is a risk factor for increased duration and number of postconcussion symptoms. Persistent symptoms occur more often in women. Prior head injury is a risk factor for persistence and number of postconcussion symptoms, consistent with the neuropathological concept of cumulative diffuse axonal injuries and contusions. A history of alcohol abuse may increase amount of symptomatology. Multiple trauma can cause additional functional impairment, depression, anxiety, and stress.

Symptoms

Most patients recover within a few months. However, a significant minority have persistent problems. Outcome studies have found persistence of symptoms in various percentages of patients (Table 9-3).

Effect of Litigation

Patients with litigation are quite similar to those without in the following aspects: symptoms that improve with time, types of headaches, cognitive test results, and response to migraine medications. Symptoms usually do not resolve with the settlement of litigation. In one study of 50 patients with posttraumatic headaches an average of 23 months after settlement, all 50 patients continued to report persistent headaches with an improvement in the headaches in only 4 patients (13). Pending litigation may increase the level of stress for some claimants and may result in an increased frequency of symptoms after settlement. Skepticism of physicians may also accentuate the level of stress and compel some patients to exaggerate so doctors will take them seriously.

However, there certainly are some patients with persistent complaints due to secondary gain, malingering, and psychological disorders. Potential indicators of malingering following mild head injury include the following: premorbid factors (antisocial and borderline personality traits, poor work record, and prior claims for injury); behavioral characteristics (uncooperative, evasive, or suspicious); neuropsychological test performance (missing random items, giving up easily, inconsistent test profile, or frequently stating, "I don't know"); postmorbid complaints (describing events surrounding the accident in great

Table 9-3.   Range of percentages of patients in different studies with persistence of symptoms at various times following mild head injury

Symptom	1 week	1 month	6 weeks	2 months	3 months	6 months	1 year	2 years	3 years	4 years
Headache	36–71	31–90	25	32	47–78	22–27	8–35	22–24	20	24
Dizziness	19–53	12–35	15	23	22	13–22	5–26	18	16	18
Memory problems		19	8		59	15–20	4			19
Irritability		25	9			20	5			

detail or reporting an unusually large number of symptoms); and miscellaneous items (engaging in general activities inconsistent with reported deficits, having significant financial stressors, resistance, and exhibiting a lack of reasonable follow-through on treatments) (14).

In a study of mild head injured litigants, Andrikopoulos compared 72 patients with no improvement or worsening headache to 39 with improving headache (15). Those with no improvement or worsening headaches performed worse on cognitive tests and had greater psychopathology on the Minnesota Multiphasic Personality Inventory (MMPI-2) than those with improving headaches, suggesting the possibility of malingering.

Lithuania has been selected to evaluate postconcussion syndrome outside the medicolegal context because there are minimal possibilities for economic gain. Fledgling insurance companies do not recognize postconcussion syndrome and there seem to be fewer expectations of persisting symptoms than in a Western society (16). Mickeviciene et al. prospectively evaluated 300 subjects with a mild head injury for 1 year in Kaunas, Lithuania, with questionnaires. The prevalence, frequency, and visual analogue scale scores of headaches both after 3 months and after 1 year did not differ significantly between the injured and the controls. After 1 year, most symptoms did not differ between the injury and the controls with the exceptions of slightly significant differences of more sporadic memory problems, concentration problems, and dizziness in the injured. The authors conclude, "Our results cast doubts on the validity of PCS as a useful clinical entity, at least for head injuries with loss of consciousness for <15 minutes." Thus no litigation, no expectation of symptoms, and no postconcussion syndrome.

However, the results of this study may not be generalizable for the following reasons: other studies have variably defined mild head injury as including loss of consciousness for up to 30 minutes; 66% of the cohort and controls were men (late symptoms occur more often in women); and 66% of the injuries were due to assaults. In addition, the prevalence of headaches more than 14 days in controls (6% at 3 months and 8% at 1 year) was higher than reported in other countries. Although I am not aware of any prevalence studies in Lithuania, compare this to population-based studies revealing the prevalence of chronic daily headache in 4.1% in the United States (5% in females and 2.8% in males). The prevalence of headaches in controls in this study is especially high when you consider that 66% of both head injured and controls were males. Although litigation and, to a much lesser extent, expectation of chronic symptoms may certainly be factors to consider in the persistence of symptoms in some cases, they clearly do not suffice to explain away persistent postconcussion syndrome.

WHIPLASH INJURIES

Whiplash is an acceleration/deceleration mechanism of energy transfer to the neck that may result from rear-end or side-impact motor vehicle collisions. An injury may or may not result.

Whiplash is best used only as a description of the mechanism of trauma and not as a description of the sequelae. The term *whiplash* was first used in 1928.

Epidemiology

In 2003 the National Safety Council estimated that there were 11.8 million motor vehicle accidents, including 3,360,000 rear-end collisions, in the United States. As many as 1 million people in the United States may have whiplash injuries yearly. Rear-end collisions are responsible for about 85% of all whiplash injuries.

Whiplash injuries occur more often in females, especially in the 20- to 40-year age group, with an overall male-to-female ratio of about 3:7. The greater susceptibility of females might be due to a narrower neck with less muscle mass supporting a head of roughly the same volume or a narrower spinal canal compared with men.

Clinical Manifestations

Table 9-4 lists the sequelae of whiplash injuries, which include neck and back injuries, headaches, dizziness, paresthesias, weakness, cognitive, somatic and psychological problems, visual symptoms, and rare sequelae (17,18).

Table 9-4. Sequelae of whiplash injuries

Neck and back injuries
    Myofascial
    Fractures and dislocations
    Disc herniation
    Spinal cord compression
    Spondylosis
    Radiculopathy
    Facet joint syndrome
    Increased development of spondylosis

Headaches
    Tension type
    Greater occipital neuralgia
    Temporomandibular joint disorder
    Migraine
    Third occipital headache

Dizziness
    Vestibular dysfunction
    Brain stem dysfunction
    Cervical origin
    Barré syndrome
    Hyperventilation syndrome

Paresthesias
    Trigger points
    Thoracic outlet syndrome
    Brachial plexus injury
    Cervical radiculopathy
    Facet joint syndrome

TABLE 9-4. *Continued*

Carpal tunnel syndrome
Ulnar neuropathy at the elbow
Trigeminal sensory impairment

Weakness
Radiculopathy
Brachial plexopathy
Entrapment neuropathy
Reflex inhibition of muscle contraction by painful cutaneous stimulation

Cognitive, somatic, and psychological sequelae
Memory, attention, and concentration impairment
Nervousness and irritability
Sleep disturbance
Fatigability
Depression
Personality change
Compensation neurosis

Visual symptoms
Convergence insufficiency
Oculomotor palsies
Abnormalities of smooth pursuit and saccades
Horner's syndrome
Vitreous detachment

Rare sequelae
Torticollis
Tremor
Transient global amnesia
Esophageal perforation and descending mediastinitis
Hypoglossal nerve palsy
Superior laryngeal nerve paralysis
Cervical epidural hematoma

Internal carotid and vertebral artery dissection

Neck Pain

About 60% of patients presenting to the emergency room after a whiplash injury complain of neck pain. The onset of neck pain is within 6 hours in 65%, within 24 hours in an additional 28%, and within 72 hours in the remaining 7%. Neck pain is usually due to myofascial or facet (zygapophyseal) joint injury. Cervical disc herniations, cervical spine fractures, and dislocations are uncommon.

Facet joint injury at different levels can produce characteristic patterns of referred pain over various parts of the occipital, posterior cervical, shoulder girdle, and scapular regions (Fig. 9-2). Neck pain may arise from at least one facet joint in 54% of patients with chronic pain from whiplash injuries.

Headaches

Up to 80% of patients complain of headaches following a whiplash injury with the following locations and frequency: occipital, 46%; generalized, 34%; other, 20%. The headaches, usually of the tension type, are often associated with greater

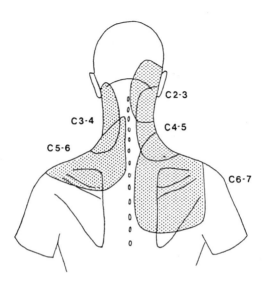

Figure 9-2. Referred pain patterns from the cervical zygapophyseal joints. (From Dwyer A, April C, Bogduk N. Cervical zygapophyseal joint pain patterns: a study in normal volunteers. *Spine* 1990; 15:453–457, with permission.)

occipital neuralgia. In a study of patients with chronic posttraumatic headaches, 37% had tension-type headaches, 27% had migraine, 18% had cervicogenic headache, and 18% did not fulfill criteria of a particular category (19).

Trigger points in muscles such as those in the suboccipital area (semispinalis capitis, obliquus capitis superior, splenius capitis, rectus capitis), splenius cervicis, upper trapezius, sternocleidomastoid, masseter, temporalis, and occipitofrontalis can also produce referred pain in the head (Figs. 9-3 and 9-4) (20). Jaw pain associated with headache can be due to temporomandibular joint (TMJ) injury. Occasionally, whiplash injuries precipitate recurring migraine with and without aura and basilar migraines de novo.

Headache may be referred from injury of the C2-3 facet joint that is innervation by the third occipital nerve, "third occipital headache" (21). C2-3 facet joint injury can result in pain complaints in the upper cervical region and extend at least onto the occiput and at times toward the ear, vertex, forehead, or eye. Fifty percent of those with persistent headaches after whiplash injury have this type of headache (22).

Dizziness

Half of patients with persistent neck pain and headaches for 4 months or longer after the injury complain of vertigo. Table 9-4 lists the various causes of the dizziness. Hyperventilation syndrome can also occur in patients who are in pain and anxious,

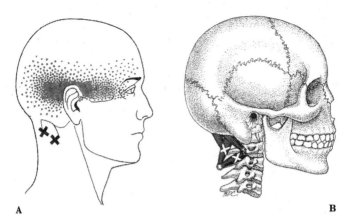

Figure 9-3.   Referred pain pattern (A) of trigger points (Xs) in the right suboccipital muscles (B). (From Travell JG, Simons DG. *Myofascial pain and dysfunction: the trigger point manual.* **Baltimore: Williams & Wilkins, 1983:322, with permission.)**

producing dizziness and paresthesias periorally and/or of the extremities either bilaterally or unilaterally (23).

Paresthesias

About one-third of patients report upper-extremity paresthesias that can be referred from trigger points, brachial plexopathy, facet joint syndrome, entrapment neuropathies, cervical radiculopathy, and spinal cord compression. Carpal tunnel syndrome can be caused by acute hyperextension of the wrist on the steering wheel.

Thoracic outlet syndrome is a common cause of aching, numbness, tingling, and burning pain usually going down the ulnar aspect of the arm and forearm into the fourth and fifth fingers. The ratio of women to men is 4:1. Following whiplash injuries, 85% of cases of thoracic outlet syndrome are of the nonspecific neurogenic type with no objective evidence of neural compression. The neurogenic type demonstrates dysfunction due to compression of the lower trunk of the brachial plexus. The nonspecific type may actually be a myofascial pain syndrome with referred pain from the scalene muscles in the anterior neck or from the pectoralis minor in the shoulder area.

The nonspecific type of thoracic outlet syndrome is a diagnosis of exclusion. Findings on physical exam that are consistent with this diagnosis include reproduction of the symptoms with the following: digital pressure on the scalene muscles; the 90-degree abduction external rotation test (the arm is abducted to a right angle and externally rotated with the forearm flexed at 90 degrees while the head is turned to the opposite side); the exaggerated military maneuver (the patient is asked to brace the shoulders downward and backward forcefully, with the chest thrust forward and the chin slightly elevated); and the hyperab-

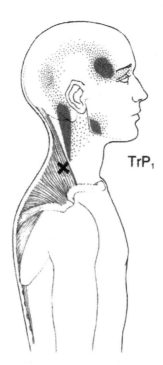

TrP₁

Figure 9-4.   Referred pain pattern and location (Xs) of trigger point 1 in the upper trapezius muscle. Solid shading shows the essential referred pain zone; stippling map shows the spillover zone. (From Travell JG, Simons DG. *Myofascial pain and dysfunction: the trigger point manual.* Baltimore: Williams & Wilkins, 1983:184, with permission.)

duction test (the arms are brought together above the head). A positive Adson's test is often not helpful because more than 50% of normal asymptomatic people will have a positive test.

Weakness

Complaints of upper-extremity weakness, heaviness, or fatigue are common even when there is no evidence of cervical radiculopathy, myelopathy, brachial plexopathy, or entrapment neuropathy. The nonspecific type of thoracic outlet syndrome can produce these complaints. Patients can also report a sensation of heaviness or weakness because of reflex inhibition of muscle due to pain that can be overcome by more central effort.

Psychological and Cognitive Symptoms

Patients often report nervousness and irritability, cognitive problems, sleep disturbances, fatigability, and depression after whiplash injuries. These symptoms are nonspecific and common in patients with postconcussion syndrome, chronic pain disorders, depression, and anxiety.

It is controversial whether persistent neuropsychological deficits following whiplash injury are evidence for mild traumatic brain injury. Subjective cognitive complaints may be due to chronic pain, depression, stressful life events, and malingering.

Other Symptoms

A variety of other problems may follow whiplash injuries. About one-third of patients complain of interscapular and low-back pain. Patients often report visual symptoms, especially blurred vision, which can be due to convergence insufficiency, although oculomotor palsies occasionally occur. Trigeminal sensory impairment, of uncertain etiology, has also been reported (24). Rare sequelae are listed in Table 9-4.

Biological Mechanisms

Animal and human studies have demonstrated structural damage from whiplash-type injuries, including muscle damage, rupture of the anterior longitudinal and other ligaments, avulsion of disc from the vertebral body, retropharyngeal hematoma, intralaryngeal and esophageal hemorrhage, cervical sympathetic nerve damage, and even various brain injuries, such as hemorrhages and contusions of the brain and brain stem. Autopsy series have demonstrated clefts in the cartilage plates of the intervertebral discs, posterior disc herniations through a damaged annulus fibrosis, and hemarthrosis in facet joints. Those with chronic pain may have central hypersensitivity.

The acute whiplash syndrome with complaints of neck stiffness, aching, and headaches is well accepted by physicians and the public. However, as the symptoms persist for months or years, some physicians argue that sprain should heal within a few months and there must be another reason that patients continue to complain. Nonorganic explanations offered for persistent complaints include emotional or psychological problems; exposure to social or medical fashions that perpetuate pain; a culturally conditioned and legally sanctioned illness, a human-made disease; a result of social and peer copying; secondary gain and malingering; and insistence on an explanation outside the realm of organic psychiatry and neurology. In addition, persistent complaints of those involved in low-speed rear-end collisions are not seen in volunteer subjects exposed to speed changes from 4 to 14 km per hour.

Diagnostic Evaluation

Cervical spine series are often obtained to exclude the occasional fracture or subluxation. In patients with abnormal neurological examinations or persistent complaints suggesting the possibility of radiculopathy or myelopathy, a cervical spine MRI study may be indicated. A cervical myelogram followed by CT scan may be useful if the MRI study demonstrates equivocal findings or if the MRI cannot be done. CT scan/myelography may be more sensitive than MRI in some cases for nerve root compression. Electromyogram and nerve conduction velocity studies can provide evidence of radiculopathy, brachial plexopathy, carpal tunnel syndrome, or ulnar neuropathy at the elbow.

Because asymptomatic radiographic findings are common, it is often difficult to determine which findings are new and which are preexisting. Cervical spondylosis and degenerative disc disease occur with increasing frequency with older age and are often asymptomatic. Cervical disc protrusions are also common in the general population. Asymptomatic disc protrusions occur in 20% of those 45 to 54 years of age and 57% of those older than 64 years.

Management

Neck pain is often treated initially with ice; then it is treated with heat, NSAIDs, muscle relaxants, and pain medications. Soft cervical collars can be used during the first 2 to 3 weeks and then avoided. Range-of-motion exercises, physical therapy, trigger point injections, and TENS units may be helpful for patients with persistent nonsurgical complaints.

In many cases, pain from trigger points may be reduced or even eliminated by trigger point injections. The injections can be performed using a local anesthetic (e.g., 3 ml of 1% lidocaine), dry needling without any injection, sterile water, or sterile saline. An injectable corticosteroid produces no more improvement than a local anesthetic alone. Based on the results of a small series, botulinum toxin may also be effective. Headaches due to greater occipital neuralgia may respond to local anesthetic blocks with or without an injectable corticosteroid.

Persistent headaches and neck pain may benefit from tricyclic antidepressants such as amitriptyline and nortriptyline. The chronic, frequent use of narcotics, benzodiazepines, butalbital, and carisprosodol should be recommended sparingly because of the potential for habituation and medication rebound headaches. Posttraumatic migraine is treated like any other migraine.

Treatment of symptomatic facet joints may be effective. The symptomatic facet joint is first identified by anesthetic blocks. Percutaneous radiofrequency neurotomy with multiple lesions of target nerves can provide at least 50% relief for a median duration of 263 days, compared with similar relief for 8 days in the control group (25). Radiofrequency neurotomy of the C2-3 facet may produce complete relief of pain from third occipital headache in 88% of patients for a median duration of 297 days (26).

Alternative Medicine Therapies

Patients with chronic complaints seek out a multitude of treatments such as chiropractic adjustments, acupuncture, prolotherapy, and pain clinics where the evidence for efficacy is suboptimal. The litigation process can also generate unnecessary consultations, testing, and treatment. In the United States, 34% of the adult population uses unconventional therapy yearly. Many of these people seek treatment for posttraumatic and other headaches. In some cases, patients will not reveal their use of alternative treatments to physicians because they anticipate being lectured or chastised. Alternative medicine users find these approaches to be more congruent with their own values, beliefs, and philosophical orientations toward health and life (27). Physicians who wish to learn more about specific alternative treatments and evidence for efficacy may read references such as Cassileth's book (28). (For example, craniosacral therapy consists of gentle massage over the bones of the head, spine, and pelvis to increase the flow of CSF. The practitioner may also claim to emit no-touch healing energy to the client.) Informed physicians can do their patients a service by providing unbiased information. Many alternative medicine treatments may have merit. Rather than getting hung up with the terms *alternative* or *conventional,* we need to understand that some medical approaches work and others do not. As Angell and Kassirer write, "Alternative treatments should be subjected to scientific testing no less rigorous than that required for conventional treatments" (29).

A compassionate, sympathetic approach by the physician may result in greater patient satisfaction and reduce unnecessary expenditures from patients' therapeutic quests. Nothing stimulates further therapeutic quests more than being told by a physician that there are no objective findings and no reason to complain of pain. If this argument is extended to nontraumatic headaches such as migraine and tension type, then no one should have headaches at all. Even if you believe there is no scientific basis for chronic pain complaints following whiplash trauma, can you read a person's mind and determine that he or she does not really have any pain? This type of physician response is the ultimate arrogance.

Prognosis (30)

Risk Factors

There are a variety of risk factors for persistent symptoms (Table 9-5). Prospective studies have demonstrated that psychosocial factors, negative affectivity, and personality traits are not predictive of persistent symptoms.

Symptoms

Numerous studies have shown persistence of symptoms in a minority of patients. Table 9-6 summarizes the results of a well-designed 2-year prospective study (31,32). Five percent of patients were disabled 1 year after the accident. Other studies have shown even higher percentages of patients with persistent symptoms. Neck pain present 2 years following the injury is still present after 10 years.

Table 9-5.   Risk factors for persistent symptoms after whiplash injuries

Accident mechanisms
 Inclined or rotated head position
 Unpreparedness for impact
 Car stationary when hit
Occupant's characteristics
 Older age
 Female gender

TABLE 9-5. *Continued*

Pretraumatic headache for injury-related headache
Significant life events unrelated to the accident

Symptoms
Intensity of initial neck pain or headache
Occipital headache
Interscapular or upper back pain
Multiple symptoms or paresthesias at presentation

Signs
Reduced range of movement of the cervical spine
Objective neurological deficit

Radiographical findings
Preexisting degenerative osteoarthritic changes
Abnormal cervical spine curves
Narrow diameter of the cervical spinal canal

Table 9-6. Percentages of patients with persistence of neck pain and headaches following a whiplash injury

Symptom	1 week	3 months	6 months	1 year	2 years
Neck pain	92	38	25	19	16
Headache	57	35	26	21	15

Effect of Litigation

Most patients who are symptomatic when litigation is settled continue to be symptomatic; they are not cured by a verdict. Litigants and nonlitigants have similar recovery rates and similar response rates to treatment for facet joint pain. However, just as with postconcussion syndrome, there are patients with pain complaints due to secondary gain, exaggeration, malingering, and psychosocial factors. The clinician should evaluate the merits of each case individually. The literature does not support bias against patients just because they have pending litigation.

REFERENCES

1. Evans RW. The postconcussion syndrome and the sequelae of mild head injury. In: Evans RW, ed. *Neurology and trauma*, 2nd ed. New York: Oxford University Press, 2006.
2. Gee JR, Ishaq Y, Vijayan N. Postcraniotomy headache. *Headache* 2003;43:276–278.
3. Headache Classification Subcommittee of the International Headache Society. The International Classification of Headache Disorders, 2nd ed. *Cephalalgia* 2004;24 (Suppl 1):59.
4. Solomon S. Posttraumatic migraine. *Headache* 1998;38:772–778.
5. Haas DC. Chronic post-traumatic headaches classified and compared with natural headaches. *Cephalalgia* 1996;16:486–493.

6. Matthews WB. Footballer's migraine. *BMJ* 1972;2:326–327.
7. Weinstock A, Rothner AD. Trauma-triggered migraine: a cause of transient neurologic deficit following minor head injury in children. *Neurology* 1995;45[Suppl 4]:A347–A348.
8. Lay CL, Newman LC. Posttraumatic hemicrania continua. *Headache* 1999;39:275–279.
9. Practice parameter: the management of concussion in sports (summary statement). Report of the Quality Standards Subcommittee. *Neurology* 1997;48:581–585.
10. Graham DI, McIntosh TK. Neuropathology of brain injury. In: Evans RW, ed. *Neurology and trauma*, 2nd ed. New York: WB Saunders, Oxford University Press, 2006.
11. Report of the Therapeutics and Technology Assessment Subcommittee of the American Academy of Neurology. Assessment: neuropsychological testing of adults. Considerations for neurologists. *Neurology* 1996;47:592–599.
12. Evans RW. The post-concussion syndrome. In: Evans RW, Baskin DS, Yatsu FM, eds. *Prognosis of neurological disorders,* 2nd ed. New York: Oxford University Press, 2000.
13. Packard RC. Posttraumatic headache: permanence and relationship to legal settlement. *Headache* 1992;32:496–500.
14. Ruff RM, Wylie T, Tennant W. Malingering and malingering-like aspects of mild closed head injury. *J Head Trauma Rehabil* 1993;8:60–73.
15. Andrikopoulos J. Post-traumatic headache in mild head injured litigants. *Headache* 2003;43:553.
16. Mickeviciene D, Schrader H, Obelieniene D, et al. A controlled prospective inception cohort study on the post-concussion syndrome outside the medicolegal context. *Eur J Neurol* 2004; 11(6):411–419.
17. Evans RW. Whiplash injuries. In: Gilman S, ed. *Medlink Neurology*. San Diego: MedLink Corp, 2004. Access at www.medlink.com.
18. Evans RW. Whiplash injuries. In: Evans RW, ed. *Neurology and trauma*, 2nd ed. New York: Oxford University Press, 2006.
19. Radanov BP, Di Stefano G, Augustiny KF. Symptomatic approach to posttraumatic headache and its possible implications for treatment. *Eur Spine J* 2001;10:403–417.
20. Travell JG, Simons DG. *Myofascial pain and dysfunction: the trigger point manual*. Baltimore: Williams & Wilkins, 1983.
21. Bogduk N, Marsland A. On the concept of third occipital headache. *J Neurol Neurosurg Psychiatry* 1986;49:775–780.
22. Lord SM, Barnsley L, Wallis BJ, et al. Chronic cervical zygapophysial joint pain after whiplash: a placebo-controlled prevalence study. *Spine* 1996;21:1737–1745.
23. Evans RW. Neurological manifestations of hyperventilation syndrome. *Semin Neurol* 1995;15:115–125.
24. Sterner Y, Toolanen G, Knibestol M, et al. Prospective study of trigeminal sensibility after whiplash trauma. *J Spinal Disord* 2001;14(6):479–486.
25. Lord SM, Barnsley L, Wallis BJ, et al. Percutaneous radiofrequency neurotomy for chronic cervical zygapophyseal-joint pain. *N Engl J Med* 1996;335:1721–1726.
26. Govind J, King W, Bailey B, et al. Radiofrequency neurotomy for the treatment of third occipital headache. *J Neurol Neurosurg Psychiatry* 2003;74:88–93.

27. Astin J. Why patients use alternative medicine: results of a national study. *JAMA* 1998;279:1548–1553.
28. Cassileth BR. *The alternative medicine handbook: the complete reference guide to alternative and complementary therapies.* New York: Norton, 1998.
29. Angell M, Kassirer JP. Alternative medicine—the risks of untested and unregulated remedies. *N Engl J Med* 1998;339:839–841.
30. Evans RW. Whiplash injuries. In: Evans RW, Baskin DS, Yatsu FM, eds. *Prognosis of neurological disorders,* 2nd ed. New York: Oxford University Press, 2000.
31. Radanov BP, Sturzenegger M, Di Stefano G, et al. Relationship between early somatic, radiological, cognitive and psychosocial findings and outcome during a one-year follow-up in 117 patients suffering from common whiplash. *Br J Rheumatol* 1994;33:442–448.
32. Radanov BP, Sturzenegger M, Di Stefano G. Long-term outcome after whiplash injury: a 2-year follow-up considering features of injury mechanism and somatic, radiologic, and psychosocial findings. *Medicine* 1995;74:281–297.

Headaches During Childhood and Adolescence

Randolph W. Evans

Headaches are common in children and teenagers. By 7 years of age, 40% of children have had headaches, with 2.5% having frequent nonmigraine types and 1.4% having migraine (1). By 15 years of age, 75% have had headaches: 15.7% with frequent tension type, 5.3% with migraines, and 54% with infrequent nonmigraine headaches.

The evaluation of the child with headaches is similar to the basic approach in adults, described in Chapter 1. A complete history is essential. Information from parents and other family members or caregivers, especially for younger children, is vital. In some adolescents, it is helpful to obtain the history from the child without family members present and then from family members. A psychosocial history is also important. For recurring or chronic headaches, what is the impact of the headaches on the child's life? Has school been missed, has homework gone undone, or have other activities been curtailed? Because of the frequent familial nature of migraine, family history is also important. When you ask the parents about their own headaches, often you will diagnose their migraines for the first time. A general physical and neurological examination is also necessary. General indications for diagnostic testing are discussed in Chapter 1. Table 1-8 focuses on indications in children and Table 1-9 gives general indications for neuroimaging.

This chapter covers the following topics: migraine, episodic tension-type headaches, chronic nonprogressive headaches, acute headaches, and chronic progressive headaches. Cluster headaches, the subject of Chapter 7, are not separately discussed because the onset usually occurs after 20 years of age and these headaches are rare in children. Some other causes of secondary headaches in children and adolescents, such as post-traumatic, ophthalmological causes, and pseudotumor cerebri, are also reviewed in other chapters.

MIGRAINE

Introduction

A variety of migraine types can occur in children and teenagers (2). Individuals may have just one type or they may have different types. In addition to obtaining the usual history, ask about possible triggers; it is also helpful to ask about a history of motion sickness or somnambulism (sleepwalking), both of which occur much more often in migraineurs. Motion sickness is reported by 45% of children with migraine and 5% of controls (3). Sleepwalking occurs in 28% of children with migraine and 5% of controls (4).

Table 10-1. The peak incidence of migraine with and without aura in males and females

Gender	Incidence (per 1000 person-years)	Peak age (years)
Male		
With aura	6.6	5
Without aura	10	10–11
Females		
With aura	14.1	12–13
Without aura	18.9	14–17

Epidemiology

The onset of migraine frequently occurs during childhood: 20% before 10 years of age and 45% before 20 years of age. Until puberty, the prevalence of migraine is the same in boys and girls. After puberty, the ratio of females to males is 3:1. The peak of new cases of migraine, the incidence, occurs during childhood (Table 10-1) (5). The onset of migraine with aura is earlier than that of migraine without aura. Migraine also begins earlier in males than in females. By 15 years of age, 5% of children have had migraines. Of these, about 1.5% have migraine with aura. The risk of a child developing migraine is 70% when both parents have migraine and 45% when one parent is affected.

Clinical Manifestations

Migraine without Aura

As in adults, migraine without aura is the most common type. However, childhood migraine can be somewhat different. The duration of headache is often much less and can last as little as 30 minutes. Pediatric migraine is more often bilateral, frontal, and temporal than unilateral (35% vs. 60% in adults). Finally, there is a higher incidence of light or noise sensitivity alone than is found in adults. Table 10-2 presents the IHS 2nd edition criteria (6).

Migraine with Aura

About 20% of children report the gradual onset of a visual aura before or during the onset of the headache. Descriptions include spots, colors, dots, or lights, which are usually found in both eyes but occasionally occur only in one eye. The aura usually lasts less than 30 minutes. Table 10-2 provides criteria for diagnosis.

"Alice in Wonderland" syndrome is a rare migraine aura in which patients experience distortion in body image characterized by enlargement, diminution, or distortion of part of or the whole body that they know is not real. The syndrome can occur at any age but is more common in children. The etiology may be migrainous ischemia of the nondominant posterior parietal lobule. Other rare visual hallucinations, distortions, and illusions

Table 10-2. IHS 2nd edition classification for migraine without aura and with typical aura

Pediatric migraine without aura (footnotes incorporated into adult classification)

A. At least five attacks fulfilling B–D

B. Headache attacks lasting 1 to 72 hours (untreated or unsuccessfully treated)

C. Headache has at least two of the following characteristics:
   1. Unilateral location. (Migraine headache is commonly bilateral in young children; an adult pattern of unilateral pain usually emerges in late adolescence or early adult life. Migraine headache is usually frontotemporal. Occipital headache in children, whether unilateral or bilateral, is rare and calls for diagnostic caution; many cases are attributable to structural lesions.)
   2. Pulsating quality
   3. Moderate or severe pain intensity
   4. Aggravation by or causing avoidance of routine physical activity (e.g. walking or climbing stairs)

D. During headache, at least one of the following:
   1. Nausea and/or vomiting
   2. Photophobia and phonophobia (may be inferred from the behavior of young children)

Typical aura with migraine headache

A. At least 2 attacks fulfilling criteria B–D

B. Aura consisting of at least one of the following, but no motor weakness: fully reversible visual symptoms including positive features (e.g., flickering lights, spots or lines) and/or negative features (i.e., loss of vision); fully reversible sensory symptoms including positive features (i.e., pins and needles) and/or negative features (i.e., numbness); fully reversible dysphasic speech disturbance

C. At least two of the following:
   1. homonymous visual symptoms and/or unilateral sensory symptoms
   2. at least one aura symptom develops gradually over ≥5 minutes and/or different aura symptoms occur in succession over ≥5 minutes
   3. each symptom lasts ≥5 and ≤60 minutes

D. Headache fulfilling criteria B–D for 1.1 Migraine without aura begins during the aura or follows aura within 60 minutes

E. Not attributed to another disorder

that have been reported in migraine include the following: zoopsia (visual hallucinations containing complex objects such as people and animals); achromatopsia (no perception of color); prosopagnosia (inability to recognize faces); visual agnosia (inability to recognize objects); akinetopsia (loss of ability to perceive visual motion); metamorphopsia (distortion of the shapes of objects); micropsia (objects appear too small); macropsia (objects appear too big); teleopsia (objects seem too far away); lilliputianism (people appear too small); multiple images; persistent positive visual phenomena (diffuse small particles such as TV static or dots in the entire visual field lasting months to years); palinopsia (the persistence or recurrence of visual images after the exciting stimulus object has been removed); cerebral polyopia (the perception of multiple images); and tilted and upside-down vision (7).

Rarely, benign occipital epilepsy can mimic migraine with aura in children and adolescents. Visual symptoms, such as amaurosis, phosphenes (flashes of light), illusions, and visual hallucinations, may be followed by usually hemiclonic movements. Other types of seizure activity can occur, such as simple partial, complex partial, and partial with secondary generalization. Headache, nausea, vomiting, and vertigo can be pre- and postictal symptoms. The electroencephalogram (EEG) usually shows occipital discharges.

Familial Hemiplegic Migraine

Familial hemiplegic migraine (8), a rare variant, is migraine with aura that includes hemiplegia or hemiparesis. At least one first- or second-degree relative has migraine aura including motor weakness. The inheritance is autosomal dominant. Familial hemiplegic migraine type 1 (FHM1) is localized to the gene CACNA1A on chromosome 19. CACNA1A encodes the alpha 1A subunit of voltage-gated P/Q-type calcium channels in neurons. Thus FHM1 is a calcium channelopathy. Familial hemiplegic migraine type 2 (FHM2) is localized to chromosome 1 where mutations occur in the ATP1A2 gene (the Na+, K+-ATPase pump gene). In approximately 50% of FHM1 families, chronic progressive cerebellar ataxia occurs independently of the migraine attacks.

The attack onset is usually in childhood, virtually always before 30 years of age, with a mean age of onset of 12 years. The frequency of attacks ranges from 1 per day to less than 5 in a lifetime with a mean of 2 or 3 per year. Long attack-free intervals from 2 to 37 years have been reported. The two most common triggers are emotional stress and minor head trauma.

Attacks may occur on the same or different side from prior episodes. The face, arm, and leg typically become paretic with a slow, spreading progression. There may be an associated alteration in consciousness that ranges from confusion to coma. When the dominant hemisphere is involved, aphasia may also be present. The headache can be ipsilateral to the paresis in one third of cases. The hemiparesis may last from less than 1 hour to days or weeks. Complete recovery usually occurs. Triptans and dihydroergotamine (DHE) should not be used during the neurological deficit because of the potential for vasoconstriction and stroke. Beta-blocker medications might be avoided because of anecdotal reports of migraine-induced stroke. Verapamil, divalproex, and topiramate can be used as preventive agents.

Depending on the availability of a family history, the evaluation is similar to that of stroke in the young and may include magnetic resonance imaging (MRI) with magnetic resonance angiography (MRA) and sometimes magnetic resonance venography, blood studies (complete blood count, with platelets, anticardiolipin antibodies, lupus anticoagulant, antithrombin III, protein S and C, factor V mutation, and others, depending on the clinical context), and cardiac evaluation, such as two-dimensional echocardiography. There are numerous causes of hemiparesis and headache, including partial seizures, congenital heart disease, acquired heart disease, infectious/inflammatory disease (e.g., HIV and varicella encephalitis), systemic vascular dysfunction (e.g., venous sinus thrombosis and hypertension), vascular disorders (e.g., carotid artery dissection; homocystinuria; mitochondrial encephalomyopathy, lactic acidosis, and strokelike episodes [MELAS] syndrome; and connective tissue disorders), hematological disorders (e.g., hemoglobinopathies, disseminated intravascular coagulation, and antiphospholipid antibody syndrome), cerebrovascular malformations (e.g., arteriovenous malformations, aneurysms, and Sturge-Weber syndrome), and head trauma.

Basilar-Type Migraine

Migraine with aura symptoms originating from the brain stem or from both occipital lobes is known as basilar-type migraine (Table 10-3) (9). The aura of basilar-type migraine usually lasts from 5 to 60 minutes but can last up to 3 days. Visual

Table 10-3.   IHS 2nd edition diagnostic criteria for basilar-type migraine (Migraine with aura symptoms clearly originating from the brain stem and/or from both hemispheres simultaneously affected, but no motor weakness.)

A. At least 2 attacks fulfilling criteria B–D
B. Aura consisting of at least two of the following fully reversible symptoms, but no motor weakness:
    1. dysarthria
    2. vertigo
    3. tinnitus
    4. hypacusia
    5. diplopia
    6. visual symptoms simultaneously in both temporal and nasal fields of both eyes
    7. ataxia
    8. decreased level of consciousness
    9. simultaneously bilateral paraesthesias
C. At least one of the following:
    1. at least one aura symptom develops gradually over ≥5 minutes and/or different aura symptoms occur in succession over ≥5 minutes
    2. each aura symptom lasts ≥5 and ≤60 minutes
D. Headache fulfilling criteria B–D for Migraine without aura begins during the aura or follows aura within 60 minutes
E. Not attributed to another disorder

symptoms–including blurred vision, teichopsia (shimmering colored lights accompanied by blank spots in the visual field), scintillating scotoma, graying of vision, or total loss of vision—may start in one visual field and spread to become bilateral. Diplopia may be present in up to 16% of cases. Vertigo (which can be present with tinnitus), dysarthria, gait ataxia, and paresthesias (usually bilateral but may alternate sides with a hemidistribution) may be present alone or in various combinations. In 50% of cases, bilateral motor weakness occurs. Impairment of consciousness often occurs, including obtundation, amnesia, syncope, and, rarely, prolonged coma.

A severe throbbing headache is present in 96% of cases, usually with a bilateral occipital location. Nausea and vomiting typically occur, with light and noise sensitivity occurring in up to 50%.

The differential diagnosis and diagnostic evaluation are similar to those in hemiplegic migraine. Partial seizures, especially of occipital and temporal lobe origin, can have features similar to basilar migraine. An EEG study may be considered part of the evaluation. EEG abnormalities are found in less than 20% of cases. Children and adolescents may have interictal occipital spike-slow-wave or spike-wave activity.

Basilar-type migraine is an uncommon disorder. The onset is typically before 30 years of age (although the first attack occasionally occurs in those over 50 years of age) with a female preponderance following puberty of 3:1, as in other forms of migraine. The age of onset peaks during adolescence. Children may also have this migraine type. Those with basilar-type migraine may also have other types of migraine, although the basilar type is the predominant one in 75% of cases.

The frequency of basilar migraine decreases as patients enter their 20s and 30s. Stroke is a rare complication. As with other forms of migraine, triggers should be avoided if possible. Analgesics or nonsteroidal antiinflammatory drugs (NSAIDs) can be used for the pain. The package inserts for triptans, ergotamine, and DHE list basilar and hemiplegic migraine as contraindications to use based on the concern over vasoconstrictive properties. Based on a small case series in which triptans were safely used in basilar-type and familial hemiplegic migraine, Klapper et al. (10) argue that triptans may actually be a safe and effective treatment for headache in this circumstance because of a neuronal mechanism of action. Beta-blockers should be avoided because of a theoretical potential for stroke (based on a small case series), but verapamil, divalproex, topiramate, and antidepressants such as amitriptyline can be tried as preventive agents.

Ophthalmoplegic Migraine

Patients with ophthalmoplegic migraine present complaining of migraine headache and diplopia. This is a rare condition. Onset is often during adolescence, although it may occur during infancy. MRI studies have been reported as demonstrating thickening and enhancement of the oculomotor nerve at its exit from the midbrain. Speculation on the pathophysiology includes a trigeminovascular migraine epiphenomenon and a recurrent demyelinating neuropathy (11).

As the intensity of an ipsilateral severe headache subsides after a day or more, paresis of one or more of cranial nerves III, IV, and VI occurs. The third cranial nerve is involved in about 80% of cases, initially with ptosis and then with oculomotor paresis that is usually complete but may be partial. Dilation of the pupil, mydriasis, is present in more than 50% of cases. Recovery of nerve function may occur in a week to 4 to 6 weeks. Recovery may be incomplete after multiple attacks. Early high-dose corticosteroid treatment may be beneficial.

The diagnosis is made by excluding, as appropriate, such conditions as Tolosa-Hunt syndrome (granulomatous inflammation in the cavernous sinus), parasellar lesions, diabetic cranial neuropathy, collagen vascular disease, and orbital pseudotumor (an idiopathic infiltration of orbital structures with chronic inflammatory cells). MRI with MRA is usually adequate, although a cerebral arteriogram may be necessary in some cases.

Benign Paroxysmal Vertigo of Childhood

The onset of benign paroxysmal vertigo of childhood (12) usually occurs between 2 and 5 years of age but can be before 1 year of age or as late as 12 years of age. Unprovoked stereotypical episodes of true vertigo (with a sensation of movement as described by verbal children) usually last for seconds or minutes but may last for hours. The child becomes pale, cannot maintain an upright posture, and wishes to remain absolutely still. There is no complaint of headache or alteration of consciousness, although nausea or other abdominal discomfort may follow the vertigo. Because the episodes are so brief, treatment is not usually needed.

As the child becomes older, the episodes of vertigo may be associated with migraine headache or may become less severe and disappear. Other types of migraine may then occur in 21% of these patients (13).

Other causes of vertigo in children should be considered. A single prolonged episode could be due to infection of the labyrinth or vestibular nerve. Partial seizures can also produce true vertigo.

Abdominal Migraine

According to the IHS 2nd edition criteria (6), the diagnostic criteria for abdominal migraine require at least five attacks of abdominal pain lasting 1 to 72 hours (untreated or unsuccessfully treated) fulfilling the following criteria. The abdominal pain has all of the following characteristics: midline location, periumbilical or poorly localized, dull or "just sore" quality, and moderate or severe intensity. During abdominal pain, at least two of the four symptoms of anorexia, nausea, vomiting, and pallor are present and not attributed to another disorder.

The prevalence peaks at ages 5 to 9 years. As with all migraine types, this is a diagnosis of exclusion. If there is alteration of consciousness, a seizure disorder should be considered. Other disorders in the differential diagnosis include urogenital disorders, ornithine transcarbamylase deficiency, peptic ulcer disease, cholecystitis, Meckel's diverticulum, partial duodenal obstruction, gastroesophageal reflux, Crohn's disease, and irritable bowel syndrome. Drugs used for migraine prevention and symptomatic treatment may be helpful.

Confusional Migraine

Confusional migraine is migraine with a headache, which can be minimal, associated with a confusional state that can last from 10 minutes to 2 days. The patient may be agitated and have impaired memory. There may be inattention, distractibility, and difficulty maintaining coherent speech or action. The diagnosis is made by excluding, as appropriate, the numerous causes of an acute encephalopathy, including partial complex seizures, metabolic disorders, infection, and subarachnoid hemorrhage (SAH).

"Footballer's" Migraine

As discussed in Chapter 9, acute minor head trauma can trigger migraine in children and adolescents. In a study of children with a mean age of 7.4 years who had mild head injuries, a history of motion sickness, migraines, and migraine in other family members is highly predictive of vomiting after a mild head injury (14).

MELAS Syndrome

Mitochondrial encephalomyopathy, lactic acidosis, and strokelike episodes (MELAS), a rare disorder, can present as episodic migraine early in the course of the disease (15). The following features must be present: strokelike episodes typically before 40 years of age; encephalopathy with seizures, dementia, or both; and evidence of a mitochondrial myopathy with lactic acidosis, ragged-red fibers, or both. At least two of the following should be present: normal early development, recurrent headache, or recurrent vomiting. Most patients have exercise intolerance, limb weakness, short stature, hearing loss, and elevated cerebrospinal fluid (CSF) protein.

The cause of 80% of cases is an A-to-G point mutation in the mitochondrial gene encoding for tRNA[Leu(UUR)] at nucleotide position 3243. The other 20% are due to 14 other mitochondrial DNA point mutations. All children of mothers with MELAS are affected because of maternal transmission of mitochondrial DNA.

Management

Nonmedication Approaches

Identification and avoidance of migraine triggers are important. Missing meals, stress, and sleep deprivation can be particularly important triggers. Elimination of caffeinated beverages can be helpful in some cases. Biofeedback, stress management, and progressive relaxation training may be beneficial (16). Education about migraine for the patient and parents or caretakers is well worthwhile.

Pharmacological Treatments

Acute or symptomatic and preventive medications are available. Many of the recommendations in this section are anecdotal because of the lack of well-designed studies of treatment of childhood and adolescent migraine.

ACUTE HEADACHES. Aspirin should be avoided before 15 years of age because of the potential for Reye's syndrome. Headaches in children 6 years of age and younger are typically brief and resolve with acetaminophen and/or sleep. For children over 6 years of age, acetaminophen (10 to 15 mg/kg) may be effective. Other options (Table 10-4) include NSAIDs such as ibuprofen (10 mg/kg) (17), naproxen sodium (10 mg/kg); isometheptene mucate (65 mg), dichloralphenazone (100 mg), and acetaminophen (325 mg) (Midrin, one capsule); butalbital (50 mg), acetaminophen (325 mg), and caffeine (40 mg) (Fioricet, 6 to 9 years, one-half tablet; 9 to 12 years, three-fourths tablet; and more than 12 years, one tablet).

Children with significant nausea and/or vomiting may benefit from the use of metoclopramide 0.2 mg/kg orally or promethazine 0.5 mg/kg orally or in suppository form. Some children and adolescents also benefit from a combination of codeine and acetaminophen or acetaminophen, butalbital, and caffeine.

Total weekly doses of symptomatic medications and caffeine should be carefully monitored because of the potential for causing rebound headaches. There are restrictions on the use of certain acute and preventive medications in hemiplegic and basilar migraine as detailed earlier.

Additional treatments are available for severe migraines in children and adolescents ages 6 and over who do not respond to these medications. In a study of 50 children between the ages of 6 and 18, Linder administered sumatriptan (Imitrex) subcutaneously (dose of 0.06 mg/kg) and reported efficacy in 78% (18). In responders, the migraine recurrence rate was 6%. Adverse events, usually transient and mild, occur in 80%.

Oral triptans are often effective in adolescents of 12 years of age and over. Sumatriptan nasal spray (ages 4–7 years, 5 mg; older than 7 years, 20 mg) and zolmitriptan nasal spray (older than 12 years, 5 mg) can also be effective. Anecdotally, triptans may be effective in children over 6 years of age. Side effects of triptans are discussed in Chapter 3. Table 10-4 provides dosages of triptans commonly used in children. Triptans are not approved by the Food and Drug Administration (FDA) for those under 18 years of age.

Alternatively, as in adults, children and adolescents with prolonged migraine often respond to an inpatient protocol of an antiemetic, metoclopramide, and DHE (Table 10-5), as reported by Linder (19). The oral metoclopramide and intravenous (IV) DHE can be given every 6 hours for a maximum of eight doses. When the headache ceases, one additional dose can be given. The dose of DHE may be increased by 0.05 mg/dose up to the point at which the patient has mild abdominal discomfort. The protocol should be continued at the dose prior to the onset of the abdominal discomfort. Triptans and DHE should not be given within less than 24 hours of each other.

These medications can have significant side effects. If metoclopramide causes an extrapyramidal syndrome, diphenhydramine can be given (1 mg/kg, maximum dose of 50 mg) orally, intramuscularly, or IV. Metoclopramide can also cause nausea and vomiting. For subsequent DHE doses, ondansetron 0.15 mg/kg IV 30 minutes prior to the DHE dose can be given as an

Table 10-4. Symptomatic treatment for migraine in children and adolescents

Medication	Dosage
Acetaminophen	10–15 mg/kg orally (po)
Pseudoephedrine HCL	30 mg po
Ibuprofen	10 mg/kg po
Naproxen sodium	10 mg/kg po
Butalbital 50 mg, acetaminophen 325 mg, caffeine 40 mg	6–9 yr, $^1/_2$ tablet
	9–12 yr, $^3/_4$ tablet
	>12 yr, 1 tablet
Isometheptene mucate, dichloralphenazone 100 mg and acetaminophen 325 mg	6–12 yr, 1 capsule
	>12 yr, 1–2 capsules
Sumatriptan	0.06 mg/kg SC
	25–mg for wt <50 lb
	25–50 mg for wt 50–100 lb
	50–100 mg for wt >100 lb
	5 mg NS 4–7 yr
	20 mg NS >7 yr
Zolmitriptan	6–8 yr, 1.25 mg po or 2.5 mg NS
	9–11 yr, 2.5 mg po or 2.5 mg NS
	>12 yr, 5 mg po or 5 mg NS
Rizatriptan	6–8 yr, 2.5 mg
	9–11 yr, 5 mg
	>12 yr, 10 mg
Almotriptan	>12 yr, 12.5 mg
Eletriptan	20 mg for wt ≤100 lb
	40 mg for wt ≥100 lb
Naratriptan	>12 yr, 2.5 mg
Frovatriptan	>12 yr, 2.5 mg
DHE IV	(see Table 10-6)

alternative, if necessary, to prevent nausea and vomiting, which can be a side effect of DHE or part of the migraine. Side effects of DHE include a flushed feeling, tingling in the extremities, leg cramping, and a transient increase in headache. DHE is not FDA approved for use in those under 18 years of age.

PREVENTIVE MEDICATIONS. Preventive medications should be considered for children and adolescents with frequent migraines that are not responsive to symptomatic medications or that significantly interfere with school or home activities (Table 10-6). In

Table 10-5. Dosing of metoclopramide and DHE for severe intractable migraine

Age in years	Metoclopramide[a]	DHE
6–9	0.2 mg/kg	0.1 mg/dose
9–12	0.2 mg/kg	0.15 mg/dose
12–16	0.2 mg/kg	0.2 mg/dose

[a]Administered orally 30 minutes prior to administration of IV DHE. Maximum dose of 20 mg.

Table 10-6. Preventive medications for migraine in children and adolescents

Medication	Dosage
Propanolol	<14 yr, initial dose 10 mg po bid. May increase by 10 mg/day/each week to 20 mg tid maximum >14 yr, initial dose 20 mg po bid. May increase by 20 mg/day each week up to 240 mg/day. Equivalent long-acting doses may be used.
Cyproheptyline HCl	≥6 yr, 4 mg po hs. May be slowly increased to 12 mg po hs or 8 mg po hs and 4 mg po q a.m.
Amitriptyline or nortriptyline	10 mg po hs. May be increased every 2 weeks to 50 mg po hs <12 yr and 100 mg po hs >12 yr
Topiramate	<12 years: week 1, 25 mg evening; week 2, 25 mg am, 25 mg evening; week 3, 25 mg am, 50 mg evening; week 4 and maintenance, 50 mg every 12 h (slow titration if side effects)
	>12 years: week 1, .25–1 mg/kg/d (no more than 25 mg); increase by initial dose each week in divided doses up to 50–100 mg total/day (slow titration if side effects)
Divalproex sodium	125–250 mg po hs, slowly increase to 500–1,000 mg in two divided doses (or once a day with ER formulation)

general, preventive medications are started at low doses and are increased slowly.

Beta-blockers such as propranolol may be effective. The initial dose for children 8 years of age or older is 10 mg two times a day, which can be increased, depending on response, by 10 mg per week or slower to a maximum of 20 mg three times a day for children under 14 years of age. Adult doses (Table 10-6) can be given to those 14 years of age and older. Those on higher doses of propranolol can be switched to or started on the long-acting preparation. Among the numerous possible side effects, beta-blockers can occasionally exacerbate asthma, cause hypotension, and cause depression. Propranolol given to diabetic children on insulin can mask symptoms of hypoglycemia. Congestive heart failure, atrioventricular conduction defects, and renal insufficiency are also contraindications to use. In some patients, nadolol or atenolol may be better tolerated, with fewer side effects, such as depression or asthenia, than propranolol.

Cyproheptadine (Periactin), an antihistamine, can also be an effective preventive medication in single doses of from 4 to 12 mg at bedtime (hs) or in divided doses, such as morning and evening for children 6 years and older (e.g., starting at 4 mg hs and, depending on effect, slowly increasing after several weeks to 8 mg hs, and later, if necessary, to 12 mg hs or 8 mg hs and 4 mg in the morning). The dose for children under 6 years of age is 1 mg hs, slowly increasing to 2 mg hs and 2 mg in the morning. Common side effects include weight gain and drowsiness. Cyproheptadine may be the preventive of first choice for those with frequent migraines and atopic allergies or sinus disease.

Tricyclic antidepressants, such as amitriptyline (Elavil) and nortriptyline (Pamelor), can also be used. For children over 8 years of age, the starting dose of either is 10 mg/day hs. Depending on the response and side effects, the total daily dose can be increased by 10 mg every 1 to 2 weeks or slower. Effective daily dosage is typically 50 mg or less in younger children and 100 mg or less in adolescents. Common side effects include sedation, weight gain, and dry mouth. Rarely, cardiac conduction abnormalities can occur with prolongation of the P-R, QRS, and Q-T intervals. Nortriptyline is less sedating than amitriptyline. The tricylics are often the preventive of choice for those with frequent migraine and tension-type headaches, chronic daily headaches, or associated depression or sleep disturbance. If a tricyclic is ineffective, a trial of trazadone (1 mg/kg a day divided into three doses) might be considered (20).

As discussed in Chapter 4, large clinical trials have demonstrated that topiramate is an effective medication for prevention for migraineurs 12 years of age or older. An open-label study also showed efficacy in younger children (21). For children 12 and older, the medication is started at 25 mg in the evening for the first week, 25 mg in the morning and 25 mg in the evening for the second week, 25 mg in the morning and 50 mg evening for the third week, and 50 mg in the morning and 50 mg in the evening (50 mg twice a day) starting for the fourth week, which is the maintenance dose. If side effects such as sleepiness, speech, or concentration problems occur, the patient may benefit from reducing the dose (e.g., starting at 12.5 mg or 15 mg) and slowing the increase of dose in the titration schedule to every 2 weeks. For children younger than 12 years, the initial dose is .25 to 1 mg/kg/day for a maximum of 25 mg hs increased by the initial dose once weekly to 50 to 100 mg. The total daily dose is given twice a day. Adverse events associated with topiramate are discussed in Chapter 4. Oligohydrosis (decreased sweating) and hyperthermia have rarely been reported in children on topiramate. Toparamate may be preferred for treatment of migraineurs with comorbidity such as epilepsy, essential tremor, or who are overweight.

Valproic acid may also be effective for migraine prevention in children and adolescents. Divalproex sodium (Depakote), the enteric coated form, is commonly used to minimize gastrointestinal side effects. According to data from adult studies, there may be efficacy for migraine prevention at doses lower than those used for epilepsy. A starting dose of 125 to 250 mg given at bedtime may be used and then slowly increased at 2-week intervals or slower. The total daily effective dose, given at bedtime and in the morning, is often 500 mg a day or less in younger children and 500 to 1,000 mg a day in adolescents. Equivalent once-daily doses may be used if the Depakote ER formulation is prescribed. This total daily dose may be less than that used for the treatment of epilepsy. There are numerous side effects, as described in Chapter 4, most commonly weight gain, tremor, hair loss, and nausea. Tremor and hair loss are fully reversible after discontinuing the medication. If nausea is persistent, the sprinkle formulation may be better tolerated. The rare complication of fatal hepatotoxicity almost always occurs in children under 10 years of age, most under the age of 2 years. (This complication has been reported for children taking the medication for epilepsy. The risk for those on polytherapy is 1:8,307 and on monotherapy, 1:16,317 (22). This drug may be especially considered for those with migraine and comorbidity of epilepsy and bipolar disease.

Prognosis

Migraine with onset before 7 years of age more commonly remits in boys than in girls. By 22 years of age, 50% of men and 60% of women still have migraine. In those with severe migraine beginning between the ages of 7 and 15, 20% are migraine free by 25 years of age and 50% continue to have it into their 50s and 60s (23).

EPISODIC TENSION-TYPE HEADACHES

The most common recurrent headache in children and adolescents is episodic tension type. Tension-type headaches typically have the following characteristics: duration of 30 minutes to many days; bilateral with a pressing or tightening quality; mild to moderate intensity; and not worsened by routine physical activity. Although nausea is absent, light or noise sensitivity may be present.

When symptomatic medication is necessary, acetaminophen, ibuprofen, or naproxen sodium may be effective. Frequent use of these or other symptomatic drugs or caffeine can lead to medication rebound headaches.

If the headaches are frequent, adequate sleep, regular exercise, and avoidance of caffeine may be beneficial. Biofeedback, stress management, and progressive relaxation training may also be helpful. Psychological or psychiatric evaluation may be worthwhile in some cases in which school or family problems, stress, depression, or anxiety is prominent. If there is a significant muscle contraction contribution, treatments such as a short-term course of muscle relaxants, NSAIDs, physical therapy, and a trial of a transcutaneous nerve stimulator unit may be warranted. Preventive medications such as amitriptyline, nortriptyline, and paroxetine (Paxil 10 to 20 mg daily) can be effective.

CHRONIC NONPROGRESSIVE HEADACHES (24)

Frequent nonmigrainous headaches occur in 2.5% of children by 7 years of age and in 15.7% by 15 years of age. The headache may be present on awakening and last all day. The history, examination, and neuroimaging, as indicated, exclude secondary headaches. Chronic pansinusitis should be considered as the cause of chronic headaches even when sinus symptoms are not present.

Depending on the specifics, the headache may be classified as chronic tension type, mixed (both distinct migraine and tension headaches or headaches with features of both), transformed migraine (a history of episodic migraine transforming into daily or near-daily headaches), or caused by medication rebound. The headache may be difficult to classify, and, in many cases, it will paroxymally worsen and accrue migrainous features (25).

Medication rebound headache is important to identify because discontinuing the analgesics alone can produce great improvement (26). These patients typically have a history of migraine and/or tension-type headache. Without a definite precipitating event or following an injury or illness, the headaches may increase in frequency; then a pattern develops of daily or almost daily analgesic use. The daily analgesic use, in susceptible individuals, can cause daily bilateral or unilateral headaches with tension and migraine features. Frequent use of caffeine may also cause or contribute to daily headaches. Episodic migraine headaches may also occur. The headaches may persist for months or years. Preventive medications may be less effective in this setting.

Medications that can cause rebound headaches include the following: acetaminophen; ibuprofen, and other NSAIDs; combination drugs with such agents as butalbital, acetaminophen, caffeine, aspirin, and codeine; propoxyphene; and ergotamine. In some cases, frequent triptan use can also cause rebound headaches. The number of doses of analgesics taken per week, in the largest study with patients from ages 5 to 17 years, ranged from 8 to 84 (27). Acetaminophen and ibuprofen were the most commonly overused medications. Discontinuing daily analgesics and taking amitriptyline 10 mg orally daily reduced the frequency of headaches by 80%.

If headaches persist despite medication withdrawal or if chronic tension-type or mixed headaches are present, a psychological or psychiatric evaluation should be considered to evaluate the presence of home and school problems, other stressors, or depression, which may contribute to headaches. Biofeedback, stress management training, relaxation training, and behavioral contingency management may be helpful in reducing the headaches. The preceding section on tension-type headaches describes preventive medications that may be effective. Divalproex sodium can also be helpful in some cases. A 3-day IV

DHE protocol administered every 8 days can be indicated for some refractory cases (Table 10-5).

New daily, persistent headaches can also occur without a history of increasingly frequent tension- and/or migraine-type headaches. The headache develops over less than 3 days. In many cases, the etiology is unknown. Other cases may reflect a postviral syndrome.

Acute infectious mononucleosis should be considered, especially when there are accompanying complaints of sore throat and findings of cervical adenopathy. (The term *infectious mononucleosis* was first used in 1920 to describe medical students at Johns Hopkins with the condition who were found to have atypical mononuclear cells.) The typical picture is a 7-day prodromal illness followed by a 4-day to 3-week acute illness with fever, headache, malaise, pharyngitis, cervical lymphadenopathy, and mononuclear leukocytosis with atypical lymphocytes (28). Transient hepatic dysfunction and splenic and hepatomegaly may be present. The diagnosis is based on a positive heterophil antibody test, the appearance of atypical lymphocytes in the blood at 1 to 4 weeks after onset of disease, and/or by changes in EBV-specific antibodies. Longer duration chronic headaches can be present with persistent Epstein-Barr infection (29).

ACUTE HEADACHES

Epidemiology

Chapter 8 reviews first or worst headaches in adults. In children and adolescents, the epidemiology is different. In a study of 150 consecutive children presenting to the emergency department with a chief complaint of acute headache, the diagnoses were as follows: viral upper respiratory infection, 39%; migraine, 18%; sinusitis, 9%; streptococcal pharyngitis, viral meningitis, and undetermined cause, each 7%; posterior fossa tumor, 2.6%; ventriculoperitoneal shunt malfunction, 2%; intracranial hemorrhage and seizure, each 1.5%; postlumbar puncture and postconcussion, each 1% (30). Upper respiratory infections with fever accounted for 54% of the cases. Viral meningitis can present without fever and with a supple neck and normal neurological examination.

In children and adolescents, aneurysmal SAH is uncommon: fewer than 2% of cases occur in those under 18 years of age. SAH is more likely due to ruptured arteriovenous malformations, which outnumber aneurysms by nearly 10 to 1 in childhood.

Brain Abscess

Brain abscess in children has a peak incidence of 4 to 7 years. Twenty-five percent of these children have cyanotic congenital heart disease with a right-to-left shunt resulting in hematogenous spread of infection. Otogenic abscesses also occur in children. Brain abscesses due to frontal or sphenoid sinusitis occur in children ages 10 and older because of the late development of these sinuses (31). Emissary veins spread infection into the brain from the paranasal sinuses, mastoids, and middle ear.

About 75% of patients with brain abscess present with symptoms of less than 2 weeks' duration. The classic clinical triad of headache, fever, and focal neurological signs occurs in only a minority of patients. Headache is present in about 75% of patients, and nausea and vomiting are found in about 50%. Signs are present as follows: fever, less than 50%; seizures, 33%; nuchal rigidity, 25%; and papilledema, 25% (32).

CHRONIC PROGRESSIVE HEADACHES

The epidemiology of chronic progressive headaches is also different in children and adolescents from that in adults (Table 10-7) (23). Causes include brain tumors, hydrocephalus, brain abscess, hematomas, pseudotumor cerebri, malformation, hypertension, and medication rebound. Pseudotumor cerebri (Chapter 14) may be present without papilledema. The diagnosis can only be made with lumbar puncture and measurement of the opening pressure. This section reviews brain tumors and hydrocephalus. The remaining causes are discussed elsewhere in this book.

Brain Tumors

Although parents and children often fear their headache is due to a brain tumor, brain tumors occur uncommonly. The clinical presentation depends on the type and location of tumor. Posterior fossa tumors that result in hydrocephalus can produce the classic brain tumor headaches with nausea, early morning vomiting, and headaches. Headaches from supratentorial tumors are less specific.

Table 10-7. Causes of chronic progressive headaches in children and adolescents

Neoplasms
    Medulloblastoma
    Cerebellar astrocytoma
    Brain stem glioma
    Ependymoma
    Pineal region tumors
    Craniopharyngioma
    Supratentorial astrocytoma
Hydrocephalus
    Obstructive
    Communicating
Brain abscess
Chronic subdural and epidural hematomas
Pseudotumor cerebri
Malformations
    Chiari malformation
    Dandy-Walker cyst
Hypertension
Medication rebound

In a study of 74 children with primary brain tumors from England, headache was present in 64%, vomiting in 65%, and changes in personality in 47% (33). Only 34% of headaches were always associated with vomiting, and only 28% occurred in the early morning. Misdiagnosis was common: migraine was diagnosed in 24% and a psychological etiology was found in 15%. Additional features of headaches due to brain tumors are discussed in Chapter 14.

Brain metastases in children and adolescents most often arise from sarcomas and germ cell tumors. A variety of primary brain tumors can occur. About 60% of primary brain tumors are infratentorial (posterior fossa) and 40% supratentorial. The annual incidence of pediatric primary brain tumors is about 2 or 3 out of 100,000.

Medulloblastoma

Medulloblastomas (primitive neuroectodermal tumors), the most common, account for 20% of childhood brain tumors and 30% to 40% of posterior fossa childhood tumors. The tumor may occur at any time of life, including adulthood, but it is most common in the first decade, with peaks at 3 to 4 years of age and 8 to 10 years. Medulloblastomas usually arise from the cerebellar vermis. Symptoms and signs are due to obstruction of the fourth ventricle and hydrocephalus, infiltration of cerebellar tissue, and leptomeningeal spread. By the time of diagnosis, 90% of patients have papilledema, headaches, vomiting (especially morning vomiting), and lethargy. Ataxia is often present early in the course of the disease.

Cerebellar Astrocytoma

The classic, or juvenile, pilocytic cerebellar astrocytoma is a slow-growing lesion arising from the lateral cerebellar hemispheres. This astrocytoma is the second most common tumor of the posterior fossa, accounting for 30% to 40% of cases, and it comprises 10% to 20% of all childhood brain tumors. The peak ages of incidence are the latter half of the first decade and the first half of the second decade of life. Initially, appendicular cerebellar symptoms may be present for weeks to months. As the tumor extends to the midline and obstructs the fourth ventricle resulting in hydrocephalus, the classic brain tumor symptoms of early morning vomiting and headaches may be present.

Brain Stem Glioma

Brain stem gliomas constitute 10% to 20% of all childhood brain tumors and are the third most common posterior fossa tumor. The median age of occurrence is between 5 and 9 years. The neurological presentation depends on the location of the tumor. The classic present is a triad of cranial neuropathies, ataxia, and long tract signs. About one third of patients have headache, nausea, and vomiting.

Ependymoma

Ependymomas comprise 5% to 10% of childhood primary brain tumors. Two thirds arise in the posterior fossa and are usually benign, whereas one third arise supratentorially and are usually malignant. Infratentorial ependymomas arise from the floor, roof, or lateral recesses of the fourth ventricle. By the time of diagnosis, most of the infratentorial tumors have blocked the third or fourth ventricle, producing hydrocephalus. Headaches, nausea, and vomiting will then occur. Depending on location of the tumor, supratentorial ependymomas can produce focal neurological findings and seizures. By the time of diagnosis, most patients have headaches and other signs and symptoms of increased intracranial pressure.

Pineal Region Lesions

Pineal region lesions include germinomas (1% of childhood primaries), pineoblastomas, glial neoplasms, meningiomas, lymphomas, and pineal cysts. Growth of the tumor causes compression of the aqueduct of Sylvius and hydrocephalus. The typical picture of hydrocephalus can occur with headaches, nausea, and vomiting. Involvement of the superior colliculus can lead to Parinaud's syndrome with paralysis of upgaze, near-light dissociation, and convergence-retraction nystagmus.

CRANIOPHARYNGIOMA. Craniopharyngiomas are benign tumors located in the parasellar region. Although they can occur at any age, the onset is before 15 years of age in 50% of cases. These are the third most common primary in children after medulloblastomas and gliomas. Growth failure is the most common sign at presentation. Visual dysfunction is present in up to 70% of patients at the time of presentation because of the prechiasmal location. Fifty percent of patients complain of severe headaches.

ASTROCYTOMA. Supratentorial astrocytomas can produce focal neurological findings and seizures (in about 25% of cases). Low-grade gliomas can produce a very gradual onset of symptoms, including headache and/or subtle neurobehavioral changes. Increased difficulty with schoolwork can be blamed on social or psychological factors. Malignant astrocytomas are more commonly seen in adults.

Hydrocephalus (34)

There are two categories of hydrocephalus, which is a heterogenous disorder. Obstructive, or noncommunicating, hydrocephalus is due to a blockage of CSF pathways at or proximal to the outlet foramina of the fourth ventricle, the foraminas of Luschka and Magendie. Communicating hydrocephalus is due to a blockage of CSF in the basal subarachnoid cisterns, in the subarachnoid spaces over the brain surface, or within the arachnoid granulations.

Table 10-8 lists the various causes of hydrocephalus in children and adults. Diagnostic testing helps define the features of hydrocephalus, including the site of blockage of CSF, the etiology, and whether the condition is arrested or progressive.

Clinical Manifestations

Small children may present with symptoms and signs of raised intracranial pressure, including headaches, vomiting, irritability, lethargy, and poor feeding. Acute hydrocephalus in older children can result in headaches, often worse in the morning; vomiting; cranial nerve VI palsies; papilledema; and altered

Table 10-8. Causes of hydrocephalus

Noncommunicating	Communicating
Aqueductal stenosis	Chiari malformation
Chiari malformation	Dandy-Walker malformation
Dandy-Walker malformation	Encephalocele
Atresia of the foramen of Monroe	Benign cysts
Skull bases anomalies	Incompetent arachnoid villi
Neoplasms	Leptomeningeal inflammation
Benign intracranial cysts	Viral infection
Inflammatory ventriculitis	Bacterial infection
Hemorrhage	Subarachnoid hemorrhage
Infection	Chemical arachnoiditis
Chemical meningitis	Carcinomatous meningitis
Ruptured arachnoid cyst	

From Kinsman SL. Hydrocephalus. In: Gilman S, ed. *MedLink neurology.* San Diego: MedLink Corp. Available at www.medlink.com., 2004. Modified, with permission.

levels of consciousness. Headaches due to hydrocephalus are often bilateral and are made worse by coughing, sneezing, straining, or head movement.

Ventriculoperitoneal shunts are appropriate treatment for many cases of hydrocephalus. Acute hydrocephalus due to shunt failure can result in headaches, vomiting, altered consciousness, and seizures. Physicians who care for children with shunts should be aware of the rare complication of slit ventricle syndrome.

Symptoms and signs of intermittent intracranial hypertension develop in a patient who has been stable for months to years with a shunt. A scan of the brain shows a smaller than normal ventricular system that could be due to acquired rigidity of the ventricular system. There are numerous other complications of shunts, including infections, subdural hematomas, and seizures.

Colloid Cysts of the Third Ventricle

Colloid cysts of the third ventricle are benign cysts that can move in and out of the foramen of Monro on its pedicle, producing intermittent obstruction of CSF. Colloid cysts are rarely diagnosed during childhood. The cysts can produce severe paroxysmal headaches that can be mistaken for migraine and can lead to sudden death in about 5% of cases (35).

Dandy-Walker Malformation

Dandy-Walker malformation is a developmental disorder characterized by partial or complete absence of the cerebellar vermis and cystlike dilatation of the fourth ventricle. Other features often present include hydrocephalus; enlargement of the posterior fossa; elevation of the tentorium, transverse sinus, or both; and lack of patency of the foramina of Luschka, Magendie, or both. The incidence is about 1 in 30,000 live births. There are a variety of clinical presentations, including mental retardation in about 50%, ataxia, brain stem dysfunction, and symptoms and signs due to hydrocephalus, which is present in about 80% of cases by 1 year of age. The initial presentation can occur as late as adulthood, with such complaints as headache, cerebellar ataxia, and progressive spastic weakness of all four extremities.

REFERENCES

1. Bille B. Migraine in school children. *Acta Pediatr Scand* 1962;51[Suppl 136]:1–151.
2. Kandt RS. Childhood migraine. In: Gilman S, ed. *MedLink Neurology*. San Diego: MedLink Corp. Available at www.medlink.com., 2004.
3. Jan MMS. History of motion sickness is predictive of childhood migraine. *J Paediatr Child Health* 1998;34:483–484.
4. Giroud M, Nivelon JL, Dumas R. [Somnambulism and migraine in children: a non-fortuitous association]. *Arch Fr Pediatr* 1987;44:263–265.
5. Stewart WF, Linet MS, Celentano DD, et al. Age and sex-specific incidence rates of migraine with and without visual aura. *Am J Epidemiol* 1993;34:1111–1120.
6. Headache Classification Subcommittee of the International Headache Society. The International Classification of Headache Disorders, 2nd ed. *Cephalalgia* 2004;24 (Suppl 1):59:1–160.
7. Liu GT, Volpe NJ, Galetta SL. Visual hallucinations and illusions. In: *Neuro-ophthalmology. Diagnosis and management*. Philadelphia: WB Saunders, 2001:401–424.
8. Peres MFP. Hemiplegic migraine. In: Gilman S, ed. *MedLink Neurology*. San Diego: MedLink Corp. Available at www.medlink.com., 2004.
9. Siow HC, Welch KMA. Basilar migraine. In: Gilman S, ed. *MedLink Neurology*. San Diego: MedLink Corp. Available at www.medlink.com., 2004.
10. Klapper J, Mathew N, Nett R. Triptans in the treatment of basilar migraine and migraine with prolonged aura. *Headache* 2001;41:981–984.
11. Carlow TJ. Oculomotor ophthalmoplegic migraine: is it really migraine? *J Neuroophthalmol* 2002;22:215–221.
12. Davidoff RA. Benign paroxysmal vertigo of childhood. In: Gilman S, ed. *MedLink Neurology*. San Diego: MedLink Corp. Available at www.medlink.com., 2004.
13. Lindskog U, Ödkvist L, Noaksson L, et al. Benign paroxysmal vertigo in childhood: a long-term follow-up. *Headache* 1999;39:33–37.
14. Jan MM, Camfield PR, Gordon K, et al. Vomiting after mild head injury is related to migraine. *J Pediatr* 1997;130:134–137.
15. Hirano M. MELAS. In: Gilman S, ed. *MedLink Neurology*. San Diego: MedLink Corp. Available at www.medlink.com., 2004.
16. Sartory G, Muller B, Metsch J, et al. A comparison of psychological and pharmacological treatment of pediatric migraine. *Behav Res Ther* 1998;36:1155–1170.
17. Hamalainen ML, Hoppo K, Valkeila E, et al. Ibuprofen or acetaminophen for the acute treatment of migraine in children: a

double-blind, randomized, placebo-controlled crossover study. *Neurology* 1997;48:103–107.

18. Linder S. Subcutaneous sumatriptan in the clinical setting: the first fifty consecutive patients with acute migraine in a pediatric neurology office practice. *Headache* 1996;36:419–422.

19. Linder S. Treatment of childhood headache with dihydroergotamine mesylate. *Headache* 1994;34:578–580.

20. Battistella PA, Ruffilli R, Cernetti R, et al. A placebo-controlled crossover trial using trazodone in pediatric migraine. *Headache* 1993;33:36–39.

21. Hershey AD, Powers SW, Vockell AL, et al. Effectiveness of topiramate in the prevention of childhood headaches. *Headache* 2002;42: 810–818.

22. Silberstein SD. Divalproex sodium in headache: literature review and clinical guidelines. *Headache* 1996;36:547–555.

23. Bille B. A 40-year follow-up of school children with migraine. *Cephalalgia* 1997;17:488–491.

24. Rothner AD, Winner P. Headaches in children and adolescents. In Silberstein SD, Lipton RB, Dalessio DJ, eds. *Wolff's headache and other head pain,* 7th ed. New York: Oxford University Press, 2001:539–561.

25. Koenig MA, Gladstein J, McCarter RJ, et al. Chronic daily headache in children and adolescents presenting to tertiary headache clinics. *Headache* 2002;42: 491–500.

26. Symon DN. Twelve cases of analgesic headache. *Arch Dis Child* 1998;73:555–556.

27. Vasconcellos E, Piña-Garza JE, Millan EJ, et al. Analgesic rebound headache in children and adolescents. *J Child Neurol* 1998;13:443–447.

28. Roos KL. Chapter 41. Viral infections. In: Goetz CG, ed. *Textbook of clinical neurology,* 2nd ed. Philadelphia: WB Saunders, 2003: 895–918.

29. Vanast WJ. New daily persistent headaches: definition of a benign syndrome. *Headache* 1987;26:318.

30. Lewis DW, Qureshi F. Acute headache in children and adolescents presenting to the emergency department. *Headache* 2000; 40:200–203.

31. Giannoni C, Sulek M, Friedman EM. Intracranial complications of sinusitis: a pediatric series. *Am J Rhinol* 1998;12:173–178.

32. Greenlee JE. Brain abscess. In: Gilman S, ed. *MedLink Neurology.* San Diego: MedLink Corp. Available at www.medlink. com., 2004.

33. Edgeworth J, Bullock P, Bailey A, et al. Why are brain tumours still being missed? *Arch Dis Child* 1996;74:148–151.

34. Kinsman SL. Hydrocephalus. In: Gilman S, ed. *MedLink Neurology.* San Diego: MedLink Corp. Available at www.medlink. com., 2004.

35. Aronica PA, Ahdab-Barmada M, Rozin L, et al. Sudden death in an adolescent boy due to a colloid cyst of the third ventricle. *Am J Forensic Med Pathol* 1998;19:119–122.

Headaches in Women

Randolph W. Evans

Women have headaches more commonly than men. The prevalence of migraine is 18% of women and 6% of men. This gender ratio increases from menarche, peaks at 42 years of age, and then declines. For young women the incidence of migraine with aura peaks between the ages of 12 and 13 (14.1/1,000 person-years), and migraine without aura peaks between the ages of 14 and 17 (18.9/1,000 person-years) (1). Table 11-1 provides the lifetime prevalence of various headaches in women and men.

Estrogen levels are a key factor in the increased prevalence of migraine in women. Evidence includes the following: migraine prevalence increases at menarche; estrogen withdrawal during menstruation is a common migraine trigger; estrogen administration in oral contraceptives and hormone replacement therapy can trigger migraines; migraines typically decrease during the second and third trimesters of pregnancy, when estrogen levels are high; migraines are common immediately postpartum, with the precipitous drop in estrogen levels; and migraines generally improve with physiological menopause. Exactly how changes in estrogen levels influence migraine is not understood. Among numerous effects, fluctuations in estrogen levels can result in changes in prostaglandins and the uterus, prolactin release, opioid regulation, and melatonin secretion. These fluctuations can also cause changes in neurotransmitters, including the catecholamines, noradrenaline, serotonin, dopamine, and endorphins (2).

This chapter reviews some important headache issues for women, including menstrual migraine, menopause and migraine, oral contraceptive use in migraineurs, and headaches during pregnancy and postpartum.

MENSTRUAL MIGRAINE

The reported prevalence of menstrual migraine varies from 4% to 73%, depending on the criteria used for the timing of the attack. According to the IHS 2nd edition appendix, pure menstrual migraine without aura are attacks that occur exclusively on day 1 ± day 2 of menstruation in at least two out of three menstrual cycles and at no other times of the cycle (3). Using this definition, about 7% (depending on the study) of female migraineurs have only menstrual migraine. Menstruation is a trigger for about 60% of migraineurs. Symptoms of the premenstrual syndrome, which occurs during the luteal phase, include depression, anxiety, crying spells, difficulty thinking, lethargy, backache, breast tenderness, swelling, and nausea. Both migraine and tension-type headaches can be associated.

Management

The symptomatic treatment is the same as for other migraines and includes nonsteroidal antiinflammatory drugs (NSAIDs),

Table 11-1.   Lifetime prevalence of headaches in women and men

Type	Women	Men
Any headache	99%	93%
Migraine	25%	8%
Tension	88%	69%

Data from Rasmussen BK, Jensen R, Schroll M, et al. Epidemiology of headache in a general population—a prevalence study. *J Clin Epidemiol* 1991;44:1147–1157.

ergotamine, dihydroergotamine, and triptans (Chapter 2) (4,5). Triptans are just as effective for menstrual migraine. Women with frequent migraines, including menstrual migraine, may benefit from preventive treatment (Chapter 2). Increasing the dose perimenstrually can be helpful in some cases.

When menstrual migraine is the only migraine or the most severe and prolonged, a variety of short-term preventive treatments may be effective starting 2 to 3 days premenstrually and continuing during the menses for women with regular cycles (Table 11-2). NSAIDs can be especially helpful when migraine occurs with dysmenorrhea or menorrhagia (6). Some patients may respond to one class of NSAIDs and not another.

Hormonal treatments that may be effective include transdermal estradiol (Table 11-2), bromocriptine 2.5 mg three times a day (continuous treatment more effective than interval) (7), danazol 200 mg two or three time a day, and tamoxifen 5 to 15 mg daily for days 7 to 14 of the luteal cycle. (There are concerns about use because of an increased risk of uterine cancer [8].) Some women on estrogen-containing combination oral contraceptives may prevent their menstrual migraine from continuous use with breaks every few months or a brand with low-dose estrogen during the menstrual week and two inert pill days (e.g., Mircette). A short, tapering dose of corticosteroids or chlorpromazine 10 to 50 mg twice a day for 4 to 7 days may be effective. Oral magnesium (360 mg of magnesium pyrrolidone carboxylic acid) may also be effective (9). Hysterectomy is not recommended for the management of menstrual migraine.

MENOPAUSE AND MIGRAINES

Two thirds of women with prior migraine improve with physiological menopause. By contrast, surgical menopause results in worsening of migraine in two thirds of cases.

Estrogen Replacement Therapy

Hormone replacement therapy has a variable effect on migraine frequency: 45% improve, 46% worsen, and 9% are unchanged (10). Table 11-3 lists changes in hormone replacement therapy that may be helpful when migraines increase (11). The usual abortive and prophylactic migraine medications can also be used (Chapter 2).

Table 11-2.   Options for interval preventative treatment of menstrual migraine starting 2–3 days before and continuing during the menses

Medication	Dose
Amitriptyline or nortriptyline	25 mg at bedtime (hs)
Propanolol long-acting	60–80 mg every day (qd)
Nadolol	40 mg qd
NSAIDs	
Naproxen sodium	550 mg twice a day (bid)
Naproxen	500 mg bid
Ibuprofen	400 mg three times a day (tid)
Mefenamic acid	500 mg bid
Ketoprofen	75 mg tid
Ergotamine	1 mg bid
DHE	1 mg SC or IM bid
Sumatriptan	50 mg qd
Naratriptan	1 mg bid
Frovatriptan	2.5 mg bid
Transdermal estradiol	100 µg on day −3 replaced on days −1 and +2

Table 11-3.   Treatment of estrogen replacement headache

Reduce estrogen dose

Change estrogen type from conjugated estrogen (Premarin) to pure estradiol (Estrace) to synthetic estrogen (Estinyl) to pure estrone (Ogen)

Convert from interrupted to continuous dosing

Convert from oral to parenteral dosing (Alora, Climara, Estraderm, or Vivelle-Dot)

Add androgens

From Silberstein SD, Merriam G. Sex hormones and headache. *J Pain Symptom Manage* 1993;8:98–114, modified with permission.

ORAL CONTRACEPTIVE USE AND MIGRAINE

Influence on Onset and Frequency

Migraines may occur for the first time following oral contraceptive (OC) use. The effect of OC use is quite variable: migraines may increase, decrease, or stay the same. Much of the data on this topic is from older studies of the use of high-dose estrogen contraception, which often increased migraine frequency. Low-estrogen-dose OCs usually have no effect or may improve migraine. When new-onset migraine occurs or migraine frequency increases, 30% to 40% of this group may improve when OCs are discontinued. However, improvement may not occur for up to 1 year.

Risk of Stroke (12)

Since the 1970s, there has been concern that OCs taken by migraineurs may increase their risk of stroke. Review of the risk of stroke in young women, in female migraineurs, and in those using OCs helps clarify this issue.

Stroke in Young Women

The annual incidence of cerebral infarction in young women is low: about 4 in 100,000 for women aged 25 to 34 and 11 in 100,000 in women aged 35 to 44. For women who do not have migraine and do not take OCs, the annual incidence is perhaps 1.3 in 100,000 for women aged 25 to 34 and 3.6 in 100,000 for women aged 35 to 44.

Hypertension, diabetes, cigarette smoking, and cocaine use are significant risk factors.

Stroke and Migraine

There is an increased risk of stroke in women with migraine (13,14). Using a variety of assumptions, Becker has calculated the approximate risk of stroke in young women not on OC with and without migraine (Table 11-4) (12).

Stroke and Use of Oral Contraceptives

Stroke and the use of OCs is a controversial topic because studies of low-dose estrogens have yielded conflicting results (15). The risk of stroke associated with OCs may vary with the estrogen dose. Based on numerous studies, OCs with different estrogen doses have an increased risk of thromboembolic stroke (odds ratio) as follows: more than 50 mg, 8 to 10; 50 mg, 2 to 4; and 30 to 40 mg, 1.5 to 2.5. However, more recent studies have not shown an increased risk of stroke in women who use low-estrogen-dose OCs (16–19). OCs containing only progesterone do not increase the risk of stroke (20).

Use of Oral Contraceptives in Migraineurs

Some evidence suggests that OC use in migraineurs increases the risk of stroke. Tzourio et al. reported the odds ratio (increase of relative risk) of ischemic stroke in young women using low-estrogen-dose OCs as follows: without migraine, 3.5, and with

Table 11-4. Approximate incidence of ischemic stroke (strokes per 100,000 women per year) in women with and without migraine who do not use oral contraceptives

| Age | Without migraine | Migraine | |
		Without aura	With aura
25–34	1.3	4	8
35–44	3.6	11	22

Data from Becker WJ. Migraine and oral contraceptives. *Can J Neurol Sci* 1997;24:16–21.

migraine, 13.9 (13). The significance of this finding is uncertain in view of the more recent OC use and stroke studies showing no increased risk.

Most women with migraine without aura can safely take low-dose-estrogen OCs when there are no other contraindications to OC use. Similarly, those with migraine with auras such as visual symptoms lasting less than 1 hour can use OCs. Women with aura symptoms such as hemiparesis or dysphasia or prolonged focal neurological symptoms and signs lasting more than 1 hour might best avoid starting low-dose-estrogen OCs and stop the medication if they are already taking it. In addition, the physician should consider other factors in prescribing OCs, such as older age, cigarette smoking, and comorbidity such as diabetes, uncontrolled hypertension, and coronary artery disease. Progesterone-only OCs and the many other contraceptive options can be considered.

HEADACHES DURING PREGNANCY AND POSTPARTUM

About 90% of headaches occurring during pregnancy and the postpartum period are benign. The frequency of tension-type headaches generally does not change. Migraine headaches usually occur less often. Management of frequent benign headaches can be challenging because of restrictions on medication use. Life-threatening causes of headache that can occur during this time include preeclampsia and eclampsia, subarachnoid hemorrhage, intracerebral hemorrhage, and cerebral venous thrombosis. There are numerous other secondary causes, including pseudotumor cerebri, brain tumors (including choriocarcinoma), and infections such as those arising from Listeria.

Neuroimaging (21)

When there are appropriate indications (Chapter 1), neuroimaging should be performed during pregnancy. With the use of lead shielding, a standard computed tomography (CT) scan of the head exposes the uterus to less than 1 mrad. A radiation dose of equal to or more than 15 rad is necessary to result in deformities that might justify termination of the pregnancy. CT scan is the study of choice for the evaluation of head trauma or acute subarachnoid hemorrhage. Magnetic resonance imaging (MRI) is more sensitive for disorders that may occur during pregnancy, such as pituitary apoplexy, cerebral venous sinus thrombosis (with the addition of magnetic resonance venography), and metastatic choriocarcinoma. There is no known risk of MRI during pregnancy, but there is some controversy because the magnets induce an electric field and raise the core temperature slightly (less than 1°C). Although there is no known risk of intravenous (IV) contrast for CT scan or gadolinium for MRI, contrast should be avoided if possible. The radiation dose to the uterus for a typical cervical or intracranial arteriogram is less than 1 mrad.

Migraine

Epidemiology

The new onset of migraine has been variably reported as occurring in 1% and 10% of migraineurs during pregnancy, usually during the first trimester. During pregnancy, preexisting migraine improves or disappears in about 60% or more, is unchanged in 20% or less, and grows more frequent in 20% or less (21). Improvement often occurs during the second or third trimester. In one study, menstrual migraine disappeared or improved in 85% and worsened in 7%, in contrast to nonmenstrual migraine, which disappeared or improved in 60% and worsened in 15% (22). When improvement occurs with the first pregnancy, improvement also occurs during subsequent pregnancies in about 50%, whereas an increased frequency occurs in the other 50% (23). Migraineurs do not have an increased risk of miscarriages, toxemia, congenital anomalies, or stillbirth.

One study reported that 38% of women had headaches during the first postpartum week, especially between days 3 and 6 (24). These headaches occurred more often in women with either a personal or family history of migraine. Many of the women described a mild to moderately severe bifrontal pain associated with photophobia and nausea. These headaches may be triggered by rapidly falling estrogen levels. In another study, 4.5% of women had the new onset of migraine during the postpartum period (25).

Management (26–30)

Fortunately, migraines usually improve or disappear during pregnancy. Nonmedication approaches include avoidance of triggers, ice, sleep, and biofeedback.

Before prescribing medication, the patient should be advised of the potential risk during pregnancy. For many drugs there is insufficient knowledge about the risks of birth defects despite the fact that perhaps 67% of women take medications during pregnancy and 50% take them during the first trimester. The Food and Drug Administration (FDA) drug-risk ratings provide some guidance for medication during pregnancy. If nonobstetricians (such as neurologists or internists) are managing the migraines, they should confer with the obstetrician about medication use.

SYMPTOMATIC MEDICATIONS. Many migraineurs want to take medication during pregnancy, especially for moderate to severe migraines. Concerns include not only the potential of risk for the fetus, but also medication rebound headaches from overuse as well as habituation with the overuse of butalbital and narcotics.

Acetaminophen, which is an FDA Class B drug (no evidence of risk in humans, but there are no controlled human studies), is the medication of choice because there is no evidence of any teratogenic effect. Aspirin is rated Class C (risk to humans has not been ruled out) during the first and second trimesters and Class D (positive evidence of risk to humans from human or animal studies) during the third trimester. Although there is no definite evidence of teratogenicity, there are multiple possible adverse effects, including the following: inhibition of uterine contraction, longer gestation and labor, increased maternal and newborn bleeding, narrowing of the ductus arteriosus, and hyperbilirubinemia. Low-dose daily aspirin is generally safe when used to prevent preeclampsia or for the treatment of antiphospholipid antibody syndrome, although there may be an increased risk of abruptio placentae.

Caffeine in small doses of less than 300 mg a day is Class B and probably safe. Although butalbital is Class C, there has been no evidence of an association with malformations. However, prolonged overuse can result in fetal dependence and severe neonatal withdrawal. If acetaminophen alone is ineffective, some patients will benefit from the addition of butalbital (Phrenillin) or butalbital and caffeine (Fioricet), which can also be combined with codeine.

Codeine in reasonable amounts is probably safe. However, indiscriminate use of codeine (Class C) during the first and second trimesters has a potential for risk because defects such as cleft lip or palate and hip dislocation have been reported. Meperidine, methadone, and butorphanol (all Class C) are probably not teratogenic.

NSAIDs such as ibuprofen and naproxen are Class B during the first two trimesters but should be avoided during the third trimester because of the potential of inhibiting labor, prolonging the length of the pregnancy, and decreasing amniotic fluid volume. There is also concern about the possibility of causing pulmonary hypertension or premature closure of the ductus arteriosus.

Ergotamine and dihydroergotamine (both Class X, contraindicated in pregnancy) should not be used during pregnancy, although the actual risk is not clear. Triptans such as sumatriptan (Imitrex) are Class C. Although there is no evidence of a large increase in birth defects at this time, the use of triptans during pregnancy should be avoided because current information is not sufficient to exclude small increases in the risk of birth defects (31).

Antiemetics may be necessary if the headache is associated with prominent nausea or vomiting, and their use may prevent dehydration that can pose a risk to both the mother and fetus. Prochlorperazine, promethazine, and chlorpromazine (available orally, parenterally, and by suppository) are all Class C. Metoclopramide and ondansetron are Class B. These drugs are generally considered reasonably safe during pregnancy, especially with occasional use. No congenital malformations have been reported with the use of metoclopramide.

Prolonged migraine may be treated with 10 mg of prochlorperazine intravenously and IV fluids. The addition of parenteral narcotics may help some patients. Migraine status may respond to the administration of intravenous corticosteroids such as dexamethasone 4 mg IV.

PREVENTIVE MEDICATIONS. Frequent severe migraines associated with nausea and vomiting may justify the use of preventive medications.

Valproic acid, which is Class D (positive evidence of risk to humans from human or animal studies), should be avoided because of the 1% to 2% risk of neural tube defects when taken between day 17 and day 30 after fertilization. Topiramate, which is Class C, should only be used if the potential benefits outweigh the potential risks because there is inadequate information on the possibility of birth defects and its use (although there are reports on birth defects in animal studies).

Beta-blockers, routinely used during pregnancy for the treatment of hypertension, are the preventive of choice if medical contraindications are not present. Atenolol, nadolol, propranolol, metoprolol, and timolol are all Class C. Although there is no evidence of teratogenicity, there may be an increased incidence of small-for-gestational-age infants. Propranolol may cause fetal and neonatal toxicity.

Antidepressants might be considered in some cases. The class rating of some tricyclic antidepressants are as follows: amitriptyline and nortriptyline, Class D; and doxepin and protriptyline, Class C. Tricyclics should be stopped at least 2 weeks before the due date. There are reports of infants with respiratory distress and feeding difficulties born to women who took tricyclics through delivery. Fluoxetine (Class C), a selective serotonin reuptake inhibitor (SSRI), is questionably effective for migraine prevention, but there is evidence of efficacy for chronic daily headache. Fluoxetine might be considered in a patient with frequent headaches and depression. None of the SSRIs or tricyclic antidepressants have been associated with an increased risk of congenital malformations, although information on long-term neurobehavioral effects remains limited (32).

Another option is the calcium channel blocker verapamil (Class C), which is probably safe during pregnancy. This drug is preferable to beta-blockers for prevention of migraine with prolonged aura. In addition, verapamil can also be considered in women with hypertension and frequent migraines who cannot take beta-blockers.

BREASTFEEDING AND MIGRAINE MANAGEMENT. The American Academy of Pediatrics Committee on Drugs has made recommendations based on their review of drug use during lactation (Table 11-5) (33). Ergotamine is contraindicated during breastfeeding. Drugs whose effect on nursing infants is unknown but may be of concern include such antidepressants as amitriptyline and fluoxetine. Their use is probably safe because there are no reported adverse effects.

Maternal medications usually compatible with breastfeeding include the following: acetaminophen; barbiturates (which may cause infant sedation); caffeine (which may cause irritability or

Table 11-5. Drug therapy in lactating women: questions and options

1. Is the drug therapy really necessary? Consultation between the pediatrician and the mother's physician can be most useful.
2. Use the safest drug—for example, acetaminophen rather than aspirin for analgesia.
3. If there is a possibility that a drug may prevent a risk to the infant, consideration should be given to measurement of blood concentrations in the nursing infant.
4. Drug exposure to the nursing infant may be minimized by having the mother take the medication just after she has breastfed the infant and/or just before the infant is due to have a lengthy sleep period.

From The American Academy of Pediatrics Committee on Drugs. The transfer of drugs and other chemicals into human milk. *Pediatrics* 1994;93:137–150.

poor sleeping pattern if the mother uses a lot of it); NSAIDs, such as ibuprofen and naproxen; beta-blockers, such as propranolol and nadolol; narcotics, including codeine, morphine, and butorphanol; valproic acid; and verapamil. Triptans (not listed in the report) should be used with caution.

Preeclampsia and Eclampsia (34)

Epidemiology

Preeclampsia occurs in up to 7% of pregnancies, and eclampsia is found in up to 0.3%. The criteria for preeclampsia include the following: proteinuria of more than 300 mg/day or two spot urines with more than 1 g protein/liter collected more than 6 hours apart; edema; hypertension persistently greater than 140/90 or relative hypertension with a rise over a first-trimester baseline blood pressure of at least 30 mm Hg systolic or 15 mm Hg diastolic; and onset after the 20th week of gestation up until 48 hours postpartum. Eclampsia occurs with the additional complications of seizures or coma. As many as 45% of cases of eclampsia have an onset postpartum, with a mean of 6 days and up to 4 weeks.

Risk factors for preeclampsia in primigravida are prepregnancy hypertension, obesity, multiple abortions or miscarriages, and cigarette smoking. The incidence of pregnancy-induced hypertension is greater in first or multiple pregnancies and in younger and older women. Black women have twice the incidence of whites.

Clinical Manifestations

Nonneurological complications include the following: renal dysfunction with oliguria, casts, and elevated serum uric acid, urea, and creatinine; pulmonary edema; vomiting and epigastric pain; subcapsular hepatic hemorrhage; and hemolysis, elevated liver enzymes, and low platelets (HELLP syndrome), which can be further complicated by disseminated intravascular coagulation (DIC) in up to 40% of patients.

Neurological complications consist of the following: headaches that are typically bilateral; dizziness; tinnitus; altered consciousness or coma; seizures; and visual disturbances, including diplopia, scotomas, blurring, and blindness. Blindness, which can occur in up to 15% of eclamptics, may be due to retinal hemorrhages, edema, or detachment or occipital ischemia.

Subarachnoid Hemorrhage

Nontraumatic subarachnoid hemorrhage (SAH) during pregnancy has an incidence of about 20 per 100,000 deliveries. This is the third most common cause of nonobstetrical mortality, accounting for 5% to 10% of all maternal deaths. This risk is five times higher than that outside pregnancy. SAH is due to ruptured saccular aneurysms and arteriovenous malformations with equal frequency. Up to 20% of aneurysmal ruptures occur during pregnancy or in the early postpartum period. The risk of aneurysmal SAH is highest during the late third trimester, during delivery, and in the puerperium (35). The most common time for hemorrhage from an arteriovenous malformation (AVM) is between 16 and 20 weeks' gestation or during parturition. About 25% of pregnant women who have already bled from an AVM will rebleed during the same pregnancy. Chapter 8 reviews the clinical manifestations of SAH.

Other causes of intracranial hemorrhage during pregnancy and the puerperium include eclampsia, cerebral venous thrombosis, choriocarcinoma, bacterial endocarditis, drug abuse, DIC, moyamoya disease, hematological disorders, tumor, ruptured spinal cord vascular malformations, and arterial hypertension.

Stroke and Cerebral Venous Thrombosis (36)

The risk of ischemic stroke is 13 times higher during pregnancy and the puerperium than expected outside of pregnancy. Either ischemic or hemorrhagic stroke occurs in up to 19 in 100,000 deliveries. Arterial occlusions account for 60% to 80% of these strokes. The headaches associated with stroke are described in Chapter 13.

The numerous causes of arterial ischemic strokes include cardioembolic disorders (rheumatic heart disease, prosthetic heart valves, atrial fibrillation, bacterial and nonbacterial endocarditis, peripartum cardiomyopathy, mitral valve prolapse, and paradoxical embolus); cerebral angiopathies (atherosclerosis; arterial dissection; fibromuscular dysplasia; cerebral vasculitis, such as systemic lupus erythematosus, Takayasu's disease, periarteritis nodosa, and isolated angiitis of the brain; and postpartum cerebral angiopathy); hematological disorders (sickle-cell anemia; Sneddon's syndrome; antiphospholipid antibodies; thrombotic thrombocytopenic purpura; homocystinuria; deficiency of antithrombin II, protein C, and protein S; and DIC); and other causes (eclampsia, choriocarcinoma, amniotic fluid embolism, air embolism, fat embolism, drug abuse, and Sheehan's syndrome).

The only three pregnancy-specific disorders are eclampsia, choriocarcinoma, and amniotic fluid embolism. Postpartum cerebral angiopathy and peripartum cardiomyopathy have also been reported apart from pregnancy.

Pregnancy and the puerperium are associated with an increased risk of cerebral venous thrombosis (Chapter 13). Ninety percent of cases occur during the puerperium, most commonly in the second or third weeks postpartum.

Sheehan's syndrome is the spontaneous ischemic necrosis of the pituitary gland in the postpartum period, resulting in hypopituitarism. Most cases are due to hypotension and shock from acute blood loss, resulting in ischemia of a hypertrophied pituitary gland of pregnancy. About 1% to 2% of women who have a significant postpartum hemorrhage will have this syndrome. In contrast to pituitary apoplexy (Chapter 14), headaches and cranial nerve abnormalities are not usually associated.

Pseudotumor Cerebri

Although pregnancy is not a risk factor, pseudotumor cerebri can develop or worsen during pregnancy. Visual outcome is the same for pregnant and nonpregnant patients (37). Subsequent pregnancy does not increase the risk of recurrent pseudotumor cerebri. This disorder is discussed further in Chapter 14.

Brain Tumors

Pregnancy does not increase the risk of developing a primary brain tumor. Meningiomas may increase in size during pregnancy and then regress postpartum. Twenty-five percent of macroprolactinomas expand enough to cause problems during pregnancy.

Choriocarcinoma is due to malignant transformation of the trophoblast. Although choriocarcinomas usually follow a molar pregnancy, they can also follow term delivery, abortion, and ectopic pregnancy. Brain metastases occur in 20% of cases.

Trophoblasts can invade blood vessels and result in thrombosis and cerebral infarctions. Neoplastic aneurysms and cerebral hemorrhage can also occur.

Infections

Pregnancy is a state of relative immunosuppression. Coccidiomycosis, tuberculosis, listeriosis, and malaria have an increased risk of spread to the central nervous system when acquired during pregnancy. Headache can certainly be a presenting or prominent symptom.

REFERENCES

1. Silberstein SD, Lipton RB, Goadsby PJ. Epidemiology and impact of headache disorders. In: *Headache in clinical practice.* London: Martin Dunitz, 2002.
2. Silberstein SD. Hormone-related headache. *Med Clin North Am* 2001;85(4):1017–1035.
3. Headache Classification Subcommittee of the International Headache Society. The international classification of headache disorders, 2nd ed. *Cephalalgia* 2004;24 (Suppl 1):59:1–160.
4. Mannix LK. Management of menstrual migraine. *Neurology* 2003;9(4):207–213.
5. Loder E. Menstrual migraine: timing is everything. *Neurology* 2004;63(2):202–203.
6. Nattero G, Allais G, De Lorenzo C, et al. Biological and clinical effects of naproxen sodium in patients with menstrual migraine. *Cephalalgia* 1991;11[Suppl 11]:201–202.
7. Herzog AG. Continuous bromocriptine therapy in menstrual migraine. *Neurology* 1997;48:101–102.
8. O'Dea JP, Davis EH. Tamoxifen in the treatment of menstrual migraine. *Neurology* 1990;40:1470–1471.
9. Facchinetti F, Sances G, Borella P, et al. Magnesium prophylaxis of menstrual migraine: effects on intracellular magnesium. *Headache* 1991;31:298–301.
10. MacGregor EA. Is HRT giving you a headache? *Br Migraine Assoc Newsletter* 1993;7:19–24.
11. Fettes I. Migraine in the menopause. *Neurology* 1999;53 (4 Suppl I):S29–S33.
12. Becker WJ. Migraine and oral contraceptives. *Can J Neurol Sci* 1997;24:16–21.
13. Tzourio C, Tehindrazanarivelo A, Iglesias S, et al. Case-control study of migraine and risk of ischaemic stroke in young women. *BMJ* 1995;310:830–833.
14. Welch KMA. Stroke and migraine—the spectrum of cause and effect. *Funct Neurol* 2003;18(3):121–126.

15. Zeitouh K, Carr PR. Is there an increased risk of stroke associated with oral contraceptives? *Drug SAF* 1999;20:467–473.
16. Petitti DB, Sidney S, Berstein A, et al. Stroke in users of low-dose oral contraceptives. *N Engl J Med* 1996;335:8–15.
17. Schwartz SM, Siscovick DS, Longstreth WT, et al. Use of low-dose oral contraceptives and stroke in young women. *Ann Intern Med* 1997;127(8,Pt 1):596–603.
18. Hannaford PC, Kay CR. The risk of serious illness among oral contraceptive users: evidence from the RCGP's oral contraceptive study. *Br J Gen Pract* 1998;48:1657–1662.
19. Siritho S, Thrift AG, McNeil JJ, et al. Risk of ischemic stroke among users of the oral contraceptive pill: the Melbourne risk factor study (MERFS) group. *Stroke* 2003;34:1575–1580.
20. Lidegaard O. Oral contraception and risk of a cerebral thromboembolic attack: results of a case-control study. *BMJ* 1993;306:956–963.
21. Silberstein SD, Lipton RB, Goadsby PJ. Pregnancy, breast feeding and headache. In: *Headache in clinical practice.* London: Martin Dunitz, 2002.
22. Bousser MG, Ratinahirana H, Darbois X. Migraine and pregnancy: a prospective study in 703 women after delivery. *Neurology* 1990;40:437.
23. Maggioni F, Alessi C, Maggino T, et al. Headache during pregnancy. *Cephalalgia* 1997;17:765–769.
24. Stein GS. Headache in the first postpartum week and their relationship to migraine. *Headache* 1981;21:201–205.
25. Granella F, Sances G, Zanferrari C, et al. Migraine without aura and reproductive life events: a clinical epidemiological study in 1300 women. *Headache* 1993:33:385.
26. Hainline B. Headache. *Neurol Clin* 1994;12:443–459.
27. Silberstein SD. Migraine and pregnancy. *Neurol Clin* 1997; 15:209–231.
28. Pfaffenrath V, Rehm M. Migraine in pregnancy: what are the safest treatment options? *Drug Safety* 1998;19:383–388.
29. Gilmore J, Pennell PB, Stern BJ. Medication use during pregnancy for neurologic conditions. *Neurol Clin* 1998;16:189–206.
30. Aube M. Migraine in pregnancy. *Neurology* 1999;53(4 Suppl I): S26–34.
31. Loder E. Safety of sumatriptan in pregnancy: a review of the data so far. *CNS Drugs* 2003;17(1):1–7.
32. Nonacs R, Cohen LS. Assessment and treatment of depression during pregnancy: an update. *Psychiatr Clin North Am* 2003; 26(3):547–562.
33. Committee on Drugs. The transfer of drugs and other chemicals into human milk. *Pediatrics* 1994;93:137–150.
34. Pleasure JR. Neurologic problems in pregnancy. In: Rosenberg RN, Pleasure DE, eds. *Comprehensive neurology,* 2nd ed. New York: John Wiley, 1998:825–847.
35. Stoodley MA, Macdonald L, Weir BKA. Pregnancy and intracranial aneurysm. *Neurosurg Clin N Am* 1998;9:549–556.
36. Sloan MA, Stern BJ. Cerebrovascular disease in pregnancy. *Curr Treat Options Neurol* 2003;5:391–407.
37. Huna-Baron R, Kupersmith MJ. Idiopathic intracranial hypertension in pregnancy. *J Neurol* 2002;249(8):1078–1081.

Headaches Over the Age of 50

Randolph W. Evans

The prevalence of headache decreases with older age (Table 12-1) (1). Although 90% of headaches in younger patients are of the primary type, only 66% of those in the elderly are primary (2).

There are numerous causes of new-onset headaches in those over 50 years of age (Table 12-2) (3). Although new-onset tension-type headaches are fairly common, migraine and cluster-type headaches uncommonly begin after 50 years of age. Temporal arteritis, hypnic headache, and headache of Parkinson's disease are secondary headaches occurring with much greater frequency in this population.

Causes of secondary headache disorders with onset or more common in later life include the following: neoplasms; subdural and epidural hematomas; head trauma; cerebrovascular disease; temporal arteritis; trigeminal neuralgia; postherpetic neuralgia; medication-related headache, including those caused by specific medications and medication rebound; systemic disease, such as infections, acute hypertension, hypoxia, or hypercarbia; and other metabolic disorders, such as hypercalcemia, severe anemia, hyponatremia, and chronic renal failure; diseases of the cranium, neck, eyes, ears, and nose, including cervicogenic headache, glaucoma, otitis, sinusitis, and dental infections; Parkinson's disease; and angina (also see Chapter 13), which may rarely present with exertional headache without chest pain.

In a study of 193 patients 65 years of age and over seen by a neurology service with new-onset headaches, the most frequent diagnoses were tension type (43%) and trigeminal neuralgia (19%) (4). Only one patient met migraine criteria. Fifteen percent had secondary headaches due to conditions such as stroke, temporal arteritis, or intracranial neoplasm. The risk of serious disorders causing headache increased 10 times after age 65, compared with younger patients.

This chapter reviews the primary headaches and some of the secondary headaches, including temporal arteritis, postherpetic neuralgia, and Parkinson's disease. The other secondary headaches are covered in Chapters 5 (medication related), 9 (subdural and epidural hematomas), and 13–15.

PRIMARY HEADACHES

Migraine

Only 2% of migraineurs have the new onset after 50 years of age. Migraine prevalence decreases with older age. The prevalence is about 5% in women and 2% in men past 70 years of age. When migraine criteria are met, computed tomography (CT) or magnetic resonance imaging (MRI) scans have a very low yield in this population (5).

Medication use presents a variety of problems in older patients. Ergotamine, dihydroergotamine (DHE), and triptans should not

Table 12-1. Prevalence of headaches at various ages

Age	Women	Men
21–34	92%	74%
55–74	66%	53%
75+	55%	22%

Table 12-2. New-onset headaches occurring over 50 years of age

Primary headaches
  Migraine
  Tension
  Cluster
  Hypnic
Secondary headaches
  Neoplasms
  Subdural and epidural hematomas
  Head trauma
  Cerebrovascular disease
  Temporal arteritis
  Trigeminal neuralgia
  Postherpetic neuralgia
  Mediation related
  Systemic disease
  Diseases of the cranium, neck, eyes, ears, and nose
  Parkinson's disease
  Exertional headache due to angina

be used in patients with coronary artery disease, cerebrovascular disease, or peripheral vascular disease. Some patients without such a history may require screening, especially if they have risk factors such as diabetes, a positive family history, smoking, or hyperlipidemia. Older patients may be more sensitive to anticholinergic, hypotensive, sedative, cognitive, and cardiac side effects of preventive medications. For example, patients with prostatism, glaucoma, or cardiac arrhythmias may need to avoid tricyclic antidepressants, whereas those with congestive heart failure, diabetes, or bronchial asthma may need to avoid beta-blockers. Drugs used for other indications, such as estrogen replacement therapy or nitrates, may trigger migraines. A variety of other medications can cause headaches, including nifedipine, phosphodiesterase inhibitors for erectile dysfunction, and nonsteroidal antiinflammatory drugs (NSAIDs) (also see Chapter 3).

Late-Life Migrainous Accompaniments

Fisher described late-life migrainous accompaniments (6,7), which are transient visual, sensory, motor, or behavioral neurological manifestations that are similar or identical to the auras of migraine with aura (8). Headache is associated with only 50%

Table 12-3.   Late-life migrainous accompaniments

1. Gradual appearance of focal neurological symptoms with spread or worsening over a period of minutes.
2. Headache is only present in 50% of cases and may be mild.
3. Positive visual symptoms such as scintillating scotoma, flashing or bright lights.
4. A history of similar episodes associated with a more severe headache.
5. Serial progression from one accompaniment to another (e.g., from flashing lights to paresthesias, paresis, or dysphasia).
6. Diagnosis facilitated with the occurrence of two or more identical episodes.
7. A duration of 15 to 25 minutes.
8. A characteristic "flurry" of accompaniments.
9. A usually benign natural history, without permanent sequelae.
10. Another cause not shown by diagnostic testing that is performed when indicated.

of cases and may be mild. These accompaniments occur more often in men than in women with a prevalence of about 1%.

Table 12-3 provides the features of this disorder. The complaints occur as follows, from most to least common: visual symptoms (transient blindness, homonymous hemianopsia, and blurring of vision); paresthesias (numbness, tingling, pins-and-needles sensation, or a heavy feeling of an extremity); brain stem and cerebellar dysfunction (ataxia, clumsiness, hearing loss, tinnitus, vertigo, and syncope); and disturbances of speech (dysarthria or dysphasia).

Other causes of transient cerebral ischemia should be considered, especially when the patient is seen after the first episode or if there are unusual aspects. The usual diagnostic evaluation for transient ischemic attacks (TIAs) or seizures (such as CT scan, MRI and magnetic resonance angiography of the brain, carotid ultrasound, electroencephalography, cardiac evaluation, and blood studies) is performed.

The following features help distinguish migraine from TIAs: a gradual buildup of sensory symptoms, a march of sensory paresthesias, serial progression from one accompaniment to another, longer duration (90% of TIAs last for less than 15 minutes), and multiple stereotypical episodes.

If the episodes are frequent, preventive treatment can be considered with medications such as topiramate, divalproex sodium, and verapamil. Beta-blockers should be avoided because of the potential for worsening vasospasm. For acute treatment, ergotamine, DHE, and triptans should be avoided because of the risk of increasing cerebral vasospasm.

Tension-Type Headaches

About 10% of those with tension-type headaches have an onset after 50 years of age. When new-onset tension-type headaches occur, the diagnosis is one of exclusion. Over the age of 65 years, the prevalence of tension-type headaches is about 27%. The patient and physician should be aware of the potential for medication-overuse headaches.

Medications for tension-type headaches are the same as those for younger people. It is often prudent to start with lower doses and to be cautious about an increased susceptibility to side effects in the elderly. Physical therapy can be helpful for cervicogenic headache.

Chronic Daily Headache

About 4% of the population age 65 years or older has chronic daily headache with a higher prevalence in women than in men. Medication overuse is a concern as a cause of rebound headache just as in younger patients.

Cluster Headaches

Cluster headaches are a rare disorder with a 5:1 male-to-female preponderance. Although the age of onset is typically between the ages of 20 and 50 years, onset can occur in the 70s.

Hypnic Headache

Hypnic headache is a rare disorder originally described by Raskin in 1988 (9), which has since been reported in men and women from the ages of 36 to 83 years. The headache only occurs during sleep when the sufferer is awakened at a consistent time. Nausea is infrequent and autonomic symptoms are rarely associated. The headache can be unilateral or bilateral, throbbing or nonthrobbing, and mild to severe in intensity. The headache can last 15 minutes to 6 hours and can occur frequently, as often as nightly, for many years. Medications that may be effective include caffeine (1 or 2 cups of caffeinated coffee or a 40- to 60-mg caffeine tablet before bedtime), lithium carbonate (300 mg at bedtime), indomethacin, atenolol, cyclobenzaprine, melatonin (6 mg at bedtime), and flunarizine (not available in the United States) (10,11).

The diagnosis is one of exclusion because secondary causes of nocturnal headaches include drug withdrawal, temporal arteritis, noctural headache-hypertension syndrome, sleep apnea, oxygen desaturation, pheochromocytomas, primary and secondary neoplasms, communicating hydrocephalus, subdural hematomas, and vascular lesions (12).

Migraine, cluster, and chronic paroxysmal hemicrania are other primary headaches that can cause awakening from sleep. Migraine typically has associated symptoms and occurs very uncommonly only during sleep. Cluster headaches have autonomic symptoms and may occur during the day as well as during sleep. Chronic paroxysmal hemicrania occurs both during the day and at night, lasts for less than 30 minutes, and occurs 10 to 30 times a day.

SECONDARY HEADACHES

Temporal Arteritis

Epidemiology

Temporal (giant cell) arteritis (TA) is a systemic panarteritis that selectively involves arterial walls with significant amounts of elastin. Approximately 50% of patients with TA have polymyalgia rheumatica, and about 15% of patients with polymyalgia rheumatica have TA. Both conditions occur almost exclusively in patients over the age of 50, with a mean age of onset of about 70. The ratio of women to men is 3:1. The disorder is more common in Scandinavia and the northern United States, and it is more common in whites than in other ethnic groups. The annual incidence is about 18 in 100,000 over 50 years of age.

Clinical Manifestations (13,14)

Headaches are the most common symptom reported by 60% to 90% of patients. The pain is most often throbbing, although many patients describe a sharp, dull, burning, or lancinating type of pain. The pain may be intermittent or continuous and is more often severe than moderate or slight. For some patients, the pain may be worse at night when lying on a pillow, while combing the hair, or when washing the face. Tenderness or decreased pulsation of the superficial temporal arteries is present on physical examination in about half of the patients with TA.

The location of the headache is variable. In one series, 65% of patients presented with temporofrontal headache (15). In another series, the following percentages of patients reported the distribution of pain in these categories: 25%, only the temple; 54%, the temple, either exclusively or inclusively; 29%, not involving the temple at all; and 8%, generalized (16). When headaches were limited to or included the temple, the headaches were bilateral in 50% of the patients. Intermittent jaw claudication was reported by 38%. Other studies have reported one-sided pain in 2%; 8% reported pain affecting the face or neck.

Temporal arteritis can present as occipital neuralgia. In a study of 46 patients with biopsy-proven TA, 17% of the patients had an initial presentation with occipital pain, which was unilateral in 38% (17). Two of the patients with unilateral pain exactly similar to greater occipital neuralgia had normal sedimentation rates but abnormal superficial temporal artery biopsies. Tenderness over the greater occipital nerve can be explained by inflammation of the occipital artery, which is adjacent to the greater occipital nerve in the suboccipital region. TA should be considered in patients over 50 years of age who present with new-onset "occipital neuralgia," even with normal sedimentation rates, especially when they do not respond to the usual treatments.

Neurological manifestations of TA are common. One series found evidence of neurological disease in 31% of the patients, including ophthalmological findings, 20%; mononeuropathies and peripheral neuropathies, 14%; carotid distribution transient ischemic events or stroke, 7%; vertebrobasilar distribution transient ischemic events or stroke, 2%; otological findings, 7%; tremor, 4%; psychiatric findings, 3%; tongue numbness, 2%; and transverse myelopathy, less than 1% (18). Depression and confusion can be associated with temporal arteritis.

There is a broad spectrum of neuroophthalmological manifestations of TA (19). Visual loss may occur because of anterior and posterior ischemic optic neuropathy; central and branch retinal artery occlusion; anterior segment ischemia; and prechiasmal, perichiasmal, and postchiasmal field defects. Ophthalmoparesis

Table 12-4.   Criteria for the diagnosis of TA of the American College of Rheumatology

Three out of the following five criteria should be satisfied:
1. Age at least 50 years
2. New onset of localized headache
3. Temporal artery tenderness or decreased pulse
4. Erythrocyte sedimentation rate of at least 50 mm/h
5. Positive histology

can be due to the following: oculomotor, abducens, and trochlear nerve palsies; orbital constriction resulting from orbital cellulitis and cavernous sinus thrombosis; and oculomotor synkinesis. Autonomic dysfunction may be caused by Horner's syndrome and parasympathetic pupillary light dysfunction/near dissociation. Rarely, complex visual hallucinations occur after infarction of the tertiary visual association cortex.

Diagnostic Evaluation

According to the American College of Rheumatology 1990 criteria, the diagnosis of TA can be established by fulfilling three out of five criteria (Table 12-4) (20). The presence of three or more of the five criteria is associated with a sensitivity of 93.5% and a specificity of 91.2%.

The diagnosis is based on clinical suspicion that is usually but not always confirmed by laboratory testing (21,22). The three best tests are the Westergren erythrocyte sedimentation rate (ESR), the C-reactive protein (CRP), and temporal artery biopsy. Elevation of plasma viscosity has a sensitivity and specificity similar to that of the ESR. Mild normochromic normocytic anemia, elevation of liver enzymes (especially alkaline phosphatase), and decreased alpha$_2$-globulin levels are fairly common.

Color duplex ultrasonography of the superficial temporal arteries may show a dark halo around the lumen of the superficial temporal arteries due to edema of the artery wall (23). However, the ultrasound may only modestly improve the probability of biopsy-proven TA and not improve the diagnostic accuracy of a careful physical examination (24).

For elderly patients, the ESR range of normal may vary from less than 20 mm/hour to 40 mm/hour. A formula for the upper limits of normal for the ESR that includes 98% of healthy people is as follows: age in years divided by 2 for men and age in years plus 10 divided by 2 for women (25). Elevation of the ESR is not specific for TA. Elevation can be seen in any infectious, inflammatory, or rheumatic disease. The level can even be affected by the length of time between the venipuncture and the laboratory testing (26). TA with a normal ESR has been reported in 10% to 36% of patients. Repeating the ESR may be helpful in some cases in which the ESR is initially normal and then rises. When abnormal, the ESR averages 70 to 80 and may reach 120 or even 130 mm/hour. When the ESR is elevated at the time of diagnosis, it can be followed to help guide the dosage of corticosteroid medication.

CRP is an acute-phase plasma protein from the liver. As with the ESR, elevation is nonspecific and can be seen with numerous disorders. The CRP is not influenced by various hematological factors or age and is more sensitive than the ESR for the detection of TA. The ESR and CRP combined give the best specificity, 97%. Levels of interleukin-6 are also a sensitive indicator of active disease.

The diagnosis is made with certainty when the superficial temporal artery biopsy demonstrates necrotizing arteritis characterized by a predominance of mononuclear cell infiltrates or a granulomatous process with multinucleated giant cells. The false-negative rate of temporal artery biopsies in various series ranges from 5% to 44%. Biopsy-negative cases may have a more benign course than biopsy-positive cases (27).

Possible reasons for negative temporal artery biopsies include noncontinuous pathological findings or skip lesions, choice of site and length of the biopsy, examination of an incomplete number of sections, involvement of other vascular territories, and initiation of corticosteroid therapy prior to the biopsy. When the biopsy is negative, a biopsy of the contralateral superficial temporal artery increases the positive yield by 5% to 15%. Pathological evidence of TA persists for at least 4 to 5 days after the start of corticosteroid treatment.

Because temporal artery biopsy is a simple, low-risk procedure, a case can be made for obtaining a biopsy in every suspected patient. However, when three or four of the American College of Rheumatology criteria are met (Table 12-4), a strong argument can be made for treatment without biopsy. The result of the CRP and/or color duplex ultrasonography may also influence the decision.

In patients in which the clinical presentation is somewhat suspicious or when there is a very high probability of corticosteroid side effects (e.g., a type I diabetic), a biopsy should be obtained. In the occasional patient with a normal or only slightly elevated ESR and a negative biopsy, the same consideration may apply in a decision to biopsy the contralateral artery.

Management

When contraindications are not present, treatment is typically started with prednisone at a dosage of 40 to 80 mg/day or 1 mg/kg/day (28,29). The headache will often improve within 24 hours. The initial dose is maintained for about 4 weeks and then slowly reduced over many months by a maximum of 10% to 20% of the total daily dose each week or every 2 weeks, depending on the clinical effect, the ESR, and occurrence of side effects. Because TA is active for at least 1 year and an average of 3 to 4 years in some series, long-term treatment is usually required. About 30% to 50% of patients have an exacerbation, especially during the first 2 years of treatment, independent of the corticosteroid regimen. There are numerous complications of long-term steroid treatment. Calcium and vitamin D supplementation should be given along with corticosteroids to help prevent osteoporosis. In patients with reduced bone mineral density, bisphosponates are also indicated. Adjunctive use of methotrexate with corticosteroids is not beneficial to control disease activity or to decrease the cumulative dose and toxicity of corticosteroids (30). Infliximab (antitumor necrosis factor onoclonal antibody) might be effective in patients unresponsive to or intolerant of corticosteroids.

Postherpetic Neuralgia (31,32)

Epidemiology

Acute herpes zoster occurs when the dormant varicella zoster virus (from a previous chickenpox infection) is reactivated in the trigeminal, geniculate, or dorsal root ganglion. The annual incidence of acute herpes zoster is approximately 400 in 100,000. The incidence dramatically increases with older age. According to various studies, the incidence ranges from 40 to 160 in 100,000 for those under 20 years of age to 450 to 1,100 in 100,000 for those 80 years of age or older. There are more than a million cases per year in the United States, most in the elderly. The lifetime risk of developing acute herpes zoster for those who live into their 70s and 80s is as high as 40%. The lifetime risk of a second or third attack in healthy people is about 5%.

Postherpetic neuralgia (PHN) is the most common neurological complication of varicella zoster infection and occurs in about 10% to 15% of those with acute zoster. PHN develops in some 50% of those older than 50 years of age and in 80% of those older than 80. Up to 200,000 people in the United States have PHN, which can persist for years. Zoster involving the face nearly doubles the risk of developing PHN, which lasts longer than PHN in other locations.

Clinical Manifestations

Radicular pain is the most common complication of zoster and may precede the eruption of grouped vesicles (shingles) by days to weeks. Zoster occurs in a trigeminal distribution, usually in the ophthalmic division, in 23% of cases. Uncommonly, an extraocular muscle paresis may be associated as a result of involvement of the third, fourth, or sixth cranial nerves. Reactivation of virus in the geniculate ganglion can result in vesicles in the external auditory canal and a facial palsy known by the eponym of Ramsay-Hunt syndrome. Occasionally, pain occurs without a rash (zoster sine herpete). The pain is usually sharp or stabbing. Typically, the vesicles crust, the skin heals, and the pain resolves within 3 to 4 weeks of the onset of the rash. However, in many people the pain can persist.

Postherpetic neuralgia is the persistence of pain after the initial rash for more than 1 to 6 months. (There are different opinions about the definition in the literature.) The involvement of the head is typically unilateral in the distribution of the ophthalmic or maxillary divisions of the trigeminal nerve or at the occipitocervical junction. Three types of pain may be present: a constant burning or deep aching; an intermittent spontaneous pain with a jabbing or lancinating quality; and a superficial, sharp, or radiating pain or itching provoked by light touch (allodynia). The types of pains vary from person to person. Allodynia is present in 90% of individuals with PHN. The pain often interferes with sleep.

Management

For the treatment of acute zoster, oral corticosteroids (prednisone starting at 60 mg/day and tapering off over 2 weeks) may reduce acute pain but may not reduce the risk of PHN. Corticosteroids should be used in combination with antiviral medication. Use of oral acyclovir (800 mg every 4 hours, 5 times daily, for 7 to 10 days) may decrease the acute pain but only modestly decreases the risk of PHN. Famciclovir (33) (500 mg every 8 hours for 1 week) and valacyclovir (1 g every 8 hours for 1 week) are more effective in reducing the incidence and duration of PHN. (The doses of both drugs are reduced in renal insufficiency.) The earlier antiviral therapy is initiated the greater the likelihood of response because in the clinical trials, antivirals were started within 72 hours of the onset of skin lesions. Although nerve blocks are a highly effective treatment for acute pain, it is uncertain if this approach will reduce the risk of PHN.

A variety of treatments are available for PHN with varying efficacies (34). Tricyclic antidepressants, including amitriptyline, nortriptyline, and desipramine, are effective treatments. Start with a low dose and then slowly increase to an optimal dose with the most pain relief and tolerable side effects. Up to 61% of patients may have pain relief with tolerable side effects. For those who can not tolerate tricyclics, venlafaxine may be more tolerable and may also be effective. Some patients may benefit from the addition of a phenothiazine medication such as fluphenazine. Gabapentin (35) and pregabalin are also effective in the treatment of pain and sleep interference associated with PHN. Anecdotally, other antidepressants such as fluoxetine may also be effective. Keppra may also be effective.

Topical agents, including capsaicin, lidocaine 5%, aspirin, and NSAIDs, may be useful. The 0.075% capsaicin cream may be more effective than lower concentrations. Some patients may have burning pain on application of the cream, which limits use.

Opioids such as sustained-release oxycodone (10 mg every 12 hours, slowly increasing as necessary to 30 mg every 12 hours) (36) and oral levorphanol may be effective when other drugs fail or cannot be tolerated. Transcutaneous electrical nerve stimulation (TENS), with the electrodes placed above and below the involved area, may help about one third of patients. Because efficacy has not been demonstrated in properly designed studies, neural destructive treatments such as neurolytic nerve blocks, nerve sectioning, and dorsal root entry zone lesions are not recommended.

Cervicogenic Headache

Cervical spondylosis and muscle spasm may cause headache in older patients. The headache may be unilateral or bilateral. Digital pressure in the suboccipital area may reproduce the headache. The headache may be due to occipital neuralgia, myofascial pain with trigger points, or referred from neck structures such as the upper cervical facets (Chapter 9). Beneficial treatments include NSAIDs, muscle relaxants, tricyclic antidepressants, and physical therapy. Occipital nerve blocks and trigger point injections may be helpful in appropriate cases.

Parkinson's Disease

Headache associated with muscle rigidity may occur more often in Parkinson's disease. Tricyclic medications such as amitriptyline or nortriptyline may be effective. Amantidine and L-Dopa, drugs for the treatment of Parkinson's, can cause headaches in some people.

REFERENCES

1. Waters WE. The Pontypridd headache survey. *Headache* 1974; 14:81–90.
2. Solomon GD, Kunkel RS, Frame J. Demographics of headache in elderly patients. *Headache* 1990;30:273–276.
3. Silberstein SD, Lipton RB, Goadsby PJ. Geriatric headache. In: *Headache in clinical practice*, 2nd ed. London: Martin Dunitz, 2002:269–283.
4. Pascual J, Berciano J. Experience in the diagnosis of headaches that start in elderly people. *J Neurol Neurosurg Psychiatry* 1994;57:1255–1257.
5. Cull RE. Investigation of late-onset migraine. *Scott Med J* 1995;40:50–52.
6. Fisher CM. Late-life migraine accompaniments as a cause of unexplained transient ischemic attacks. *Can J Neurol Sci* 1980; 7:9–17.
7. Fisher CM. Late-life migraine accompaniments: further experience. *Stroke* 1986;17:1033–1042.
8. Purdy RA. Late-life migrainous accompaniments. In: Gilman S, ed. *MedLink neurology*. San Diego: Arbor, 2004. Available at www.medlink.com.
9. Raskin NH. The hypnic headache syndrome. *Headache* 1988; 28:534–536.
10. Dodick DW, Mosek A, Campbell JK. The hypnic ("alarm clock") headache syndrome. *Cephalalgia* 1998;18:152–156.
11. Evers S, Goadsby PJ. Hypnic headache: clinical features, pathophysiology, and treatment. *Neurology* 2003 25;60(6):905–909.
12. Gould JD, Silberstein SD. Unilateral hypnic headache: a case study. *Neurology* 1997;49:1749–1750.
13. Myklebust G, Gran JT. A prospective study of 287 patients with polymyalgia rheumatica and temporal arteritis: clinical and laboratory manifestations at onset of disease and at the time of diagnosis. *Br J Rheumatol* 1996;35:1161–1168.
14. Wyand CM, Goronzy JJ. Giant-cell arteritis and polymyalgia rheumatica. *Ann Intern Med* 2003;16;139(6):505–515.
15. Jonasson F, Cullen JF, Elton RA. Temporal arteritis: a 14-year epidemiological, clinical and prognostic study. *Scot Med J* 1979;24:111–117.
16. Solomon S, Cappa KG. The headache of temporal arteritis. *J Am Geriatr Soc* 1987;35:163–165.
17. Jundt JW, Mock D. Temporal arteritis with normal erythrocyte sedimentation rates presenting as occipital neuralgia. *Arthritis Rheum* 1991;34:217–219.
18. Caselli RJ, Hunder GG, Whisnant JP. Neurologic disease in biopsy-proven giant cell (temporal) arteritis. *Neurology* 1988;38:352–358.
19. Mehler MR, Rabinowich L. The clinical neuro-ophthalmologic spectrum of temporal arteritis. *Am J Med* 1988;85:839–844.

20. Hunder GG, Bloch DA, Beat AM, et al. The American College of Rheumatology 1990 criteria for the classification of giant cell arteritis. *Arthritis Rheum* 1990;33:1122–1128.

21. Lee AG, Brazis PW. Temporal arteritis: a clinical approach. *J Am Geriatr Soc* 1999;47:1364–1370.

22. Smetana GW, Shmerling RH. Does this patient have temporal arteritis? *JAMA* 2002;287:92–101.

23. Schmidt WA, Kraft HE, Voker L, et al. Color duplex ultrasonography in the diagnosis of temporal arteritis. *N Engl J Med* 1997;337:1336–1342.

24. Salvarani C, Silingardi M, Ghirarduzzi A, et al. Is duplex ultrasonography useful for the diagnosis of giant-cell arteritis? *Ann Intern Med* 2002;137(4):232–238.

25. Miller A, Green M, Robinson D. Simple rule for calculating normal erythrocyte sedimentation rate. *BMJ* 1983;286:266.

26. Hayreh SS, Podhajsky PA, Raman R, et al. Giant cell arteritis: validity and reliability of various diagnostic criteria. *Am J Ophthalmol* 1997;123:285–296.

27. Duhant P, Pinede I, Bornet H, at al. Biopsy proven and biopsy negative temporal arteritis: differences in clinical spectrum at the onset of the disease. *Ann Rheum Dis* 1999;58:335–341.

28. Nesher G, Rubinow A, Sonnenblick M. Efficacy and adverse effects of different corticosteroid dose regimens in temporal arteritis: a retrospective study. *Clin Exp Rheumatol* 1997;15:303–306.

29. Salvarani C, Cantini F, Boiardi L, et al. Polymyalgia rheumatica and giant-cell arteritis. *N Engl J Med* 2002;347(4):261–271.

30. Hoffman GS, Cid MC, Hellmann DB, et al. A multicenter, randomized, double-blind, placebo-controlled trial of adjuvant methotrexate treatment for giant cell arteritis. *Arthritis Rheum* 2002;46(5):1309–1318.

31. Gnann JW Jr, Whitley RJ. Herpes zoster. *N Engl J Med* 2002;347:340–346.

32. Cluff RS, Rowbotham MC. Pain caused by herpes zoster infection. *Neurol Clin* 1998;16:813–832.

33. Dworkin RH, Boon RJ, Griffin DR, et al. Postherpetic neuralgia: impact of famciclovir, age, rash severity, and acute pain in herpes zoster patients. *J Infect Dis* 1998;178[Suppl 1]:S76–S80.

34. Pappagallo M, Haldey EJ. Pharmacological management of postherpetic neuralgia. *CNS Drugs* 2003;17(11):771–780.

35. Stacey BR, Glanzman RL. Use of gabapentin for postherpetic neuralgia: results of two randomized, placebo-controlled studies. *Clin Ther* 2003;25(10):2597–2608.

36. Watson CP, Babul N. Efficacy of oxycodone in neuropathic pain: a randomized trial in postherpetic neuralgia. *Neurology* 1998;50:1837–1841.

Vascular Disorders and Headaches

Randolph W. Evans

Vascular disorders are commonly associated with headaches. Topics covered in this chapter are migraine and stroke, stroke, carotid endarterectomy, unruptured arteriovenous malformations and migraine, carotid and vertebral dissections, cerebral venous thrombosis, hypertension, carotidynia, and anginal headache. Vascular disorders reviewed in other chapters are subarachnoid hemorrhage (Chapter 8), subdural and epidural hematomas (Chapter 9), preeclampsia and eclampsia (Chapter 11), and temporal arteritis (Chapter 12).

MIGRAINE AND STROKE

Relationships

Between 1% and 17% of cerebral infarctions in young persons, especially women, have been attributed to migrainous infarction in various studies (also see Chapter 11). Migraineurs with aura have a greater stroke risk than those without aura. The strokes are often in the distribution of the posterior cerebral artery (1). Welch et al. consider four relationships (2).

1. Migraineurs can have a stroke due to another mechanism that occurs remotely in time from a typical attack of migraine.
2. A structural lesion (such as an arteriovenous malformation [AVM] or carotid dissection) unrelated to migraine can present with clinical features typical of migraine with neurological aura. A nonstructural mimic is pseudomigraine with temporary neurological symptoms and lymphocytic pleocytosis, which is also termed HaNDL ("headache with neurological deficits and cerebrospinal fluid lymphocytosis") (3). This condition affects those between 15 and 40 years of age who often have a history of migraine. Twenty-five percent report a viruslike illness up to 3 weeks prior to symptoms. Patients may have 1 to 12 episodes of changing variable neurological deficits (including sensory and motor symptoms and dysphasia) associated with a throbbing, bilateral moderate to severe headache and occasional fever. The duration of the neurological deficit ranges from 5 minutes to 1 week with a mean of 5 hours. Sensory (78% of episodes), aphasic (66%), and hemiparetic (56%) are the most common focal presentations. Migrainelike visual symptoms occur in 18% of cases. Patients are asymptomatic between episodes and following the symptomatic period, which can last up to 84 days. Complete recovery always occurs. The cerebrospinal fluid (CSF) typically reveals a CSF lymphocytic pleocytosis (10 to 760 cells mm^3) and elevated protein with-

out evidence of oligoclonal bands. Studies for infectious causes are negative. Computed tomography (CT) and magnetic resonance imaging (MRI) scans of the brain are normal.

3. Migrainous infarction is defined by the International Headache Society (IHS) 2nd edition classification as one or more aura symptoms associated with an ischemic brain lesion in an appropriate territory demonstrated by neuroimaging (4). The present attack is typical of previous attacks except that one or more aura symptoms persists for more than 60 minutes. Possible causes of migraine-induced stroke are decreased regional cerebral blood flow and platelet dysfunction.

There are types of migraine that can mimic other disorders that cause cerebral ischemia. Examples include hemiplegic migraine, basilar migraine, and rare genetic disorders such as mitochondrial encephalomyopathy, lactic acidosis, and strokelike episodes (MELAS) (Chapter 10) and cerebral autosomal dominant arteriopathy with subcortical infarcts and leukoencephalopathy (CADASIL).

CADASIL (5) is a rare inherited arterial disease of the brain due to a mutation of the Notch 3 gene, which is located on chromosome band 19q12. The systemic angiopathy is characterized by the replacement of the smooth muscle cells of the arterial media in small vessels by an unidentified granular, electron-dense, osmiophilic, and eosinophilic material. The resulting concentric thickening of the arterial wall presumably leads to ischemia and culminates in the infarctions and demyelination that underlie the clinical signs and symptoms of CADASIL.

The classic phenotype is for migraine to develop in the third and fourth decades in 40% to 60% of patients, strokes in the fourth and fifth decades, dementia in the sixth and seventh decades, and death usually in the seventh decade. However, increasing awareness and testing for this disease has identified patients who have relatively mild disease or may even be clinically unaffected in the seventh and eighth decades.

In one study, MRI demonstrated variable lesions at different ages: 20 to 30 years of age, hyperintense lesions in the anterior temporal lobe and subcortical lacunar lesions; 30 to 40 years, lacunar infarcts and areas of hyperintensity often in the external capsule, basal ganglia, and brain stem; 41 to 50 years, microbleeds in 19%; and over 50 years, areas of hyperintensity, subcortical lacunar lesions, lacunar infarcts, and microbleeds frequently present (5). In another study, moderate or severe involvement of the anterior temporal pole on MRI had a sensitivity of 89% and specificity of 86% for diagnosis; external capsule involvement had a high sensitivity of 93% but a low specificity of 45% (6).

Diagnosis can be made by genetic testing and by detection of granular osmiophilic material on skin biopsy. Both techniques have false negatives. Patients with CADASIL are treated empirically for migraine (with avoidance of triptans, DHE, and ergotamine) and lacunar stroke because treatment trials have not been performed.

4. Many migraine-related strokes cannot be categorized with certainty. Complex or multiple factors can interact with migraine and lead to stroke. Examples include medications (ergots, triptans, and oral contraceptive use); smoking; stroke occurring when cerebral angiography is performed during a migraine episode; and late-life migrainous accompaniments (Chapter 12).

   Another interesting example is livedo reticularis, which is present more often in migraineurs (7). Livedo reticularis is a dermatopathy characterized by an irregular, violaceous, net-like pattern that spares the face resulting from narrowing of small and medium arteries at the dermis-subcutis border. A subset of patients with livedo reticularis develop stroke in the absence of other vascular risk factors, which has been termed Sneddon syndrome.

5. Cardiac abnormalities that can result in embolic stroke are more common in migraine with aura. Persons with migraine with aura have an increased frequency of cardiac and pulmonary right-to-left shunts (about 45%) compared to those with migraine without aura (23%) and normal controls (about 18%) (8). The shunt is usually across a persistent foramen ovale but may involve an atrial septal defect or a pulmonary arteriovenous malformation. Transcatheter closure of atrial right-to-left shunts improves frequency and severity of attacks of migraine with aura in about half of migraineurs who undergo the procedure and abolishes attacks altogether in most of the remainder. The shunt can be a cause of paradoxical embolus and stroke as well as decompression sickness. It is hypothesized that vasoactive chemicals and microemboli in the venous circulation, which are not filtered by the lung, trigger migraine with aura. An atrial septal aneurysm, another potential cause of stroke, was detected by transesophageal echocardiogram in 28.5% of those with migraine with aura as compared to 3.6% of those with migraine without aura and 1.9% of controls (9).

White-Matter Abnormalities

White-matter abnormalities (WMA) are foci of hyperintensity on both proton density and T2-weighted images in the deep and periventricular white matter due to either interstitial edema or perivascular demyelination. WMA are easily detected on MRI but are not seen on CT scan. WMA have been reported in 12% to 46% of migraineurs, compared with 2% to 14% of controls (10).

Kruit et al. evaluated WMA and silent infarcts in patients with migraine from the population from the ages of 30 to 60 as compared to controls (11). Their results suggested that patients with migraine from the general population are at increased risk of subclinical cerebellar infarcts (5.4% in migraineurs vs. 7% in controls). Patients with migraine with aura and a high attack frequency are at greatest risk. In addition, women, but not men, with migraine with and without aura are at increased risk of high deep white-matter lesions load, and this risk also increases with increasing attack frequency. There was no association between periventricular white-matter lesions and migraine.

Although this was a well-done study, the finding of such a relatively high percentage of silent cerebellar infarcts has not been my experience or that of other neurologists or neuroradiologists I have discussed this with who have obtained numerous MRIs on migraineurs.

Although the cause of WMA in migraine is uncertain, various hypotheses have been advanced, including increased platelet aggregability with microemboli, abnormal cerebrovascular regulation, and repeated attacks of hypoperfusion during the aura. The presence of antiphospholipid antibodies might be a risk factor for WMAs in migraine, but the antibodies may not be an additional risk factor for stroke in migraineurs (12).

Retinal Migraine

Retinal migraine (13) is a rare disorder of at least two attacks of monocular visual disturbance including scintillations, scotoma, or blindness, associated with migraine headache often lasting 10 to 20 minutes. There should be a normal ophthalmological examination outside of an attack, and embolism and arteritis should be ruled out by appropriate investigations. (Because the retinal and ciliary circulations may be affected, the terms *ocular* or *anterior visual pathway migraine* have been proposed as more accurate.) The symptoms include unilateral quadrantic; altitudinal; or total grayout, whiteout, or blackout visual loss. Some patients report a concentric constriction of the monocular visual field proceeding from the periphery to the center, with spots and splotches of darkness that look like ink spots running together. There may be total loss of vision or a small piece of normal central vision remaining. Retinal migraine can also cause posterior ischemic optic neuropathy, mimicking retrobulbar optic neuritis. The retinal vessels appear to be in spasm during an attack. Permanent visual loss can occasionally occur with altitudinal field loss (especially nasal inferior loss), small blind spot extensions, and total visual loss (14).

Persistent Positive Visual Phenomena

Persistent positive visual phenomena in migraine are visual disturbances such as dots or flashes in both visual fields that persist indefinitely without evidence of infarction (15). Persistent migraine aura may respond to divalproex sodium (16) or lamotrigine.

Management

Preventive treatment that may be beneficial for patients with prolonged migraine aura or migrainous infarction include antiplatelet agents (e.g., aspirin and clopidogrel) and verapamil. Beta-blockers should be avoided because they may worsen intracranial vasoconstriction (17). Ergots and triptans should not be used for treatment of headache associated with prolonged migraine aura because of the potential for increased vasoconstriction.

STROKE

Epidemiology

Headaches due to stroke may be caused by electrochemical or mechanical stimulation of the trigeminovascular afferent system. Headaches commonly accompany stroke (18). In a prospective study of 163 patients with stroke, headache occurred in 29% with bland infarcts, 57% with parenchymal hemorrhage, 36% with transient ischemic attacks, and 17% with lacunar infarcts (19). Patients with a history of prior recurrent throbbing headaches and women were more likely to have headaches associated with stroke. The headache began prior to the event in 60% and at its onset in 25%. The quality, onset, and duration of the headaches varied widely. The headaches are equally likely to be abrupt or gradual in onset.

Clinical Manifestations

Various studies report a usually unilateral and focal headache of mild to moderate severity, although up to 46% of patients may have an incapacitating headache. The headache may be throbbing or nonthrobbing and may rarely be stabbing. The headache is more often ipsilateral than contralateral to the side of the cerebral ischemia. Headache is more common in ischemia of the posterior than the anterior circulation and in cortical than subcortical events. The duration of the headache is longest in cardioembolic infarcts and thrombotic infarcts, of medium duration in lacunar infarction, and shortest in transient ischemic attacks (20). Associated symptoms in one study include nausea in 44%, vomiting in 23%, and light and noise sensitivity in 25% (21). Bending, straining, and jarring the head usually increases the intensity. A sentinel or warning headache has been reported in 10% to 43% of patients before ischemic strokes, especially before cardioembolic stroke. The headache is usually unilateral and focal and lasts more than 24 hours (22). The occurrence may be hours to days before the stroke. Sentinel and other headaches due to subarachnoid hemorrhage (SAH) are reviewed in Chapter 8.

CAROTID ENDARTERECTOMY

A benign ipsilateral frontotemporal intense headache may follow endarterectomy with a latency of 36 to 72 hours. The headache may recur intermittently for up to 6 months. Headache can also develop postoperatively due to intracerebral hemorrhage, which is a complication of 0.75% of operations (23). The hemorrhage occurs at a median of 3 days after surgery with a range of 0 to 18 days.

UNRUPTURED AVM AND MIGRAINE

The prevalence of AVMs is about 0.5% in postmortem studies. In contrast to saccular aneurysms, up to 50% present with symptoms or signs other than hemorrhage. Migrainelike headaches with and without visual symptoms can be associated with arteriovenous malformations, especially those in the occipital lobe, which is the predominant location of about 20% of parenchymal AVMs (24). Although headaches always occurring on the same side (side locked) are present in 95% of those with AVMs, 17% of those with migraine without aura and 15% of patients with migraine with aura have side-locked headaches (25). Typical migraine due to an AVM is the exception, as there are usually distinguishing features. Bruyn reported the following features in patients with migrainelike symptoms and AVM: unusual associated signs (papilledema, field cut, bruit), 65%;

short duration of headache attacks, 20%; brief scintillating scotoma, 10%, absent family history, 15%; atypical sequence of aura, headache, and vomiting, 10%; and seizures, 25% (26).

CAROTID AND VERTEBRAL ARTERY DISSECTIONS (27–29)

Epidemiology

Of all patients with a first stroke, 2.5% have an internal carotid artery (ICA) dissection, with 90% involving the cervical carotid and 10% the intracranial. The frequency of vertebral artery (VA) dissections is about one third that of carotid. Twenty percent of spontaneous ICA dissections and almost half of VA dissections are bilateral. Combined ICA and VA dissections occasionally occur. Rarely, headache can be the initial manifestation of aortic dissection type A extending into the cervical arteries.

Dissections occur due to penetration of circulating blood through an intimal tear into the subintimal, medial, and, less commonly, adventitial layers of the vascular wall that extends for varying distances along the vessel. Risk and predisposing factors for spontaneous dissections include migraine, hypertension, oral contraceptives, fibromuscular dysplasia (found in about 15% of cases), temporal arteritis, polyarteritis nodosa, meningovascular syphilis, Ehlers-Danlos syndrome, Marfan syndrome, cystic medial necrosis, and moyamoya disease. Traumatic dissections due to penetrating or nonpenetrating injuries have even been associated with minor or trivial trauma, including coughing, blowing the nose, turning the head, sleeping in the wrong position, sports activities, chiropractic manipulation, yoga exercises, sexual activity, and whiplash injuries. More than 70% of the patients are younger than 50 years of age, with a mean age of approximately 45. Dissections occur slightly more often in women.

Clinical Manifestations

Head, face, orbital, or neck pain, usually ipsilateral to the site of the dissection, is the initial manifestation in about 80% of patients with extracranial ICA dissection. Focal cerebral ischemic symptoms occur in about 60% of patients and may follow the headache by up to 4 weeks or may precede it. The presence of deficits is as follows: neurologically normal, 50%; mild deficits only, 21%; moderate to severe deficits, 25%; and death, 4%. An incomplete ipsilateral Horner's syndrome with ptosis and miosis but not anhidrosis is present in about 50% of cases due to damage of the sympathetic fibers. Either subjective or objective bruits or both are present in about 45% of patients.

Uncommon symptoms and signs of extracranial ICA dissection include syncope, amaurosis fugax, scalp tenderness, neck swelling, positive visual phenomena (e.g., scintillations), sixth cranial nerve palsies, lower cranial nerve palsies (e.g., ipsilateral tongue paresis and dysgeusia from involvement of the hypoglossal nerve and chorda tympani), and a sensation of pulsation in the neck. Transient symptoms resembling migraine with aura (30) and cluster headache (31) have been reported.

Intracranial ICA dissection typically presents with a severe ipsilateral headache and a major stroke. SAH can occur in 20%

of cases. Rarely, prolonged isolated orbital pain can be the only symptom of intrapetrous ICA dissection (32).

The most common symptom of VA dissection is headache and neck pain (present in 88%) followed by vertebrobasilar distribution stroke or transient ischemic attacks (TIAs)—especially lateral medullary syndrome—from within hours to 2 weeks. Less frequently, the patients may present with vertebrobasilar stroke or TIAs only or with only headache and/or neck pain. The presence of deficits is as follows: neurologically normal or mild deficits only, 83%; moderate to severe deficits, 11%; and death, 6%. SAH can occur with dissection of the intracranial portion of the VA. Rare symptoms and signs of VA dissection include vertigo and upside-down vision, hemifacial spasm, upper-extremity pain that can mimic myocardial ischemia, acute cervical epidural hemorrhage, bilateral distal upper-limb amyotrophy, respiratory arrest, and transient amnesia.

The onset of headache is gradual in about 75% of patients with ICA and VA dissections. More than 10% of those with ICA and more than 20% of those with VA dissections report a thunderclap headache, a severe sudden headache usually without associated SAH. The headaches in both dissections are usually described as constant, steady aching or steady sharp pain and, less commonly, as throbbing. Facial pain, including ear pain, is reported by about one third, and orbital and eye pain occurs in about 40% of patients with ICA dissection. This pain is always ipsilateral to the dissection. Neck pain (usually anterolateral) is reported by about 25% of those with ICA dissection. About half of those with VA dissection report posterolateral neck pain, which is bilateral in one third of patients.

Diagnostic Evaluation

Arteriograms are the standard study for evaluating ICA and VA dissections and may reveal stenosis, often irregular and tapered, dissecting aneurysms, intimal flaps, and occlusion of distal branches. ICA dissections usually begin 2 cm or more distal to the origin and extend rostrally for a variable distance. Irregular narrowing may give a "wavy ribbon" appearance, and severe narrowing may produce a "string sign."

Axial MRI may demonstrate the abnormal lumen and the intramural clot. Magnetic resonance angiography (MRA) increases the yield of MRI studies. Table 13-1 gives the sensitivity and specificity of MRI and MRA compared with conventional angiography according to the study of Levy et al. (33). The sensitivity for detection of VA dissections is less than that for ICA dissections because of technical artifacts due to the smaller size and the broad variation in the normal caliber of the vertebral arteries. MRA is particularly useful for follow-up of patients. Occasionally, MRI and MRA may detect dissections not seen on conventional angiography due to undetectable narrowing of the lumen by intraluminal hematomas. Helical (spiral) CT angiography may have a similar sensitivity and specificity to MRA.

Carotid duplex ultrasound may show a tapering luminal stenosis and a double lumen. Extracranial Doppler may show reduced or absent distal carotid artery flow at the level of the bifurcation. Limitations of duplex ultrasound include anatomical factors

Table 13-1. Sensitivity and specificity of MRI and MRA for the evaluation of internal carotid and vertebral artery dissections compared to conventional angiography

Artery	Study	Sensitivity (%)	Specificity (%)
Carotid	MRI	84	99
	MRA	95	99
Vertebral	MRI	60	98
	MRA	20	100

(e.g., a short or fat neck and a high bifurcation) and not detecting intracranial ICA involvement. Extracranial vertebral duplex ultrasound has only fair sensitivity and specificity and does not image the intracranial portions.

Management

In the absence of SAH, intracranial hemorrhage, or a massive stroke, the standard treatment for dissection is anticoagulation with heparin followed by warfarin to prevent thrombus propagation and embolic stroke. The optimal time for treatment is unknown. Because most arteries heal within 3 months, a follow-up study such as MRA is typically done. Then a decision is made on whether to continue warfarin or not. Many patients do well with or without treatment: a complete or excellent recovery occurs in about 85% of those with ICA and VA dissections. Antiplatelet agents are being studied as an alternative to anticoagulation. The recurrence rate for second dissections is 2% for the first month and then about 1% per year. Occasionally, resection of a residual dissecting aneurysm that has been a source of embolization or the source of SAH is performed. Another occasional surgical option is superficial temporal artery-middle cerebral artery bypass for those with tight ICA stenosis and hemodynamic ischemic symptoms.

CEREBRAL VENOUS THROMBOSIS

Introduction and Epidemiology

Cerebral venous thrombosis (CVT) (34,35) is commonly associated with headaches. There are numerous causes and predisposing conditions. Local infectious causes include direct septic trauma, intracranial infection (e.g., abscess or meningitis), and regional infections (such as otitis, tonsillitis, and sinusitis). Systemic infections that can be causative include bacterial infections (e.g., septicemia and endocarditis), viral infections (e.g., herpes, HIV, CMV), parasitic infections (malaria, trichinosis), and aspergillosis. There are many noninfectious causes. Local pathology includes head injury, neurosurgical operations, cerebral infarcts and hemorrhages, tumors, porencephaly, arachnoid cysts, dural AVMs, and internal jugular vein infusions. Any type of surgery with or without deep venous thrombosis has been associated. Pregnancy and the puerperium as a cause is discussed in Chapter 11. Oral contraceptives are also a risk factor.

There are numerous medical associations, including cardiac disease, malignancies, red blood cell disorders (e.g., polycythemia, sickle-cell disease), thrombocythemia, coagulation disorders (protein C and protein S deficiency and antiphospholipid antibody deficiency), severe dehydration, ulcerative colitis and Crohn's disease, connective tissue disorders, venous thromboembolic disease, Behçet's disease, sarcoidosis, nephrotic syndrome, androgen therapy, homocystinuria, and thyrotoxicosis. Increased resistance to activated protein C with factor V Leiden mutation may be found in up to 20% of cases. Despite this extensive list of associations and causes, up to 35% of causes are idiopathic.

The incidence of CVT is not known. All age groups may be affected. Postpartum women appear to have the greatest risk of this disease. Neonates or young infants with severe dehydration are also a high-risk group.

Clinical Manifestations (35)

In 75% of cases, multiple veins or sinuses are involved. The superior sagittal sinus (SSS), which drains the major part of the cerebral cortices and reabsorbs CSF, is involved in about 70% of cases of cerebral venous thrombosis (CVT). Thrombotic obstruction of the SSS elevates intracranial pressure by increasing intravenous and CSF pressure. The presentation of raised intracranial pressure is often headaches and papilledema. Extension of the thrombus into the superficial cortical veins can result in cerebral edema, infarction, hemorrhage, and seizures. The lateral sinus, which drains blood from the sagittal sinus, cerebellum, brain stem, and posterior part of the cerebral hemispheres, is involved in about 70% of cases. Patients usually present with symptoms and signs of raised intracranial pressure.

The deep cerebral veins and sinuses, which drain the deep white matter of the cerebral hemispheres and the basal ganglia, are involved in more than 10% of cases. Headache and alterations in the level of consciousness are present with extensive thrombosis of these structures. More severe cases may result in findings such as hemorrhagic infarction of the thalami and basal ganglia, dysphasia, and hemiparesis. The cavernous sinuses, which drain blood from the orbits and the anterior part of the base of the brain, are involved in less than 5% of cases. Headache, chemosis, proptosis, and painful ophthalmoplegia (initially unilateral but often becomes bilateral) are the usual presentations of cavernous sinus thrombosis.

Headache, present in 80%, is the earlier symptom in two thirds of cases. The headaches, usually due to raised intracranial pressure, are typically diffuse, progressive, and rather constant. However, a sudden severe thunderclap headache can result if CVT leads to SAH. The headache of CVT is almost always associated with the following signs: papilledema in up to 80% of cases, which can cause transient visual obscurations (visual clouding in one or both eyes lasting seconds) when severe; focal deficits, which are present at some time during the course of the disease in 50% of patients; and partial and/or generalized seizures, which are present at some time during the disease in 40% of cases.

There are some important patterns of symptoms and signs that can simulate other disorders. Isolated intracranial hypertension, with headache, papilledema, and sixth cranial nerve palsy, occurs in up to 40% of patients. This presentation can exactly mimic pseudotumor cerebri (see later). Subacute encephalopathy, with an altered level of consciousness and no focal findings similar to a metabolic encephalopathy, often occurs in either very young or very old patients. During the postpartum period, some presentations of CVT can mimic other disorders as follows: headache alone can be mistaken for postpartum migraine; headache and seizures can be taken for eclampsia; and depression, irritability, anxiety, and lack of interest can be misdiagnosed as postpartum depression.

Diagnostic Evaluation

CT scan of the brain, which can exclude associated findings such as cerebral infarction or hemorrhage, has limited sensitivity for the detection of CVT. The "empty delta sign" on an enhanced study, which is due to the opacification of collateral veins in the wall of the SSS surrounding the nonenhancing clot within the sinus, is present in only 35% of cases. In addition, false positives can occur because the posterior sagittal sinus divides into two channels in about 25% of normal patients.

MRI, especially when combined with MR venography, is the best way to detect CVT (36). The studies can demonstrate flow void, the thrombus, and, later, recanalization. Cerebral angiography can certainly reveal partial or complete lack of filling of a sinus. However, false positives can occur due to normal variants such as absence of the anterior part of the sagittal sinus or partial or total agenesis of one lateral sinus.

In settings where CT is normal and MRI and cerebral angiography is not available, the d-dimer test may be helpful. A level of more than 500 μg/mL has a sensitivity of 83% and negative predictive value of 95% (37).

Lumbar puncture, which should be avoided if there is a large cerebral infarction or hemorrhage, can document elevated intracranial pressure and help exclude infectious or leptomeningeal malignancy as the cause of CVT. CSF findings include mild to moderate elevation of CSF protein in two thirds of patients, more than 20 red cells in two thirds, and a mild pleocytosis in one third of cases. An abnormal CSF protein and cell count can help diagnose CVT in cases of isolated intracranial hypertension simulating pseudotumor cerebri where only a CT scan of the brain is obtained with normal findings.

Management

The treatment of CVT includes the following: the limitation or elimination of thrombus; treatment of an underlying cause, if present; control of seizures; treatment of raised intracranial pressure; and management of cerebral infarctions and hemorrhages.

Intravenous or subcutaneous heparin is the treatment of choice (except for neonates) with prolongation of the partial thromboplastic time (PTT) to 2 to 2.5 times normal. Some authorities recommend prolongation of the PTT to only 1.25 to

1.5 times normal in patients with associated hemorrhagic infarction. Heparin is continued until the patient improves or stabilizes. Warfarin then replaces heparin and is usually continued for at least 3 months. The dosage of warfarin is adjusted to obtain an international normalized ratio (INR) between 2.5 and 3.5. Serial MRI and magnetic resonance venography studies are useful in determining the duration of warfarin therapy. In a study of 33 patients followed with serial MRI, recanalization only occurred within the first four months following cerebral venous thrombosis and not thereafter, irrespective of oral anticoagulation (38).

Management of symptomatic raised intracranial pressure is controversial. Treatments sometimes used, depending on the clinical picture, include lumbar puncture before starting anticoagulation, steroids, mannitol, glycerol, acetazolamide, furosemide, shunting, optic nerve fenestration (in cases of progressive visual loss), intracranial pressure monitoring, and pentobarbital-induced coma. There is concern, however, that use of diuretics might lead to additional thrombus extension. If patients worsen despite optimal symptomatic and heparin treatment, some authorities recommend local urokinase infusion through the internal jugular route or tissue plasminogen activator via catheter at the site of the clot (39).

The mortality rate of CVT in recent series ranges from 6% to 30%. Full recovery occurs in more than 75% of survivors.

HYPERTENSION

Although mild or moderate hypertension does not usually cause headache, hypertension due to the following can cause headache: acute pressor response to exogenous agents; pheochromocytoma; malignant hypertension; and preeclampsia and eclampsia (Chapter 11). Headaches due to severe hypertension are usually a biocciptal throbbing but can be generalized or a frontal throbbing (especially in children). The headache is often present in the morning on awakening. The diastolic blood pressure is usually elevated to 120 mm Hg or higher.

Acute Pressor Responses

A sudden severe headache can occur due to a rapid increase in blood pressure when patients taking monoamine oxidase inhibitors drink red wine or eat foods such as cheese, chicken livers, or pickled herring, which have a high tyramine content, or also take sympathomimetic medications such as pseudoephedrine. Use of illicit drugs with sympathomimetic actions such as cocaine, methamphetamine, and methylenedioxymethamphetamine ("ecstasy") can also cause acute hypertension (sometimes leading to strokes) and headache.

Pheochromocytoma

Epidemiology

Pheochromocytoma (40,41), a rare tumor, arises from the chromaffin cells of the adrenal medulla and is named for the color of its cut surface (from the Greek *phaios,* meaning "dusky"). The tumor usually secretes norepinephrine and epinephrine with a ratio of 4:1 or more. Ten percent to 20% are associated with genetic disorders such as multiple endocrine neoplasia syndromes, von Hippel-Lindau complex, neurofibromatosis type I, Sturge-Weber syndrome, tuberous sclerosis, and Zollinger-Ellison syndrome. Of the 80% to 90% of sporadic cases, 10% are malignant, 10% are bilateral, and 10% are found outside the adrenal gland. Ninety percent of the extraadrenal tumors are located within the abdomen, typically in the sympathetic ganglia between the diaphragm and the lower poles of the kidneys (paragangliomas), in the urinary bladder (where micturition can trigger attacks), and in the organ of Zuckerkandl (at the bifurcation of the aorta). Extraabdominal locations are the chest (pericardium, myocardium, and posterior mediastinum) and neck (in the carotid body, vagus nerve, or jugular bulb).

Clinical Manifestations

The most common symptom of pheochromocytoma is a rapid-onset headache that is reported by up to 92% of patients. The headache, which lasts less than 1 hour in 70%, is bilateral, severe, and throbbing, and it may be associated with nausea in 50% of cases. Some patients may not get headaches even with blood pressures as high as 260/100 mm Hg. Hypertension, which is paroxysmal in 50% and sustained in 50%, is found in 90% of patients. The paroxysmal hypertension may show elevations to 300/160 mm Hg. Symptoms and signs of adrenergic stimulation are common with sweating, palpitations, and tachycardia with palpitations each reported by about 70% of patients. Anxiety, dizziness, abdominal pain, chest pain, weight loss, heat intolerance, nausea/vomiting, pallor (less often flushing), syncope, and orthostatic hypotension may also occur. Many patients have spells lasting between 15 and 60 minutes occurring from several times per day to once or twice a year. Paroxysms can begin spontaneously or be triggered by physical exertion, certain medications, emotional stress, changes in posture, and increases in intraabdominal pressure.

Diagnostic Evaluation

Laboratory and imaging studies are required to make the diagnosis. A 24-hour urine collection reveals elevations and sensitivity for diagnosis as follows: metanephrine and normetanephrine, up to 98%; vanillylmandelic acid, 60% to 70%; and total catecholamines, 60% to 79%. MRI of the abdomen, pelvis, chest, and neck is almost 100% sensitive in detecting pheochromocytomas. CT scans have a sensitivity of 95% and specificity of 65% for detection of adrenal tumors. Scintigraphic imaging with I-131 metaiodobenzylguadnidine has a sensitivity of 88% and specificity of 99%. Indications include evaluation of extraadrenal, recurrent, or metastatic pheochromoctyomas or those with silent adrenal masses and borderline catecholamine levels.

Management

The hypertension due to pheochromocytoma is treated first with slow upward titration of an alpha-blocker (e.g., prazosin, terazosin, and phenoxybenzamine) and later addition of a beta-blocker for rate control after full alpha-blockade. A combination drug such as labetalol can sometimes be useful. Direct vasodilators, calcium channel blockers, and angiotensin-converting enzyme inhibits are sometimes used cautiously when the hypertension is resistant to initial therapy. Surgical removal can be curative, especially in benign tumors.

Malignant Hypertension

Hypertensive encephalopathy is an acute cerebral syndrome due to sudden, severe hypertension. The rate and extent of the rise of the blood pressure are the most important factors in the development of this condition. In those with chronic hypertension, hypertensive encephalopathy may not result unless the blood pressure is 250/150 mm Hg or higher. A previously normotensive person may develop the encephalopathy with a lower elevation. The presenting symptoms can be headache, nausea, and vomiting. Complaints of blurred or dim vision, scintillating scotoma, or visual loss may also be reported. Anxiety, agitation, and then decreased levels of consciousness and sometimes seizures can follow. Papilledema and focal neurological deficits can be present.

CAROTIDYNIA

Carotidynia is neck pain associated with carotid artery tenderness, especially near the bifurcation (42). Facial pain may also occur alone or with the neck pain. Symptomatic causes of carotidynia include disorders of the carotid artery, including dissection (see earlier), occlusion or stenosis, aneurysm, fibromuscular dysplasia, temporal arteritis (Chapter 12), and following endarterectomy. In the acute presentation, these disorders should be excluded with appropriate studies such as carotid ultrasound, MRI and MRA, angiography, and a sedimentation rate. In idiopathic cases, MRI has been reported as showing abnormal enhancing tissue centered at the carotid artery within the carotid sheath (43).

Acute monophasic carotidynia, which may have a viral basis, typically occurs in young or middle-aged adults and persists for an average of 11 days. Structural abnormalities and temporal arteritis are excluded by appropriate testing. Analgesics, nonsteroidal antiinflammatory drugs such as indomethacin, or a short course of corticosteroids may relieve the pain (44).

Chronic or recurrent carotidynia, which occurs in adults, is characterized by recurring pain lasting minutes to hours with episodes occurring daily or weekly. This form, which may be related to migraine, may respond to treatment with indomethacin, a short course of corticosteroids, triptans (45), and migraine preventive medications. This is a diagnosis of exclusion. Evaluation by an ENT physician to exclude nonvascular abnormalities including thyroiditis and Eagle's syndrome (Chapter 14) may be useful.

ANGINAL HEADACHE

Cardiac ischemia can rarely cause a unilateral or bilateral headache brought on by exercise and relieved by rest (46,47). The headache can occur alone or be accompanied by chest pain. The mechanism of the referral of cardiac pain to the head is obscure. Angina is generally believed to be due to afferent impulses that traverse cervicothoracic sympathetic ganglia, enter the spinal cord via the first and the fifth thoracic dorsal roots, and produce the characteristic pain in the chest or inner aspects of the arms. Cardiac vagal afferents, which mediate anginal pain in a minority of patients, join the tractus solitarius. A potential pathway for referral of cardiac pain to the head would be convergence with craniovascular afferents (48).

REFERENCES

1. Suchurkova D, Moreau T, Lemesle M, et al. Migraine history and migraine-induced stroke in the Dijon Stroke Registry. *Neuroepidemiology* 1999;18:85–91.
2. Welch KMA. Stroke and migraine—the spectrum of cause and effect. *Funct Neurol* 2003;18:121–126.
3. Pascual J, Valle N. Pseudomigraine with lymphocytic pleocytosis. *Curr Pain Headache Rep* 2003;7(3):224–228.
4. Headache Classification Subcommittee of the International Headache Society. The international classification of headache disorders, 2nd ed. *Cephalalgia* 2004;24 (Suppl 1):59:1–160.
5. van den Boom R, Lesnik Oberstein SA, Ferrari MD, et al. Cerebral autosomal dominant arteriopathy with subcortical infarcts and leukoencephalopathy: MR imaging findings at different ages—3rd–6th decades. *Radiology* 2003;229(3):683–690.
6. Markus HS, Martin RJ, Simpson MA, et al. Diagnostic strategies in CADASIL. *Neurology* 2002;59:1134–1138.
7. Tietjen GE, Gottwald L, Al-Qasmi MM, et al. Migraine is associated with livedo reticularis: a prospective study. *Headache* 2002;42(4):263–267.
8. Evans RW, Wilmshurst P, Nightingale S. Is cardiac evaluation for a possible right-to-left shunt indicated in a scuba diver with migraine with aura? *Headache* 2003;43:294–295.
9. Carerj S, Narbone MC, Zito C, et al. Prevalence of atrial septal aneurysm in patients with migraine: an echocardiographic study. *Headache* 2003;43(7):725–728.
10. Evans RW. The evaluation of headaches. In: Evans RW, ed. *Diagnostic testing in neurology*. Philadelphia: WB Saunders, 1999.
11. Kruit MC, van Buchem MA, Hofman PA, et al. Migraine as a risk factor for subclinical brain lesions. *JAMA* 2004;28;291(4): 427–434.
12. Chapman J, Rand JH, Brey RL, et al. Non-stroke neurological syndromes associated with antiphospholipid antibodies: evaluation of clinical and experimental studies. *Lupus* 2003;12(7): 514–517.
13. Moore KL, Corbett JJ. Retinal migraine. In: Gilman S, ed. *Medlink neurology*. San Diego: Medlink, 2004. Available at www. medlink.com.
14. Beversdorf D, Stommel E, Allen C, et al. Recurrent branch retinal infarcts in association with migraine. *Headache* 1997;37: 396–399.
15. Liu GT, Schatz NJ, Galetta SL, et al. Persistent positive visual phenomena in migraine. *Neurology* 1995;45:664–668.
16. Rothrock JF. Successful treatment of persistent migraine aura with divalproex sodium. *Neurology* 1997;48:261–262.

17. Alvarez SJ, Molins A, Turon A, et al. Migraine-infarct in patients treated with beta-blockers. *Rev Clin Esp* 1993;192:228–230.
18. Mitsias P, Welch KMA. Headache associated with ischemic cerebrovascular disease. In: Gilman S, ed. *Medlink neurology*. San Diego: Medlink, 2004. Available at www.medlink.com.
19. Portenoy RK, Abissi CJ, Lipton RB, et al. Headache in cerebrovascular disease. *Stroke* 1984;15:1009–1012.
20. Arboix A, Massons J, Oliveres M, et al. Headache in acute cerebrovascular disease: a prospective clinical study in 240 patients. *Cephalalgia* 1994;14:37–40.
21. Vestergaard K, Andersen G, Nielsen MI, et al. Headache in stroke. *Stroke* 1993;24:1621–1624.
22. Gorelick PB, Hier DB, Caplan LR, et al. Headache in acute cerebrovascular disease. *Neurology* 1986;36:144–150.
23. Ouriel K, Shortell CK, Illig KA, et al. Intracerebral hemorrhage after carotid endarterectomy: incidence, contribution to neurologic morbidity, and predictive factors. *J Vasc Endovasc Surg* 1999;29:82–87.
24. Kupersmith MJ, Vargas ME, Yashar A, et al. Occipital arteriovenous malformations: visual disturbances and presentation. *Neurology* 1996;46:953–957.
25. Leone M, D'Amico D, Frediani F, et al. Clinical considerations on side-locked unilaterality in long lasting primary headaches. *Headache* 1993;33:381–384.
26. Bruyn GW. Intracranial arteriovenous malformation and migraine. *Cephalalgia* 1984;4:191–207.
27. Mokri B. Headache in cervical artery dissections. *Curr Pain Headache Rep* 2002;6(3):209–216.
28. Saver JL, Easton JD. Dissections and trauma of cervicocerebral arteries. In: Barnett HJM, Mohr JP, Stein BM, et al., eds. *Stroke: pathophysiology, diagnosis, and management,* 3rd ed. New York: Churchill Livingstone, 1998:769–786.
29. Silverman IE. Spontaneous carotid artery dissection. In: Gilman S, ed. *Medlink neurology*. San Diego: Medlink, 2004. Available at www.medlink.com.
30. Silverman IE, Wityk RJ. Transient migraine-like symptoms with internal carotid artery dissection. *Clin Neurol Neurosurg* 1998;100:116–120.
31. Rosebraugh CJ, Griebel DJ, DiPette DJ. A case report of carotid artery dissection presenting as cluster headache. *Am J Med* 1997;102:418–419.
32. Guillon B, Biousse V, Massiou H, et al. Orbital pain as an isolated sign of internal carotid artery dissection: a diagnostic pitfall. *Cephalalgia* 1998;18:222–224.
33. Levy C, Laissy JP, Reveau V, et al. Carotid and vertebral dissections: three dimensional time-of-flight MR angiography and MR imaging versus conventional angiography. *Radiology* 1994;190:97.
34. Crassard I, Bousser MG. Cerebral venous thrombosis. *J Neuroophthalmol* 2004;24(2):156–163.
35. Kasner SC, Morales X, Broderick JP. Cerebral venous thrombosis. In: Gilman S, ed. *Medlink neurology*. San Diego: Medlink, 2004. Available at www.medlink.com.
36. Bianchi D, Maeder P, Bogousslavsky J, et al. Diagnosis of cerebral venous thrombosis with routine magnetic resonance: an update. *Eur Neurol* 1998;40:179–190.

37. Lalive PH, de Moerloose P, Lovblad K, et al. Is measurement of D-dimer useful in the diagnosis of cerebral venous thrombosis? *Neurology* 2003;61(8):1057–1060.
38. Baumgartner RW, Studer A, Arnold M, et al. Recanalisation of cerebral venous thrombosis. *J Neurol Neurosurg Psychiatry* 2003;74(4):459–461.
39. Frey JL, Muro GJ, McDougall CG, et al. Cerebral venous thrombosis: combined intrathrombus rtPA and intravenous heparin. *Stroke* 1999;30:489–494.
40. Pleet AB. Neuroendocrine disorders. In: Evans RW, ed. *Diagnostic testing in neurology.* Philadelphia: WB Saunders, 1999:419–435.
41. Rose-Innes AP. Pheochromocytoma. In: Gilman S, ed. *Medlink neurology.* San Diego: Medlink, 2004. Available at www.medlink. com.
42. Wesselmann U, Reich SG. The dynias. *Semin Neurol* 1996;16: 63–74.
43. Burton BS, Syms MJ, Petermann GW, et al. MR imaging of carotidynia. *Am J Neuroradiol* 2000;21:766–769.
44. Emmanuelli JL, Gutierrez JR, Chiossone JA, et al. Carotidynia: a frequently overlooked or misdiagnosed syndrome. *Ear Nose Throat J* 1998;77:462–469.
45. Valle N, Gonzalez-Mandly A, Oterino A, et al. A case of carotidynia with response to almotriptan. *Cephalalgia* 2003;23(2): 155–156.
46. Lipton RB, Lowenkopf T, Bajwa ZH, et al. Cardiac cephalalgia: a treatable form of exertional headache. *Neurology* 1997;49: 813–816.
47. Grace A, Horgan J, Breathnach K, et al. Anginal headache and its basis. *Cephalalgia* 1997;17:195–196.
48. Lance JW, Lambros J. Unilateral exertional headache as a symptom of cardiac ischemia. *Headache* 1998;38:315–316.

Headaches and Neoplasms, High and Low Pressure, and HEENT Disorders

Randolph W. Evans

NEOPLASMS

Introduction and Epidemiology

Many patients with frequent or severe headaches are concerned they may have a brain tumor. Fortunately, brain tumors are an uncommon cause of headaches. In the United States, about 18,000 primary brain tumors are diagnosed per year, including the following types: glioblastomas, 50%; astrocytomas, 10% (about 50% of these present with headache); meningiomas, 17%; pituitary adenomas, 4%; neurilemoma, 2%; ependymoma, 2%; and oligodendroglioma, 3%. At least 100,000 new cases of metastatic brain tumors are diagnosed per year in the United States (1). Eighty percent occur after the diagnosis of the primary site, and 70% have multiple cerebral lesions. The frequency by primary site in adults is as follows: lung, 64%; breast, 14%; unknown primary, 8%; melanoma, 4%; colorectal, 3%; hypernephroma, 2%; and other, 5%. The average interval between the diagnosis of the primary carcinoma and the development of brain metastasis is 4 months for lung carcinoma and 3 years for breast cancer. By contrast, slow-growing cancers of the ovary, uterus, or breast can result in cerebral metastasis up to 15 years after the diagnosis of the primary. Neoplasms in children and adolescents are discussed in Chapter 10.

The prevalence of adults with primary and metastatic brain tumors who complain of headaches at the time of diagnosis has been variably reported as 31% (2), 48% (3), 50% (4), and 71% (5). The median duration of headache at the time of diagnosis has been variably reported as from 3.5 weeks to 15.7 months. Headaches have been reported variably as equally frequent with primary and metastatic tumors and as more frequent with primary than with metastatic tumors.

Clinical Manifestations

Eight percent of patients with headaches and brain tumors have a normal neurological examination. Papilledema, which is usually associated with headaches, is present in 40% of patients with brain tumors. The presence of headache is related to the size of the tumor and the amount of midline shift. Patients with previous headaches are more likely to have a headache with a brain tumor. The brain tumor headache may have an identical character to prior headaches but is more severe or frequent, and it is usually associated with other problems, such as seizure, confusion, prolonged nausea, hemiparesis, or other focal findings.

The most common location of headaches is bifrontal, although patients may complain of pain in other locations of the head as well as the neck. Unilateral headaches are usually on the same side as the neoplasm. Although the quality of the headache is usually similar to the tension type, occasional patients have headaches similar to migraine without aura and rarely migraine with aura and cluster headaches. Most of the headaches are intermittent with moderate to severe intensity, but a significant minority report only mild headaches relieved by simple analgesics. The so-called classic brain tumor headache—severe, worse in the morning, and associated with nausea and vomiting—occurs in a minority of patients with brain tumors.

Headaches as a Complication of Treatment of Brain Tumors (6)

Headaches can have an iatrogenic origin. Radiotherapy may cause headaches. Acute radiation encephalopathy presents within 2 weeks of the onset of radiation with new or worsening headache, focal neurological symptoms and signs, and nausea and vomiting. Corticosteroids usually relieve symptoms. Subacute (early delayed) radiation encephalopathy can present between 1 and 6 months after completion of radiation with headache, lethargy, and new or worsening neurological symptoms and signs. Imaging usually shows increased edema and may show new contrast enhancement that can be difficult to differentiate from tumor, although the lesion is typically hypometabolic on PET scanning. Temporary use of corticosteroids may improve symptoms. When headaches develop as corticosteroids are tapered after treatment due to corticosteroid withdrawal syndrome, subacute radiation encephalopathy should be excluded.

Chemotherapeutic agents used to treat brain tumors may also cause headache. Temozolomide, used to treat malignant gliomas and brain metastases, has been reported to cause headache in up to 25% of patients. Aseptic meningitis with headache, nausea, vomiting, lethargy, and nuchal rigidity results from intrathecal chemotherapy with methotrexate or cytosine arabinoside (Ara C), especially its sustained-release version DepoCyt, in about 10% and 25% of patients, respectively. Thalidomide, cisplatinum, etoposide, imatinib, and hydroxyurea may also cause headache.

Other medications may also cause headaches. The selective serotonin receptor antagonists, ondansetron and granisetron, used as antiemetics during chemotherapy, cause headache in 14% to 39% of patients. Bromocriptine, which is used for treatment of prolactinomas, has an 18% incidence of headache.

Pituitary Adenomas

The incidence of headaches in patients with pituitary adenomas has been reported as between 33% and 72%. The headache, which may be intermittent or continuous, is usually bilateral and occurs more frequently in the anterior half of the head (7). In contrast, Sheehan's syndrome (the spontaneous ischemic necrosis of the pituitary gland in the postpartum period resulting in hypopituitarism) does not usually result in headache (Chapter 11).

Pain due to pituitary tumors can mimic seemingly benign disorders. Pituitary macroadenomas can present with trigeminal neuralgia, short-lasting unilateral neuralgiform headache attacks with conjunctival injection and tearing (SUNCT) (8), hemicrania continua, clusterlike headaches (9), and Raeder's syndrome (10). Raeder's syndrome is a rare disorder characterized by ptosis, miosis, impairment of sweating over the medial aspect of the forehead, and sudden onset of severe frontotemporal burning, aching pain often in a periorbital or trigeminal distribution. Episodic pain is usually due to cluster headaches (Chapter 7), and those with more constant pain can be due to lesions involving the internal carotid artery and impinging on the first division of the trigeminal nerve. In addition, other lesions than pituitary tumors include aneurysms, trauma, infections, and internal carotid artery dissection (11).

Acute pituitary apoplexy is an uncommon syndrome due to hemorrhage of a pituitary macroadenoma with compression of neighboring neural and vascular structures. Signs and symptoms occur in the following percentages of patients: headache, 83%; visual disturbance, 59%; ocular palsies, 48%; nausea/vomiting, 38%; altered mentation, 22%; meningismus, 15%; and fever, 7% (12). Rarely, entrapment of the internal carotid artery within the cavernous sinus can lead to hemiparesis (13). The incidence of pituitary apoplexy in patients with known pituitary adenomas is reported as 2% to 5%, usually occurring in adenomas of more than 1 cm.

Pituitary hemorrhage can be clinically silent or present as a migrainelike headache without associated signs or as aseptic meningitis (14). The headache may even temporarily respond to a triptan (15). Pituitary hemorrhage even in a macroadenoma can be overlooked and underimaged on a routine computed tomography (CT) scan of the head for acute headache using 10-mm cuts. A magnetic resonance imaging (MRI) scan even without pituitary views routinely identifies the pathology.

Pituitary macroadenomas with hemorrhage can result in a migrainelike headache with a III nerve palsy (16) and a migrainelike headache without aura with a normal examination (17). Although uncommon, pituitary hemorrhage with and without apoplexy should be considered in the differential diagnosis of acute headache (also see Chapter 8).

Leptomeningeal Metastasis

The term *leptomeningeal metastasis* is favored over the older term *meningeal carcinomatosis* because it includes malignancies other than carcinoma and excludes dura metastasis. Meningeal involvement (18) occurs in about 5% of all patients with cancer. The primary sites in cases of leptomeningeal metastasis due to solid non–central nervous system (CNS) tumors are breast (41.5%), lung (31.8%), melanoma (9.2%), gastrointestinal (5%), genitourinary (4.8%), head and neck (1.4%), miscellaneous (0.9%), and unknown (5.5%). In addition, for every 100 patients with disease from these primaries, one can expect to see about 42 patients with leukemia, 33 patients with lymphoma, and 18 patients with primary CNS tumors metastatic to leptomeninges.

Symptoms and signs of leptomeningeal metastasis include cerebral involvement in 50% (headache, mental status alteration, seizures, nausea, and vomiting), cranial nerve dysfunction in 56% (most commonly involved are III, IV, and VI followed by VII, VIII, and II), and spinal involvement in 82% (symptoms and signs due to spinal roots, spinal cord, and meningeal disease, including neck and back pain [19]). Headache, which is present in 33% to 62% of patients, is usually not severe.

A CT scan of the brain is usually normal in leptomeningeal metastasis, although meningeal enhancement with contrast administration is sometimes present. Hydrocephalus can be present in some cases. An MRI scan with contrast often demonstrates dura and arachnoid enhancement. Initial CSF examination demonstrates elevated white blood cells in 51%, elevated protein in 73%, and hypoglycorrhachia or decreased CSF glucose in 28%. CSF cytology is positive in 54% on the first lumbar puncture, in an additional 30% after the second, and in 1% more after the third. Sending a relatively large volume of approximately 10 mL or more of CSF for cytology may increase the yield. CSF biochemical markers, such as beta-glucuronidase, carcinoembryonic antigen, and lactic dehydrogenase isoenzyeme 5, may be present in cases of meningeal involvement from breast and lung carcinoma and melanoma but are nonspecific.

Colloid Cysts of the Third Ventricle

Colloid cysts (20) account for up to 1% of primary intracranial mass lesions and are usually asymptomatic until between 20 and 50 years of age. Colloid cysts usually present with one of the following: headache, bilateral papilledema, and, occasionally, false localizing focal, motor, and sensory signs; progressive or fluctuating dementia and raised intracranial pressure with or without headache; or paroxysmal severe headaches (21), nausea, vomiting, syncope, stupor, or coma. Episodic positional headaches, which occur in a minority of cases, may be due to movement of the colloid cyst on its pedicle in and out of the foramen of Monro with intermittent obstruction of CSF. Acute neurological deterioration, including coma in 15% and sudden death in 5%, is usually due to acute CSF obstruction by cysts 15 mm or greater in diameter (22).

Because of the risk of sudden death, surgery is generally recommended even in asymptomatic persons. Options include shunting of CSF, stereotactic cyst aspiration, transcortical-transventricular microsurgery, transcollosal microsurgery, and endoscopic surgery.

PSEUDOTUMOR CEREBRI

Introduction and Epidemiology

Pseudotumor cerebri (PTC) (23,24) is a syndrome of increased intracranial pressure without a space-occupying lesion. PTC can be diagnosed using the following criteria: the neurological examination is normal with the exceptions of papilledema, visual loss, and cranial nerve VI palsy; CSF pressure is increased (more than 20 cm H_2O in nonobese and more than 25 cm H_2O in obese patients); CSF analysis is normal with the exception of decreased protein; no hydrocephalus or mass lesions exist; and there are no other identifiable causes. When no secondary cause is identified, the syndrome is termed *idiopathic intracranial hypertension (IIH)*.

More than 90% of patients with PTC are young obese women. Obesity is present in 66% of adult men with PTC. The female-to-male ratio is 8:1, and the mean age at the time of diagnosis is 30 years. The average annual incidence per 100,000 population is as follows: 0.9 cases in the general population; 3.3 cases for women ages 15 to 44; and 19 cases for obese (20% above ideal body weight) women ages 20 to 44 years. In children, PTC affects boys and girls equally. Obesity occurs in 43% of patients with PTC ages 3 to 11, 81% in ages 12 to 14, and 91% in ages 15 to 17 (25). Associated conditions or secondary causes are common in children with PTC (26).

PTC is usually primary or idiopathic. There are numerous secondary causes and associations (Table 14-1). Medications associated with PTC include nalidixic acid, vitamin A (oversupplementation with vitamins or use of isotretinoin [Accutane] for acne), tetracycline and minocycline (27), quinolones, nalidixic acid, lithium, growth hormone, levonorgestrel, danazol, leuprolide acetate, stanazol, anabolic steroids, and corticosteroid withdrawal. Oral contraceptives are probably not associated with this disorder. Other causes include obstructive sleep apnea, head trauma, meningitis/encephalitis, intracranial and extracranial venous outflow obstruction and hypertension (cerebral venous thrombosis [Chapter 13], surgical ligation of extracranial veins, radical neck dissection, chronic otitis, hypercoaguable states, cerebral edema, cardiac failure, and chronic respiratory disease), systemic disease (renal disease and hypoparathyroidism), diseases with elevated CSF protein concentration (Guillain-Barré syndrome, systemic lupus erythematosis, and spinal tumors, especially oligodendrogliomas), hypertensive disorders (hypertensive encephalopathy, preeclampsia, and eclampsia) and large arteriovenous malformations. Other considerations in children include acute frontal sinusitis (28), Lyme disease (29), and parameningeal infections. Patients with optic drusen and a primary headache condition such as chronic daily headache might be confused with PTC. Optic neuritis and central retinal venous thrombosis are almost always unilateral.

Clinical Manifestations

Table 14-2 summarizes the features of idiopathic PTC. Headache is present in 75% or more of idiopathic cases of PTC. The headaches, which may be the patient's worst ever, are usually pulsatile, daily, and continuous. The headache can be unilateral, bilateral, frontal, or occipital, although a bifrontotemporal location is the most common. Nausea occurs in about 60%; vomiting in 40%; and orbital pain in about 40%. Pain on eye movement, retrobulbar and bilateral, is reported by up to 20% of patients. Many patients have coexistent migraine. Patients taking daily symptomatic medications are at risk of developing medication rebound headaches.

Papilledema is present in about 95%. Visual symptoms include transient visual obscuration (TVO, an episode of visual

Table 14-1. Etiologies of papilledema and headache

Intracranial mass

Obstruction or deformity of the ventricular system

Cerebral venous thrombosis

Extracranial venous obstruction
  Radical neck dissection
  Cardiac failure
  Chronic respiratory disease

Hypertensive encephalopathy

Preeclampsia and eclampsia

Meningitis/encephalitis

Leptomeningeal metastasis

Obstructive sleep apnea

Elevated CSF protein concentration
  Guillain-Barré syndrome
  Systemic lupus erythematosus
  Spinal tumors, especially oligodendroglioma

Large arteriovenous malformations

Optic neuritis (usually unilateral)

Central retinal venous thrombosis (usually unilateral)

In children
  Lead toxicity
  Lyme disease
  Parameningeal infection

Head trauma

Medications
  Vitamin A and derivatives (iroretinoin)
  Minocycline and tetracycline
  Quinolones
  Nalidixic acid
  Lithium
  Growth hormone
  Levonorgestrel
  Danazol
  Leuprolide acetate
  Stanazol
  Anabolic steroids
  Steroid withdrawal
  Nalidixic acid

Other medical conditions
  Renal disease
  Hypoparathyroidism
  Hypercoaguable states

Table 14-2. Features of idiopathic pseudotumor cerebri

Ninety percent of patients are young obese women

Headache present in 75% or more

Papilledema in 95%

Cranial nerve VI palsy in 25%

Transient visual obscurations in 70%

Visual loss in 30%

Secondary causes or associations are excluded

Diagnostic testing
    CT or MRI scans show no evidence of intracranial mass, hydrocephalus, or cerebral venous thrombosis
    Lumbar puncture reveals an elevated opening pressure
    CSF analysis is normal except for decreased CSF protein concentration in some cases

clouding in one or both eyes usually lasting seconds) in 70%, diplopia in 40%, and visual loss in 30%. Cranial nerve VI palsy, a nonlocalizing sign of raised intracranial pressure, is present in 25% of patients. Visual field testing may show early enlargement of the blind spot and peripheral constriction, especially nasal inferior.

PTC without papilledema should be considered in patients with chronic daily headache with any of the following features: obesity, pulsatile tinnitus, an empty sella, a history of head trauma or meningitis, or a headache unrelieved by standard therapy (30). In patients with pseudopapilledema, headaches, and/or TVO (which can also be due to pseudopapilledema), a lumbar puncture is required to exclude PTC (31).

Other symptoms and signs include unilateral or bilateral tinnitus, often pulsatile, in 60%; back and shoulder pain; arthralgias of the shoulders, wrists, and knees; ataxia; vomiting; and a cranial bruit over the mastoid or the temporalis (due to turbulence in the major venous sinuses). Uncommon manifestations include hearing loss, Lhermitte's sign, facial nerve paralysis in children, and facial pain. In infants and young children, PTC may present with nausea, vomiting, lethargy, and focal neurological deficits. Papilledema may not occur when there is an open fontanelle.

Biological Mechanisms

The cause of idiopathic PTC is unknown. Postulated mechanisms include an increased rate of CSF formation, an increased intracranial venous pressure, a decreased rate of CSF absorption, and an increase in brain interstitial fluid.

Diagnostic Evaluation

A number of causes of papilledema and headache need to be excluded (Table 14-1). A CT scan or MRI scan of the brain is first obtained to exclude a tumor or hydrocephalus. MRI is more sensitive than CT scans for the detection of some intracranial neoplasms and for the detection of cerebral venous thrombosis, especially with the addition of MR venography (Chapter 13). In some settings, MRI scans may be unavailable or impossible because the patient may be too obese, may be claustrophobic, or may have a contraindication. Elevation of intracranial pressure in PTC produced the following MRI findings in one study: empty sella, 70%; flattening of the posterior sclera, 80%; distension of the perioptic subarachnoid space, 45%; enhancement of the prelaminar optic nerve, 50%; vertical tortuosity of the orbital optic nerve, 40%; and intraocular protrusion of the prelaminar optic nerve, 30% (32). The scan may also show small ventricles.

If the scan shows no other explanation for the papilledema, a lumbar puncture is mandatory. The opening pressure should be carefully measured in the lateral decubitus position with the legs partially extended. If the patient is not relaxed, increased intraabdominal pressure can raise the opening pressure. The CSF analysis should be normal except for a low protein level in some cases. An ophthalmologist usually sees the patient to evaluate the fundus, visual acuity, and visual fields, which are then followed periodically to help prevent visual loss.

Management

Symptomatic causes of PTC should be treated or eliminated as appropriate. The treatment of idiopathic PTC depends on the clinical presentation. Obese patients should be encouraged to lose weight. In a study comparing obese women with weight loss of more than or equal to 2.5 kg during any 3-month interval, those who lost weight recovered more rapidly from both papilledema and visual field dysfunction (33).

Repeated lumbar punctures, withdrawing enough fluid to reduce the pressure to 12 to 17.5 cm H_2O, may benefit some patients. Many patients, especially obese ones for whom the lumbar puncture may be difficult or those who develop low back pain, do not want repeated lumbar punctures. Performance of the procedure using fluoroscopy can make the lumbar puncture easier. In some cases, the lumbar puncture may cause a low-CSF-pressure headache.

Medications may be effective (34). Diuretics may be of benefit. Acetazolamide, which inhibits carbonic anhydrase and reduces CSF production, may be effective, starting with a dose of 500 mg twice daily and increasing up to 4 g depending on the response. When PTC occurs during pregnancy, acetazolamide may be used after 20 weeks' gestation. Side effects include numbness and tingling of the hands and feet and periorally, nausea, and kidney stones. Furosemide, at a dose of 40 to 160 mg per day along with potassium supplementation, may also be effective. For patients who can not take acetazolamide or furosemide due to sulfa allergies, spironolactone or triamterene might be effective.

Patients with persistent headache may benefit from preventive medications used for migraine. Frequent use of analgesics may complicate the picture if medication rebound headaches develop. For some cases, there may be value in combining migraine-preventive drugs with a diuretic (with the exception of topiramate). Topiramate, using a migraine titration schedule and going up to

100 to 200 mg depending on effect (see Chapter 4), can be quite effective for PTC because of its effect on headache, weak carbonic anhydrase inhibition, and frequent weight loss (35). Corticosteroids are typically used for emergent treatment of impending visual loss. Disadvantages of corticosteroids include a rebound rise in intracranial pressure when steroids are withdrawn and weight gain and fluid retention, especially in already obese patients.

There are surgical treatments for papilledema and headache. Optic nerve sheath fenestration usually improves or stabilizes visual fields and acuity (36) and even improves headaches in up to 65% (37). The operation might be effective due to improved optic nerve axoplasmic flow and continuous intraorbital CSF drainage. However, this procedure may fail any time postoperatively and has a small risk of visual loss. Lumboperitoneal shunting is often effective for treatment of patients with severe visual loss at presentation or with intractable headache (with or without visual loss) (38). Disadvantages include the need for frequent shunt revisions in a few patients, low-pressure headaches, lumbar radiculopathies, and headaches from an acquired Chiari I malformation (see later). Recently, high pressures found in the intracranial venous sinuses in some idiopathic PTC cases have been associated with focal stenotic lesions in the lateral sinuses obstructing cranial venous outflow. The role of venous sinus dilatation and stenting for venous stenosis is being defined (39).

LOW-CEREBROSPINAL-FLUID-PRESSURE HEADACHES

Epidemiology

Low-CSF-pressure headaches are most often due to the following: post–lumbar puncture, the most common cause; spontaneous occurrence; and CSF shunt overdrainage (40–42). Infrequent causes include those that are traumatic, postoperative (following craniotomy or spinal surgery), and associated with other medical conditions (e.g., severe dehydration, diabetic coma, uremia, hyperpnea, meningoencephalitis, and severe systemic infection). The features of low-CSF-pressure headaches of any cause are the same as those of post–lumbar puncture headaches (PLPH) or spontaneous intracranial hypotension headaches. Rarely, intracranial hypotension can present with a severe encephalopathy (43).

SPONTANEOUS INTRACRANIAL HYPOTENSION SYNDROME (40)

Etiology

Almost all cases of spontaneous intracranial hypotension syndrome (SIH) result from spontaneous CSF leaks and most leaks occur in the spine, especially the thoracic spine. The precise cause is often not certain. A minority of patients report a trivial trauma such as coughing, lifting, pushing, falls, sports activity, and so on, which could be a cause. Uncommonly, a dural tear and CSF leak may result from a spondylotic spur or disc herniation. Single or multiple meningeal diverticula are often present in those with spontaneous CSF leaks and heritable disorders of connective tissue such as Marfan's syndrome. Weakness of the dural sac in others with SIH may be due to disorders of fibrillin and elastin.

Clinical Features

An orthostatic headache, a headache when upright that is relieved when lying down, is the most common clinical feature. The headache is usually but not always bilateral and may or may not be throbbing. Distributions include frontal, frontal-occipital, generalized, and occipital. In some chronic cases, a chronic daily headache is present without orthostatic exacerbation. In other cases, second half of the day headaches often with some orthostatic features may be present. Other types reported include exertional headaches without any orthostatic features, acute thunderclap onset, parodoxical orthostatic headaches (present in recumbency and relieved when upright), intermittent headaches due to intermittent leaks, the acephalgic form, or no headaches. Neck or interscapular pain may precede the onset of headache in some cases by days or weeks.

A variety of other clinical features have been reported: pain or stiff feeling of the neck that may be orthostatic; radicular upper limb symptoms; nausea and sometimes vomiting that is often orthostatic; unilateral or bilateral sixth cranial nerve palsy; less often than sixth nerve, third and fourth cranial nerve palsies; dizziness; muffled, distant, distorted, or echoed hearing; orthostatic tinnitus; blurred vision; photophobia; a superior binasal field cut; interscapular or low back pain; facial numbness or weakness; galactorrhea; labyrinthine hydrops; encephalopathy; stupor; coma; Parkinsonism, ataxia, bulbar weakness; paroxysmal ataxia of gait; frontotemporal dementia; bowel or bladder control difficulty; and subdural hematomas that may or may not be symptomatic.

Diagnostic Evaluation

A repeat lumbar puncture usually demonstrates an opening pressure from 0 to 70 cm H_2O (and can even be negative), although the pressure can be in the normal range (44), especially if the procedure is performed after a period of bed rest. The CSF analysis may be normal or can demonstrate a moderate, primarily lymphocytic pleocytosis (50 cells/mm^3 are common and values may be as high as 220 cells/mm^3), the presence of red blood cells, and elevated protein levels that can rarely be as high as 1,000 mg/dl. CSF glucose concentration is never low.

Table 14-3 summarizes MRI abnormalities of the brain and spine that are variably present. SIH can be present with normal MRI with contrast of the brain and spine. An MRI scan of the brain may reveal diffuse pachymeningeal (dural) enhancement with gadolinium without leptomeningeal (arachnoid and pial) involvement and, in some cases, subdural fluid collections, which return to normal with resolution of the headache. An interesting finding is reversible descent of the cerebellar tonsils below the foramen magnum (acquired Chiari I malformation), which can be due to SIH and also due to lumbar puncture and overdraining CSF shunts (45). The diffuse meningeal enhancement on MRI may be explained by dural vasodilation and a greater concentration of gadolinium in the dural microvasculature and in the

Table 14-3. MRI abnormalities in CSF leaks

Head MRI

Diffuse pachymeningeal (dural) enhancement

Descent ("sagging" or "sinking") of the brain

Descent of cerebellar tonsils (may mimic Type I Chiari)

Obliteration of some of the subarachnoid cisterns (i.e., prepontine or perichiasmatic cisterns)

Crowding of the posterior fossa

Enlargement of the pituitary

Flattening or "tenting" of the optic chiasm

Subdural fluid collections (typically hygromas, infrequently hematomas)

Engorged cerebral venous sinuses

Decrease in size of the ventricles (ventricular collapse)

Increase in anteroposterior diameter of the brain stem

Spine MRI

Extraarachnoid fluid collections (often extending across several levels)

Extradural extravasation of fluid (extending to paraspinal soft tissues)

Meningeal diverticula

Identification of level of the leak (not uncommonly)

Identification of the actual site of the leak (very uncommonly)

Spinal pachymeningeal enhancement

Engorgement of spinal epidural venous plexus

From: Mokri B. Low cerebrospinal fluid pressure syndromes. *Neurol Clin N Am* 2004;22:55–74, with permission.

interstitial fluid of the dura. (Before the characteristic picture of the postural headache and diffuse pachymeningeal enhancement on MRI was recognized, some patients underwent extensive testing, including meningeal biopsy, to exclude other conditions such as meningeal carcinomatosis and neurosarcoidosis.) The pleocytosis and elevated protein in the CSF and the subdural fluid collections are probably due to decreased CSF volume and hydrostatic pressure changes resulting in meningeal vasodilation and vascular leak.

CT myelography is more sensitive than other studies for determining the actual site of a CSF leak. Because the leaks can be high or low flow, early and delayed CT may be helpful. The study may demonstrate extraarachnoid fluid, meningeal diverticula, and extradural leak of contrast into the paraspinal soft tissues.

Radioisotope cisternography using indium-111 may demonstrate an absence or paucity of activity over the cerebral convexities at 24 or 48 hours. Less commonly, parathecal activity at the approximate level of the leak may be apparent.

Management

In some patients, the leak stops without treatment. Many of the treatments are the same as the treatment of post–lumbar puncture headache (see next section) including bed rest, hydration, overhydration, caffeine, theophylline, and lumbar epidural blood patches. There are a few case reports of the resolution of SIH with a short course (e.g., 10 days) of corticosteroids. If conservation treatment fails, an epidural blood patch may be effective; the success with each patch in spontaneous CSF leaks is about 30%. Thus many patients require more than one. Intrathecal fluid infusions or epidural infusions of crystalloids such as saline or colloids (e.g., dextran) have been reported with variable results. Epidural injection of fibrin glue might also be effective. Surgery may be effective for cases where the site of the leak is located.

POST–LUMBAR PUNCTURE HEADACHE

Epidemiology

Headache is the most common complication of lumbar puncture (46), occurring in up to 40% of patients after diagnostic lumbar puncture. There are a variety of unmodifiable and modifiable risk factors (Table 14-4). The five following demographic features increase the risk of post–lumbar puncture headache (PLPH): female gender, age (greatest in those 18 to 30 years of age), lesser body mass index, prior chronic or recurrent headaches, and prior PLPH. PLPH occurs twice as often in women as in men. The highest incidence is in the 18- to 30-year-old age group. Younger women may be at greater risk because of increased dural fiber elasticity, which could maintain a patent dural defect better than a less elastic dura. Estrogens might also increase substance P receptor sensitivity. The incidence is much less in children younger than 13 years and adults older than 60. Decreased dural fiber elasticity, a smaller epidural space, and decreased sensitivity of pain structures in the dura and blood vessels may explain the lower incidence in those over age 60. The incidence is greater

Table 14-4.   Risk factors for developing post–lumbar puncture headache

Patient demographics
  Female gender
  Age (greatest in range of 18-30 years)
  Lesser body mass index
  Prior chronic or recurrent headache
  Prior post–lumbar puncture headache
Quincke lumbar puncture needle
  Larger-diameter needle
  Perpendicular orientation of the bevel
Sprotte lumbar puncture needle
  Not reinserting the stylet

in patients with lesser body mass index (wt/ht^2). Younger female patients with a low body mass index may have the highest risk in developing PLPH.

Patients with a headache before the lumbar puncture are at greater risk for PLPHs, which are more severe and last longer than headaches of those with no preceding headache. Patients with chronic or recurrent headaches are three times more likely to develop PLPH as those without. Patients with a prior history of PLPH are also at increased risk. Risk factors related to the lumbar puncture needle are discussed later.

Clinical Manifestations

PLPH is a bilateral, frontal, occipital, or generalized pressure or throbbing occurring in the upright position and decreasing or resolving when supine. The headache is worse with head movement, coughing, straining, sneezing, and jugular venous compression. The headache begins within 48 hours in about 80% and within 72 hours in about 90% of patients. The onset can be immediately after the lumbar puncture or delayed for as long as 14 days. The headache lasts for less than 5 days in about 80%, although it can persist for 12 months. In one study, the headaches were reported as mild in 11%, moderate in 22%, and severe in 69% (47). Additional symptoms were present in the following percentages: neck stiffness, 43%; nausea, 66%; vomiting, 27%; cochlear symptoms, 15%; and ocular symptoms, 12%. In another series, nausea was present in 22% and vomiting occurred in 2%.

Dysfunction of cranial nerves III, IV, V, VI, VII, and VIII, usually transient, can also occur after lumbar puncture. Abducens paresis may follow as often as 1 in 400 lumbar punctures or spinal anesthetics and can be unilateral or bilateral. The paresis usually occurs 4 to 14 days after the procedure and usually resolves over 4 to 6 weeks. Reversible hearing loss may be symptomatic in up to 8% of patients.

Other complications of lumbar puncture include the following: uncal or tonsillar herniation; reversible tonsillar descent; spinal coning in patients with rostral subarachnoid block; nerve root irritation, herniation, and transection; low back pain; implantation of epidermoid tumors if a stylet is not used; infections; bleeding complications, including intracranial bleeding, traumatic lumbar puncture, and spinal hematomas; other complications include vasovagal syncope, cardiac arrest, seizures, and incorrect laboratory analysis of CSF.

Biological Mechanisms

Although the cause of PLPH is not entirely certain, the best explanation is low CSF pressure due to CSF leakage through a dural and arachnoid tear produced by the puncture that exceeds the rate of CSF production. CSF hypotension can produce headache and cranial nerve symptoms through downward descent of the brain and stretching of pain-sensitive structures, including the dura, nerves (cranial nerves V, IX, and X and the upper three cervical nerves), and bridging veins. Traction on cranial nerves can also result in cranial neuropathies. Intracranial venous dilatation and increased brain volume occur secondarily as the veins passively dilate in response to decreased extravascular pressure.

Diagnostic Evaluation

The diagnosis is usually made based on the typical history. MRI of the brain may show pachymeningeal enhancement just as in SIH. Lumbar MRI may also be abnormal following lumbar puncture. In one study of 11 patients, all had evidence of CSF leakage ranging from 1 to 460 mL (46). The CSF may be abnormal as in SIH.

Prevention (47,48)

Activity

Although many physicians recommend bed rest of varying durations for prevention, controlled prospective studies show no benefit for prevention of PLPH from bed rest for up to 24 hours in the supine, prone, or head-down position (49–51). There may be an increased incidence of PLPH in those recumbent as compared with patients immediately mobilized (52). An increased intake of oral fluids after the lumbar puncture does not prevent PLPH (53).

Diameter of Quincke Needle

The incidence of PLPH decreases with a smaller diameter of the Quincke (standard) needle. A smaller diameter needle produces a smaller tear in the dura and less potential for leakage. The incidence of PLPH decreases from up to 40% with use of a 20-gauge (G) needle down to 5% to 12% with use of a 24- to 27-G needle. Although smaller diameter needles can be used for spinal anesthesia and myelography, they are not a practical choice for diagnostic lumbar puncture. The CSF flow rate is very slow with smaller diameter needles. The flow rate in milliliters per hour for various needles is as follows: 20 G, 133; 22 G, 30.4; and 25 G, 10.5. In addition, the time needed to measure the CSF opening pressure with the manometer is increased from 43 seconds with a 20-G needle to 225 seconds with a 22-G needle, and 336 seconds with one of 25 G.

Parallel Insertion of the Bevel

Insertion of the bevel parallel to the longitudinal dural fibers reduces the incidence of PLPH by about 50% (54). Parallel insertion means that a plane passing through the flat part of the bevel, going through both edges of the bevel, is parallel to the long or vertical axis of the spine. This reduction of PLPH occurs because puncturing the dura with the bevel parallel to the fibers severs fewer fibers than when the bevel is perpendicular. The dural fibers run parallel to the long axis of the spine.

Atraumatic Needles

Atraumatic or pencil-point needles such as the Whitacre or Sprotte (Fig. 14-1) significantly reduce the incidence of PLPH when used for diagnostic lumbar puncture, myelography (55), and spinal anesthesia (56). This reduction is probably due to atraumatic needles spreading rather than cutting dural fibers.

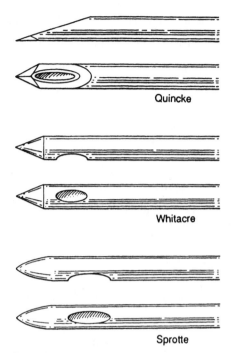

Figure 14-1. Three types of spinal needle tips: the Quincke, Whitacre, and Sprotte. (From Peterman SB. Postmyelography headache rates with Whitacre versus Quincke 22-gauge spinal needles. *Radiology* 1996;200:771–778, with permission.)

Based on one study using the Sprotte 21-G needle, the incidence is also reduced by replacing the stylet and rotating the needle 90 degrees before withdrawing it (57). (This is thought to be beneficial because a strand of arachnoid may enter the needle with the CSF, and when the needle is removed, the strand may be threaded back through the dural defect and produce prolonged CSF leakage.) Following diagnostic lumbar puncture with a Sprotte 21-G needle, for example, the incidence of PLPH is about 5% (58,59), compared with about 30% with a Quincke 20-G (standard) needle. In another study, the incidence of PLPH was 12.2% with a Sprotte 22-G needle as compared to 24.4% with a Quincke 22-G needle (60). The physician should consider use of an atraumatic needle in patients with risk factors (Table 14-4) for PLPH.

A few lumbar punctures with the Sprotte needle are usually necessary for the physician to feel comfortable. Because the tip of the needle is relatively dull, a sharp, short introducer is provided with the Sprotte needle. The introducer should be inserted to two thirds of its length before inserting the Sprotte needle. Unlike the Quincke needle, which can be wiggled and where the direction can be easily changed, the direction of the introducer has to be changed if the needle is not in the proper location. The procedure can be performed without the introducer by using the anesthetic needle to make a skin entry first, but use of the introducer is simpler for most physicians and may result in less damage to the needle tip. The feel of the atraumatic needle is different from the Quincke needle, and the physician must push harder with the introduction of the needle. Occasionally, the lumbar puncture cannot be performed with the Sprotte needle and the physician will have to change to the Quincke.

Management

Table 14-5 lists the treatments available for PLPH. Recumbent position relieves the headache but is inconvenient. Relief usually occurs within 20 seconds but can be delayed for up to 15 minutes. The longer the patient is upright, the longer the headache takes to resolve when supine. For more severe or persistent headaches, there are other effective treatments for PLPH (61). Analgesics are usually not helpful.

Caffeine and Theophylline

The methylxanthines caffeine and theophylline may relieve PLPH. The mechanism may be blockade of cerebral adenosine receptors leading to intracerebral arterial constriction, resulting in a decrease of cerebral blood flow and intracranial pressure or increased CSF production by stimulating the sodium-potassium pump. Oral caffeine, 300 mg every 4 to 6 hours (in tablet form or in beverages), is worthwhile trying initially for PLPH (62), although the relief may be transient. In a study of postpartum women with PLPH as a complication of epidural anesthetics, a single oral dose of 300 mg of caffeine reduced headache intensity within 4 hours in 90% of patients, with improvement persisting for 24 hours in 70% (63). A slow intravenous (IV) bolus of 500 mg of caffeine sodium benzoate may initially relieve headache in 75%, but permanent relief occurs in only about 50% (64). IV caffeine should be used with caution in patients with coronary artery disease and seizure disorders. In a pilot study, sustained-release theophylline (281.7 mg of theophylline) given orally three times per day also reduced the intensity of PLPH (65).

Table 14-5. Treatments for post–lumbar puncture headaches

Initial or for mild headache
    Bed rest
    Caffeine 300 mg orally every 6 to 8 hours or theophylline 300 mg
        orally every 8 hours
Moderate to severe headache present for more than 24 hours
    Bed rest
    Caffeine sodium benzoate 500 mg slow IV bolus
    Epidural blood patch

Epidural Blood Patch

The epidural blood patch (EBP) is the most effective treatment for PLPH and indicated for patients with moderate to severe headache present for more than 24 hours. The success rate is about 85% after one injection and near 98% after a second (66). The EBP is performed by slowly injecting 10 to 20 mL of the patient's blood into the lumbar epidural space at the same interspace or the interspace below the prior puncture. Following the procedure, the patient should stay in the decubitus position for at least 1 hour, and preferably for 2 hours, to obtain maximum benefit.

Based on a MRI study, the EBP has a mass effect that compresses the dural sac and displaces the conus medullaris and cauda equina (67). The mass effect disappeared after 7 hours. The main bulk of the clot occupied four or five vertebral levels with a thinner spread cephalad and caudad. The presumed mechanism of action is an immediate gelatinous tamponade of the dural hole (68). Alternative hypotheses include a sudden increase in CSF pressure that antagonizes adenosine receptors and compression of the dural sac, leading to activation of adrenergic, cholinergic, or peptidergic fibers (69).

Side effects of EBP are usually mild and transient. In a retrospective study of 196 patients, the following percentages reported various side effects: 37%, pain at the site of injection; 12%, pain in the lower extremities; 10%, sensory disturbances in the lower extremities; 8%, walking disturbances; and 8%, weakness in the lower extremities (70). The low back pain usually resolves from within 1 to 3 days. Potential complications include infection and arachnoiditis. Spinal subdural hematoma is a rare complication of EBP.

HEAD, EAR, EYES, NOSE, AND THROAT (HEENT) DISORDERS

Migraine and Vertigo (71)

Migraineurs report about 2.5 times more episodes of vertigo and about 2.5 times more spells of dizziness during headache-free periods than nonmigraineurs. Chapter 10 describes benign paroxysmal vertigo of childhood.

Migrainous Vertigo

Migrainous vertigo (also termed *vertigo as a migraine equivalent, migraine-associated dizziness, migraine-related vestibulopathy,* and *vestibular migraine*) has a female-to-male ratio of 1.5–5:1 and is more common in persons with migraine without aura than migraine with aura. Spontaneous or positional vertigo (rotational vertigo or other illusory sensations of movement) may occur; 40% to 70% have positional vertigo at some point. Head motion intolerance (episodic imbalance and illusory motion aggravated or provoked by head movements) is common. The duration of vertigo ranges from seconds to 5 minutes (20% to 30%), 5 to 60 minutes (10% to 30%), and hours to several days (20% to 50%). Occasionally, full recovery can take up to several weeks. Nausea and imbalance often accompany the vertigo; light and noise sensitivity may also occur. The frequency is highly

Table 14-6. Recurrent vertigo in patients with migraine: differential diagnoses for migrainous vertigo

Disorder	Key features
Benign paroxysmal positional vertigo (BPPV)	Vertigo lasting seconds to 1 min provoked by changes in head position. Positive positional test with typical torsional nystagmus.
Ménière's disease	Vertigo lasting 20 min to 3 hrs with concurrent hearing loss, tinnitus, and aural fullness. Progressive hearing loss over years is a diagnostic criterion.
Central positional vertigo	History similar to BPPV but latency, duration, and direction of positional nystagmus not typical for BPPV. Frequently additional neurological or neurotological signs.
Vertebrobasilar TIA	Attacks lasting mostly minutes, with brain-stem symptoms including vertigo, ataxia, dysarthria, diplopia, or visual field defects (not long-standing recurrent vertigo alone). Usually elderly patients with vascular risk factors.
Vascular compression of the 8th nerve	Brief attacks of vertigo (seconds) several times per day with or without cochlear symptoms, response to carbamazepine.
Perilymph fistula	Vertigo after head trauma, barotrauma, stapedectomy provoked by coughing, sneezing, straining, or loud sounds.
Autoimmune inner ear disease	Frequent attacks of variable duration, often bilateral with rapidly progressing hearing loss.
Insufficient compensation of unilateral vestibular loss	Brief and mild spells of vertigo during rapid head movements, oscillopsia with head turns to affected ear. Positive head thrust test to affected side.
Schwannoma of the 8th nerve	Rarely presents with attacks of vertigo. Key symptoms are slowly progressive unilateral hearing loss and tinnitus. Abnormal BAER.

From: Neuhauser H, Lempert T. Vertigo and dizziness related to migraine: a diagnostic challenge. *Cephalalgia* 24(2):83–91, with permission.

variable. Episodes of vertigo without headache can occur in persons who also have the same vertigo with migraine episodes as an aura or during the headache. Occasionally, mild and transient hearing loss and tinnitus can occur with the episodes of vertigo.

Table 14-6 summarizes some other causes of recurrent vertigo in migraineurs. The pathophysiology is not certain, but possibilities include spreading depression of cortical areas involved in vestibular processing and vestibular neuronal dysfunction. Migraine preventative medications may be helpful in reducing frequent episodes of migrainous vertigo. Triptans and vestibular suppressants such as promethazine, dimenhydrinate, benzodiazepines, and meclizine might be beneficial for prolonged acute attacks. Better treatment studies are needed.

Migraine and Ménière's Disease, Benign Paroxysmal Positional Vertigo, and Motion Sickness

The prevalence of migraine is twice as high in those with Ménière's disease as in controls. Thirty-six percent of patients with Ménière's disease have migraine and always experience at least one migrainous symptom (migrainous headache, photophobia, aura symptoms) along with their Ménière's disease attacks. Thus it can be somewhat difficult early on to distinguish migrainous vertigo from Ménière's disease. However, hearing loss is only an occasional, mild, and nonprogressive feature of migrainous vertigo, whereas hearing loss typically accompanies Ménière's disease progressing to severe hearing loss within a few years.

Migraine is two times more common in patients with idiopathic benign paroxysmal positional vertigo (BPPV) than controls. BPPV presents with recurrent short (usually 10 to 20 seconds; never more than 60 seconds) episodes of rotational vertigo provoked by changes in head position such as looking up or turning over in bed. Following frequent attacks, patients may report nonspecific dizziness or imbalance. The diagnosis can be confirmed by the Dix-Hallpike maneuver in 80% to 95% of cases that involve the posterior semicircular canal. The head down to the symptomatic side reproduces the vertigo sometimes after a latency of a few seconds and is associated with torsional nystagmus, often with a smaller upbeating vertical component, beating toward the undermost ear. Positional exercises such as those of Epley or Semont are curative in about 90% of cases. Approximately 5% to 20% of cases involve the horizontal canal. Attacks of vertigo are provoked by turning the head to either side in the supine position, whereas sitting up or lying down produces only minimal symptoms. Appiani's maneuver may be curative. BPPV may be best explained by the effects of mobile otoconia, canalolithiasis.

Motion sickness occurs more frequently in migraineurs (30% to 50%) than controls without headache or tension headache (about 20%). Motion sickness is especially common in children with migraine and in migraine with aura. Migrainous vertigo can be triggered by motion stimuli. Although not yet studied, I suspect that mal de débarquement is more common in migraineurs also. (Mal de débarquement is an inappropriate sensation of movement after termination of motion accompanied by disequilibrium but not vertigo. Mal de débarquement is usually experienced after a sea voyage but can also occur following other types of travel by car, train, air, or space travel. Most cases have an immediate onset but the onset may be delayed by up to several days. The duration of most cases is 24 hours, but a small minority may have persistent symptoms.)

Migraine and Other Causes of Dizziness

Dizziness due to orthostatic changes is much more common in migraineurs than in controls, which may be due to hypersensitivity to dopaminergic stimulation. Syncope during migraine attacks has been reported in 5%. Dizziness in migraineurs can also be due to hyperventilation (see Chapter 15) as well as panic attacks and generalized anxiety disorder, which are comorbid with migraine. Dizziness is also a side effect of many medications used to treat migraine including beta-blockers, tricyclic antidepressants, divalproex sodium, topiramate, and triptans.

Painful Ophthalmoplegias

With the exceptions of myasthenia gravis and chronic progressive external ophthalmoplegia, ophthalmoplegias (72,73) can cause unilateral orbitofrontal pain. The possible causes are extensive and include lesions from the midbrain to the orbit (Table 14-7). Ophthalmoplegic migraine is further discussed in Chapter 10.

Clinical Manifestations

Orbital pseudotumor and Tolosa-Hunt syndrome, which are inflammatory disorders of unknown etiology, have overlapping features. Orbital pseudotumor may be diffuse or localized to extraocular muscles, sclera, or the lacrimal gland and may cause uveitis or optic neuropathy. Unlike Tolosa-Hunt syndrome, orbital signs are often present in orbital pseudotumor, including unilateral lid swelling or ptosis, globe protrusion or displacement, and a palpable or visible orbital mass. Tolosa-Hunt syndrome is a recurrent granulomatous inflammation in the cavernous sinus and superior orbital fissure. The ipsilateral optic, oculomotor, trochlear, abducens, and first two divisions of the trigeminal nerve may be involved either singly or in different combinations. The pupil may be dilated or sluggish. The pain in both, which is ipsilateral to the involved side, is most intense in the orbit, brow, or directly in or behind the eye. The pain of Tolosa-Hunt may radiate to the ipsilateral frontal, temporal, or occipital areas. Both conditions respond to corticosteroids.

Diagnostic Evaluation

The diagnosis of both is one of exclusion using CT and MRI scans of the brain and orbit. Orbital pseudotumor may demonstrate infiltration of retrobulbar fat, enlargement of extraocular muscles, thickening of the optic nerve sheath complex, and proptosis. Imaging studies in Tolosa-Hunt syndrome may show soft tissue infiltration in either the orbital apex or the cavernous sinus without bony changes.

Ophthalmological Disorders

Refractive errors, imbalance of the extraocular muscles, diplopia, and a new refraction can cause tension-type headaches

Table 14-7.   Conditions causing painful ophthalmoplegia[a]

Vascular
   Arterial: hypertension, diabetes, carotid dissection, internal
      carotid aneurysm, posterior communicating aneurysm,[b]
      pituitary apoplexy, midbrain infarction[b]
   Venous: cavernous sinus thrombosis, carotid-cavernous fistula,
      dural-cavernous shunt
   Inflammatory
      Granulomatous: sarcoid, Wegener's granulomatosis, Tolosa-
         Hunt syndrome
      Dysimmune: systemic lupus erythematosus, rheumatoid arthri-
         tis,[b] mixed connective-tissue disorder, necrotizing vasculitis,
         temporal arteritis, multiple sclerosis,[b] segmental Guillain-
         Barré syndrome, chronic inflammatory demyelinating
         polyneuropathy[b]
      Parainfectious/postinfectious: Epstein-Barr virus,[b] mycoplas-
         ma,[b] herpes simplex,[b] herpes zoster, idiopathic cranial
         polyneuropathy
      Infectious: mucormycosis, aspergillosis, syphilis, tuberculosis,
         Lyme disease
Neoplastic
   Solid: epidermoid, meningioma, craniopharyngioma, chordoma,[b]
      chondrosarcoma, hemangioma, hemangiopericytoma, pituitary
      adenoma, metastases
   Hematological: lymphoma, macroglobulinemia, lymphoid
      hyperplasia
   Meningeal carcinomatosis
Other
   Ophthalmoplegic migraine

From: Averbuch-Heller L, Daroff RB. Painful ophthalmoplegias, Tolosa-Hunt
syndrome, and ophthalmoplegic migraine. In: Goadsby PJ, Silberstein SD, eds.
Headache. Boston: Butterworth-Heinemann, 1997:287, with permission.
[a]All may result in combined painful ophthalmoplegia.
[b]This condition usually involves a single ocular motor nerve.

(74–76). However, the eye is rarely responsible for headache
localized to the eye and orbit without obvious signs, such as a
red eye; symptoms, such as decreased vision; or a history of eye
trauma. The exceptions to the maxim that a white eye is not the
cause of a monosymptomatic painful eye or headache are the following: optic neuritis, in which pain on eye movement may precede visual loss; the first 30 minutes of acute angle-closure glaucoma, in which the eye may hurt before the cornea clouds;
subacute angle-closure glaucoma; posterior scleritis; uveitis;
corneal disease; intraocular or intraorbital tumor; and orbital
myositis (Table 14-8).

Clinical Manifestations

   Pain in or behind the eye or brow occurs in 77% of cases of
optic neuritis and can precede visual loss. The pain can be present at rest, with voluntary movement, and with pressure on the
globe. Eye movement worsens the pain because of traction of the

Table 14-8.   Causes of a white eye and monosymptomatic ocular pain or headache

Optic neuritis when pain on eye movement precedes visual loss

The first 30 minutes of acute angle-closure glaucoma

Subacute angle-closure glaucoma

Posterior scleritis

Uveitis

Corneal disease

Intraocular or intraorbital tumor

Orbital myositis

superior and medial recti on the optic nerve sheath at the orbital apex.

Acute angle-closure glaucoma presents with the rapid onset of severe orbitofrontal pain, nausea, vomiting, photophobia, visual halos, and loss of vision. A decreased level of consciousness may be present. Examination reveals a red eye, hazy cornea, fixed and mid-dilated pupil, and markedly elevated intraocular pressure. Chronic angle-closure glaucoma does not cause headache or a red eye. The presentation is visual loss due to a gradual elevation of intraocular pressure.

Subacute angle-closure glaucoma (SACG) is uncommon. Episodes of nausea, vomiting, blurred vision, facial pain, or headache last 1 to 4 hours and may occur at any time of the day or night. The headache may be in or over the eye or temporal. The eye is usually normal in appearance. Intraocular pressure measurement is normal between attacks. Gonioscopy (use of a mirrored prism on the surface of the eye) makes the diagnosis and reveals peripheral anterior synechiae, pathological adhesions between the iris and trabecular meshwork tissue, which close the outflow chamber of the eye and raise intraocular pressure. The symptoms of SACG can be misdiagnosed as due to migraine, cluster headache, or temporal arteritis.

In addition to acute angle-closure glaucoma, there are many other causes of a red eye (Table 14-9). The uveal tract is the pigmented middle ocular tissue, the iris, ciliary body, and choroid. About 50% of patients with uveitis have pure anterior involvement, iritis. The presentation of acute disease includes ocular pain, photophobia, miosis, and decreased vision. A subacute onset is often asymptomatic. Causes include rheumatological disorders (psoriatic arthritis, Reiter's syndrome, juvenile chronic arthritis), sarcoidosis, postoperative trauma, Kawasaki disease, Behçet's syndrome, syphilis, and herpesvirus.

About 50% of patients with uveitis have posterior involvement, chorioretinitis, with inflammation of the ciliary body and/or choroid. Posterior uveitis is more likely to cause visual loss than anterior disease and produces blurred vision, scotomas, and floaters. Toxoplasmosis is the most common cause. There are numerous infectious causes of panuveitis. Pars planitis is associated with multiple sclerosis.

Table 14-9.   Differential diagnosis of red eye

Conjunctivitis, the most common cause
Infectious (bacterial and viral), allergic, and sicca syndromes
Trauma
Iritis
Keratopathy, including corneal ulcer
Scleritis
Episcleritis
Subconjunctival hemorrhage
Periocular or orbital cellulitis
Angle-closure glaucoma
Blepharitis, inflammation of the lid margins

Inflammation of the sclera (scleritis) produces a violaceous hue of the sclera, a tender globe to touch, and fixed blood vessels to the globe. Severe and piercing referred pain to the jaw and forehead is usually present. About 50% of cases are idiopathic with other causes, including herpes simplex virus, herpes zoster, and collagen vascular disease. Posterior scleritis, a rare disorder, usually presents with pain, proptosis, ptosis, lid edema, and decreased vision but can present with only ocular pain. Episcleritis presents more acutely and with milder pain than scleritis.

Preseptal cellulitis involves the lids and structures anterior to the orbital septum. Orbital cellulitis, which is an infection of tissues posterior to the septum, can cause conjunctival infection and chemosis; proptosis with restricted ocular motility and pain; and optic nerve findings with decreased acuity and color vision and an afferent pupillary defect.

Ophthalmodynia

More than 60% of patients with ophthalmodynia (benign, brief, jabbing, unilateral eye pain) are migraineurs. Similar pain can occur with cluster headaches and temporal arteritis.

Nose and Paranasal Sinus Disorders

Introduction and Epidemiology

Nose and paranasal sinus disorders (77–80) are often misdiagnosed as the cause of headaches by laypersons and some physicians, perhaps the result of the ubiquitous sinus medication commercials and ads. Many of the 60% of persons with unrecognized migraines attribute their symptoms to sinusitis. However, disorders of the nose and paranasal sinuses are common and can cause headaches. The term *rhinosinusitis* may be more accurate than *sinusitis* because rhinitis usually precedes sinusitis, the mucosa of the nose and sinuses are contiguous, symptoms of nasal obstruction and discharge are common in sinusitis, and sinusitis without rhinitis is rare.

The lifetime prevalence of headaches associated with disorders of the nose and sinuses is 15%. About 50% of patients presenting to ear, nose, and throat (ENT) physicians with symptoms of sinusitis complain of severe headaches. About 70% of patients with chronic sinusitis requiring surgery have headaches. Sinusitis affects more than 30 million people per year in the United States. It is a complication of about 0.5% of upper respiratory infections in adults. Sinusitis is more common in children than in adults. It rarely involves the frontal and sphenoid sinuses in children because of the late development of these sinuses (the sphenoid sinus starts to pneumatize at 8 years of age, and the frontal sinuses develop from the anterior ethmoid sinus at about 6 years of age) but is involved in teenagers. Radiographical evidence of sinusitis is present in about 40% of adults without symptoms as an incidental finding.

Clinical Manifestations

Acute sinusitis lasts from 1 day to 4 weeks; subacute sinusitis, from 4 to 12 weeks; and chronic sinusitis, for more than 12 weeks. The headaches associated with sinusitis are usually continuous.

The location of the pain and the position that improves the headache vary, depending on the sinus involved (Table 14-10). Nasal congestion, purulent nasal drainage, and facial tenderness and pain are commonly present in acute sinusitis. Fever is present in 50% of adults and 60% of children. Anosmia, pain on mastication, and halitosis may also be present.

The pain of acute maxillary sinusitis is usually in the cheek, the gums, and the maxillary teeth. Less often, the pain is in the periorbital, supraorbital, or temporal areas. The pain is improved when supine and worse when the head is upright. The maxillary sinus is tender to palpation. Maxillary sinusitis is usually accompanied by rhinitis.

Acute frontal sinusitis causes severe frontal headaches with tenderness over the frontal sinus on percussion or palpation. The pain is less when the head is upright and worse when it is

Table 14-10.   Possible locations of pain and position that improves pain in acute sinusitis

Paranasal sinus	Possible locations of pain	Position that improves pain
Maxillary	Cheek, gums, maxillary teeth	Lying supine
	Periorbital, supraorbital, temporal	Head upright
Frontal	Frontal	Head upright
Ethmoid	Periorbital, retroorbital, temporal, inner canthal area, midline behind the nose	Head upright
Sphenoid	Retroorbital, occipital, frontal, temporal, vertex	Head upright

supine. Frontal sinusitis can result in brain abscess, meningitis, subdural or epidural abscess, osteomyelitis, subperiosteal abscess, orbital edema, orbital cellulitis, and orbital abscess.

Acute sphenoid sinusitis is responsible for 3% of all cases of acute sinusitis and usually associated with pansinusitis. Headache is always present and may be frontal, occipital, temporal, or a combination and periorbital. Vertex headache is rare. The pain is less when upright and worse when the head is supine. The headache may be aggravated by standing, walking, bending, or coughing; it is frequently associated with nausea and vomiting; and it may interfere with sleep. Nasal discharge and drainage are present in only about 30% of patients. Fever occurs in more than 50% of patients. Photophobia and eye tearing may be present. The headache and associated symptoms may lead to a misdiagnosis of migraine, meningitis, trigeminal neuralgia, or brain tumor. Complications of sphenoid sinusitis include bacterial meningitis, cavernous sinus thrombosis, subdural abscess, cortical vein thrombosis, ophthalmoplegia, and pituitary insufficiency. A parameningeal focus may cause an aseptic meningitis.

Acute ethmoid sinusitis typically produces pain in the periorbital, retroorbital, temporal, inner canthal area or between the eyes. Coughing, straining, or lying supine can worsen the pain, whereas keeping the head upright lessens it. Ethmoid sinusitis is usually associated with rhinitis. Complications of ethmoid sinusitis include meningitis, orbital cellulitis, cavernous sinus thrombosis, and cortical vein thrombosis.

Headaches associated with chronic sinusitis are usually low grade and diffuse and often accompanied by nasal obstruction, congestion, and fullness. Symptoms often increase during the day. A nighttime cough can be present.

Numerous anatomical variants in the nose and paranasal sinuses can be seen on endoscopic examination, CT scan, or both and are reported as causing headaches that improve with surgery (Table 14-11) (81). For example, the headache associated with a septal spur is reported as mild to moderate, frontal or facial, and dull or deep with fullness or heaviness. Anatomical variants as a cause of headaches including migraine are controversial. Because both anatomical variants and primary headaches are common, a primary headache can be misattributed as due to an anatomical variant. In addition, daily headaches can develop from overuse of decongestants or analgesics. Surgery can also have a powerful placebo effect.

A mucocele or mucous retention cyst is a mucus-containing cyst in the sinus. Those in the frontal, sphenoid, and ethmoid sinuses can enlarge and erode into surrounding structures. Mucoceles are most common in the maxillary sinus, where they are usually benign.

Biological Mechanisms

Normal sinuses contain anaerobic bacteria, and more than one third have a mix of anaerobes and aerobes. Aerobes present include Gram-positive streptococci (alpha, beta, and *Streptococcus pneumoniae*) and *Staphylococcus aureus*, and Gram-negative *Moraxella catarrhalis, Hemophilus influenzae,*

Table 14-11.   Anatomical variations in the nose and paranasal sinuses reported as causes of headaches

Septal deviation/spurs

Agger nasi cells

Uncinate process
  Medially or laterally bent
  Curved anteriorly
  Contacting middle turbinate
  Pneumatized

Middle turbinate
  Concha bullosa (pneumatized middle turbinate)
  Paradoxically bent
  Bulging into lateral nasal wall

Ethmoid bulla
  Large, filling middle meatus
  Anterior growth, overlapping hiatus semilunaris or protruding
    from middle meatus

Sphenoid sinus lesions
  Cysts, polyps, or mucoceles
  Mycotic infection

Maxillary sinus disease
  Cysts, polyps, or mucosal disease in contact with infraorbital
    nerve

From: Close LG, Aviv J. Headaches and disease of the nose and paranasal sinuses. *Semin Neurol* 1997;17:351–354.

and *Escherichia coli.* Anaerobes include Gram-positive pepto-cocci and *Propionibacterium* species. The *Bacteroides* and *Fusobacterium* species can cause chronic sinusitis. Obstruction of the ostia can result in ciliary dysfunction and retention of secretions, bacterial proliferation, and sinusitis.

Risk factors for sinusitis include systemic diseases (cystic fibrosis, immune deficiency, bronchiectasis, and the immobile cilia syndrome) and local factors (upper respiratory infection, allergic rhinitis, overuse of topical decongestants, hypertrophied adenoids, deviated nasal septum, nasal polyps, tumors, and cig-arette smoke). The sinuses are involved in nearly 90% of viral upper respiratory infections and usually clear spontaneously.

Diagnostic Evaluation

Plain sinus radiographs can diagnose acute maxillary or frontal sinusitis but are often inadequate for ethmoid or sphe-noid sinusitis. CT scans of the sinuses without contrast in the coronal plain are highly sensitive for the detection of nasal and paranasal sinus disease, including the ethmoid and sphenoid sinuses. Routine CT scan of the head may inadequately cover these structures. Because a MRI scan of the brain will also visu-alize nasal and paranasal sinus structures, MRI is the study of choice for the evaluation of headaches.

MRI is more sensitive than CT scan for the detection of fungal infection and the evaluation of nasal or paranasal sinus neoplasms. MRI is highly sensitive on T2-weighted images for the detection of retained fluid and inflamed tissue of the sinuses and may lead to an exaggeration of the significance of minimal sinus disease such as mild inflammation, small polyps, and retention cysts. In some cases on MRI, chronic sinusitis can mimic a tumor or an air-filled sinus. CT scan is the preferred examination when inflammatory sinus disease is suspected.

Transillumination and ultrasonography of the sinuses have low sensitivity and specificity. Diagnostic endoscopy with the flexible fiberoptic rhinoscope permits direct visualization of the nasal passages and sinus drainage areas. This procedure is complementary to a CT or MRI scan.

Management

Treatment of acute sinusitis includes a decongestant (phenylpropanolamine), mucoevacuant (guiafenesine), steam, saline, and appropriate antibiotics for at least 10 to 14 days. Intranasal steroids may improve the symptoms of nasal obstruction, but antihistamines are not helpful. Acute frontal and sphenoid sinusitis require immediate referral to an otolaryngologist for appropriate treatment to avoid intracranial complications.

The initial treatment of chronic sinusitis is the same as that for acute sinusitis. Otolaryngology consultation should be considered when the symptoms are not relieved with at least two consecutive 2-week courses of treatment.

Temporomandibular Disorders

Introduction and Epidemiology

The pain of migraine, cluster headache, chronic paroxysmal hemicrania, trigeminal neuralgia, and cough headache can be referred to oromandibular structures, including the teeth (82,83). Conversely, pain from the temporomandibular joint (TMJ) and associated musculature and ligaments—temporomandibular disorders (TMD)—can be referred to the head. TMD are common in the general population, with at least one sign present in 75% and at least one symptom in 33%. The lifetime prevalence of TMD is up to 69%. Women report symptoms of TMD 2.1 times more often than men. Only 5% of patients with signs of TMD require treatment, and fewer than 5% have associated headache.

Clinical Manifestations

Pain—usually localized in the muscles of mastication, the preauricular area, or the TMJ—is the most common presenting symptom of TMD. It is usually aggravated by jaw function. Because both the ear and TMJ have sensory innervation from the auriculotemporal nerve, otalgia is a common initial symptom of TMD. Signs include limited or asymmetrical jaw movements, joint noise on movement, and locking on opening. Joint noises, such as clicking and crepitus on movement (caused by poor lubrication in the joint associated with inflammation, arthritis, or a slipped disc), are also very common in asymptomatic subjects. TMJ joint displacement also occurs in up to 38%

of asymptomatic people. Because TMD and headache are both so common, it can be easy to misattribute headache as due to TMD.

The extraoral examination includes palpation of the TMJ both laterally (the lateral capsule of the TMJ) and endaurally (the posterior recess and capsule of the TMJ) for tenderness. Mandibular range of motion can be measured vertically and laterally. The maximum vertical opening, measured with a ruler from the incisal edge of the upper and lower central incisors, normally ranges from 35 to 55 mm. Deviation of the mandibular midline to one side is usually due to a failure of the condyle to slide forward on the side to which the chin is deviating. Lateral excursion distance to the right and left, measured from the midline of the maxillary central incisors to the midline of the mandibular central incisor teeth, usually ranges from 8 to 15 mm. Protrusive or forward mandibular movements can also be measured.

Biological Mechanisms

The TMJ is a diarthrodial synovial joint with two compartments separated by a fibrous disc. Rotation of the condyle within the fossa occurs with the first 25 mm of mouth opening. Then translation of the disc condyle complex along the articular complex allows for the second 25 mm of mouth opening.

Numerous disorders can cause TMD, including the following: synovitis, which can be due to excessive loading of the joint; myofascial pain, which can be associated with stress, grinding the teeth, and bruxism; osteoarthritis with roughened articular surfaces and worn-away cartilage; anterior disc displacement; adhesions, which can be due to trauma, synovitis, and lack of mobility; bony ankylosis, which can be due to trauma, infection, previous placement of TMJ implants or arthropathies; systemic arthropathies, including rheumatoid arthritis, Lyme disease, systemic lupus erythematosis, psoriatic arthritis, and gouty arthritis; and other conditions, such as tumors of the mandibular condyle, trigeminal neuropathy, parotid tumors, carcinoma with invasion of the pterygoid muscles, and traumatic condylar or subcondylar fractures.

Myofascial pain is the most common cause of pain arising from the TMJ. Malocclusion as a cause of TMD and headache is a controversial topic, with proponents arguing for and against an etiological role.

Diagnostic Evaluation

Tomograms of the maxilla and mandible, including open and closed position views of bilateral TMJs and a panoramic radiograph, are useful for diagnosing bony pathology. CT scan of the TMJs is useful for further defining bony pathology, such as tumors, bony/fibrous ankylosis, and osteoarthritis. MRI can diagnose soft tissue and other pathology, including synovial joint effusion, osteoarthritis, and disc displacement.

Management

TMD usually responds to conservative reversible therapies. An oral appliance or bite plate, which fits between the upper and lower teeth, relieves pressure or unloads the TMJ by creating a space between the upper and lower teeth. Forces are distributed throughout the dental arch. The appliance is placed in the mouth at night and sometimes during the day. A soft diet and the application of moist heat help relieve exacerbations of TMD. Physical therapy may be worthwhile initially; then the patient can continue passive jaw motion exercises and apply moist heat, ice, or both at home. Clenching or grinding habits may be reversed in some cases with patient education. Other patients may benefit from stress reduction techniques, such as biofeedback. Medications such as nonsteroidal antiinflammatory drugs (NSAIDs), muscle relaxants, tricyclic antidepressants, and the judicious use of narcotics can also be helpful.

When conservative treatment fails and the patient's TMJ symptoms are significant, surgery is indicated for a small percentage of cases. TMJ arthroscopy can be used for removal of fibrous adhesions and osteoarthritic cartilage, in cases of an anterior displaced disc without reduction (closed lock) and for steroid injection of inflamed synovial membranes. TMJ arthrotomy or open-joint surgery may be indicated for more advanced cases with obliteration of the joint space with adhesions and/or bone and for neoplasia.

Dental Disease

Dental disease uncommonly causes headache. Pericoronitis, infection or traumatic irritation around a partially erupted tooth, usually a molar, is the most common periodontal inflammation causing headache. Less often, pulpitis causes headache. Apical root infection or dental caries can cause a neuralgic pain in the second or third trigeminal divisions, with a constant aching and paroxysmal, jabbing pains. Hot or cold liquids in the mouth worsen the pain. Maxillary pain can be due to dental disease and maxillary sinusitis. Atypical odontalgia is pain in a tooth or tooth site in the absence of a detectable organic cause.

Atypical Facial Pain

Atypical facial pain (84) often affects patients in their fourth and fifth decades and is more common in women than in men. The pain has a steady, diffuse quality—described as deep, aching, pulling, boring, or gnawing—and can last hours or days. The pain is usually not limited to the distribution of the fifth or ninth cranial nerves and can spread over the areas supplied by the cervical root. The most common locations are the nasolabial fold or the chin overlying the lower gum. Atypical facial pain often begins after a dental procedure or insignificant facial trauma. Trigger zones are rare. The attacks are not precipitated by swallowing, cold water in the mouth, talking, or chewing. The pain is often refractive to analgesics, nerve blocks, and surgical intervention.

The diagnosis is made after excluding disorders of the eyes, nose, teeth, sinuses, and pharynx, including nasopharyngeal cancer as well as neuralgias and facial migraine. Depending on the symptoms, evaluation may include examinations by ophthalmologists, ENT physicians, dentists, and neurologists, and imaging studies, such as panorama radiographs and MRI scans of the head. A variety of medications can be used, such as antidepressants and baclofen, as well as behavioral and pain clinic approaches.

Gradenigo's Syndrome

Lesions of the apex of the petrous temporal bone, such as middle ear infections and tumors, can cause pain referred to the frontotemporal region and ear associated with a sixth cranial nerve palsy.

Eagle's Syndrome

Eagle's syndrome (85) is an uncommon disorder due to an elongated styloid process. (Either the styloid process alone or the combined lengths of the process and stylohyoid or stylomandibular ligaments exceed 40 mm.) Symptoms include dysphagia and unilateral pharyngeal pain radiating to the ear, which is worse with swallowing. Digital palpation (either through the pharynx or externally in the region of the mandibular angle) of an elongated styloid process can precipitate or increase pain.

There are numerous conditions in the differential diagnosis, including the following: neuralgias (glossopharyngeal, superior laryngeal, occipital, and nervus intermedius), migraine, cervicogenic headache, carotidynia, oromandibular disorders (TMJ disorders, unerupted or distorted third molar, faulty dental prostheses, and sialolithiasis), and ENT disorders (chronic tonsillitis, tonsillar calculi, otitis, mastoiditis, fracture of the hyoid bone, spasm of the pharyngeal constrictor muscle, Ernest syndrome, pterygoid hamulus bursitis, elongated pterygoid uncinus), and others (psychosomatic, foreign bodies, inflammatory and neoplastic diseases, nuchal cellulitis and fibrositis, and neck-tongue syndrome).

Some patients with Eagle's syndrome may respond to transpharyngeal injection of steroid and local anesthetic at the hyoid bone's inferior cornu or into the inferior tonsillar fossa. Surgical excision (there are advocates for both an intraoral and extraoral approach) often relieves the pain. In some cases, the styloid process may regenerate.

Neck-Tongue Syndrome

Neck-tongue syndrome is an uncommon disorder characterized by acute unilateral occipital pain and numbness of the ipsilateral tongue lasting seconds to 1 minute precipitated by sudden movement, usually rotation, of the head (86,87). The symptoms are due to transient subluxation of the atlantoaxial joint that stretches the joint capsule and the C2 ventral ramus (which contains proprioceptive fibers from the tongue originating from the lingual nerve to the hypoglossal nerve to the C2 root). Although neck-tongue syndrome can occur without obvious abnormalities, associated disorders include degenerative spondylosis, ankylosing spondylitis, psoriatic arthritis, and genetically determined laxity of ligaments of joint capsules. A benign, familial form of neck-tongue syndrome has been described without anatomical abnormality that spontaneously resolves during adolescence.

Nummular Headache

Nummular headache (a coin-shaped cephalalgia) is a rare, chronic, mild to moderate, pressurelike pain in a rounded or elliptical scalp area (most often the parietal region) of about 2 to 6 cm in diameter (88). Typically, the pain is continuous and persists for days to months with exacerbations described as lancinating pains lasting for several seconds or gradually increasing for 10 minutes to 2 hours. The affected area may show a combination of hypoesthesia and touch-evoked paresthesias. Spontaneous remissions may occur but the pain usually recurs. Diagnostic testing, including MRI of the brain and blood work, is normal. Although the cause is not known, the disorder is benign and may be due to a localized terminal branch neuralgia of the trigeminal nerve. Medication is often not required but, if needed, gabapentin may be effective.

The Red Ear Syndrome

Lance first described the red ear syndrome in 1995 and also proposes the term *auriculo-autonomic cephalalgia* (89,90). The disorder is characterized by episodic burning pain usually in one earlobe associated with flushing or reddening of the ear with a duration of less than 30 minutes to 3 hours in children and adults. In an individual, one ear or alternating ears or occasionally both ears can be involved in attacks, which can occur rarely or up to six times a month. The redness can occur without pain. The syndrome can be primary, occur during migraine headaches, or be in association with upper cervical spine pathology. The cause is uncertain. Lance postulates that the cause might be ABC (angry backfiring C-nociceptor) syndrome with pain and increased ear temperature due to antidromic release of vasodilator peptides or localized sympathetic dysfunction.

Burning Mouth Syndrome

Burning mouth syndrome (BMS) is characterized by a burning, tingling, hot, scalded, or numb sensation in the oral cavity in patients with a clinically normal oral mucosal examination (91). Synonyms include glossodynia, glossopyrosis, glossalgia, stomatodynia, stomatopyrosis, sore tongue and mouth, burning tongue, oral or lingual paresthesia, and oral dysesthesia. This pain most commonly occurs on the anterior two thirds and tip of the tongue but may also occur on the upper alveolar region, palate, lips, and lower alveolar region. Less commonly, the buccal muscosa, floor of the mouth, and the throat are affected. The pain may be constant or absent in the morning and progress during the day or intermittent with symptom-free intervals. The prevalence in the general population is 3.7% with a 7:1 female-to-male ratio usually in a middle-aged and elderly population with a mean age of 60 years.

The diagnosis is one of exclusion. Although perhaps one third may have a psychiatric disorder, often depression or anxiety, other causes should be considered. The following are causes: xerostomia or dry mouth, which can be due to medications such as tricyclic antidepressants or systemic disease such as Sjogren's; nutritional deficiency such as iron deficiency anemia, vitamin B_{12}, zinc, or B complex vitamins; allergic contact dermatitis due to food and oral preparation, which may be detected by patch testing; denture related; parafunctional behavior such as clenching or grinding the teeth, thrusting the tongue, or running the tongue along the teeth; candidiasis in up to 30% of cases that can be present with a normal exam; diabetes mellitus may be present in 5% of cases; and angiotensin-converting enzyme inhibitors (e.g., enalapril, captropril, and lisinopril).

If an underlying cause can not be found and treated, treatments that might be tried include empirical anticandidal agents, B complex vitamins, tricyclic antidepressants, oral clonazepam, and topical clonazepam (suck a 0.5 to 1 mg tablet for 3 minutes and then spit it out three times a day).

Ice Cream Headache

Ice cream headache (cold stimulus headache) can result from swallowing or holding in the mouth a cold food, beverage, or ice. This can cause short-lasting moderate to severe pain in the palate and throat that can be referred to the forehead, temple, or ears. The pain is usually bilateral but can be unilateral. The average onset of the pain is 12.5 seconds after the cold stimulus, and the average duration is 21 seconds (92). Occasionally, later onset and longer duration pain can occur. Ice cream headache may be more common in migraineurs. The mechanism might be cold stimulus–induced cerebral vasoconstriction followed by vasodilation causing pain. Anecdotally, treatments reported as effective include the following: drinking water without ice, placing the hand over the throat, burping, placing the tongue or pad of the thumb against the roof of the mouth, lowering the head below the level of the heart, massaging the carotid bifurcation, swallowing a pinch of salt, and placing a cold object on the inner wrist (93).

Hot Bath–Related Headache

Hot bath–related headache is provoked by pouring hot water over the patient or by soaking in a hot bath (94). The onset may be immediate or with a delay of up to 10 minutes. The headaches are bilateral with a gradual onset progressing to moderate to severe intensity over 10 to 15 minutes without associated aura, nausea, light, or noise sensitivity and a duration of 30 minutes to 6 hours. Those with hot bath–related headache are often migraineurs and may also have ice cream headaches (cold stimulus headaches). Bathing in hot water may also provoke a primary thunderclap headache (see Chapter 8).

External Compression Headache

An external compression headache results from continued stimulation of cutaneous nerves by application of pressure from a band around the head, a tight hat, sunglasses, or swim goggles. If the stimulus is prolonged, a migraine headache may be triggered (95). During a migraine headache associated with cutaneous allodynia, some migraineurs do not wear hats, headbands, or sunglasses due to discomfort.

Glossopharyngeal neuralgia

Glossopharyngeal neuralgia is a rare disorder with an incidence of 1.3% or less of trigeminal neuralgia with onset typically after the sixth decade. Glossopharyngeal neuralgia and trigeminal neuralgia occur in a combined form in 10% of patients. Paroxysmal pain occurs in the throat, tonsillar fossa, tongue, and ear lasting for several seconds to one minute. Triggers include swallowing, particularly cold liquids, and, occasionally, yawning or sneezing. Up to 2% of patients have syncope during pain paroxysms, probably the result of bradycardia or asystole.

The evaluation of a patient who has glossopharyngeal neuralgia should include an MRI scan with contrast. Secondary glossopharyngeal neuralgia may be the result of an oropharyngeal malignancy, a peritonsillar infection, or vascular compression by a loop of a posterior fossa vessel compressing the nerve.

Glossopharyngeal neuralgia is treated with anticonvulsant medications, such as carbamazepine, phenytoin, baclofen, and gabapentin. Patients who are refractory to medical therapy can be treated surgically with intracranial sectioning of the glossopharyngeal nerve and the upper rootlets of the vagus nerve as well as microvascular decompression of the ninth cranial nerve.

REFERENCES

1. Patchell RA. Metastatic brain tumors. *Neurol Clin* 1995;13: 915–925.
2. Vasquez-Barquero A, Ibanez FJ, Herrera S, et al. Isolated headache as the presenting clinical manifestation of intracranial tumors: a prospective study. *Cephalalgia* 1994;14:270–272.
3. Forsyth PA, Posner JB. Headaches in patients with brain tumors: a study of 111 patients. *Neurology* 1993;43:1678–1683.
4. Pfund Z, Szapary L, Jaszbernyi O, et al. Headache in intracranial tumors. *Cephalalgia* 1999;19:787–790.
5. Suwanwela N, Phanthumchinda K, Kaoropthum S. Headache in brain tumor: a cross-sectional study. *Headache* 1994;34:435–438.
6. Purdy RA, Kirby S. Headaches and brain tumors. *Neurol Clin N Am* 2004;22:39–53.
7. Abe T, Matsumoto K, Kuwazawa J, et al. Headache associated with pituitary adenomas. *Headache* 1998;38:782–786.
8. Matharu MS, Levy MJ, Merry MT, et al. SUNCT syndrome secondary to prolactinoma. *J Neurol Neurosurg Psychiatry* 2003;74: 1590–1592.
9. Milos P, Havelius U, Hindfelt B. Clusterlike headache in a patient with a pituitary adenoma. With a review of the literature. *Headache* 1996;35:184–188.
10. Friedman AH, Wilkins RH, Kenan PD, et al. Pituitary adenoma presenting as facial pain: report of two cases and review of the literature. *Neurosurgery* 1982;10:742–745.
11. Selky AK, Pascuzzi R. Raeder's paratrigeminal syndrome due to spontaneous dissection of the cervical and petrous internal carotid artery. *Headache* 1995;35:432–435.
12. Rose-Innes AP. Pituitary apoplexy. In: Gilman S, ed. *MedLink neurology*. San Diego: MedLink Corp, 2004. Available at www.medlink.com.
13. Rolih CA, Ober KP. Pituitary apoplexy. *Endocrinol Metab Clin North Am* 1993;22:291–302.
14. Haviv YS, Goldschmidt N, Safadi R. Pituitary apoplexy manifested by sterile meningitis. *Eur J Med Res* 1998;12:263–264.
15. Krimsky W, Weiss H. Cryptic pituitary hemorrhage presenting with headache. *Headache* 2002;42:291–293.
16. Silvestrini M, Matteis M, Cupini LM, et al. Ophthalmoplegic migraine-like syndrome due to pituitary apoplexy. *Headache* 1994;34:484–486.

17. Evans RW. Migraine-like headaches associated with pituitary hemorrhage. *Headache* 1997;37:455–456.
18. Junck L. Leptomeningeal metastasis. In: Gilman S, ed. *MedLink neurology.* San Diego: MedLink Corp, 2004. Available at www.medlink.com.
19. Wasserstrom W, Glass J, Posner J. Diagnosis and treatment of leptomeningeal metastases from solid tumors: experience with 90 patients. *Cancer* 1982;49:759–772.
20. Shaikh ZA. Colloid cysts. In: Gilman S, ed. *MedLink neurology.* San Diego: MedLink Corp, 2004. Available at www.medlink.com.
21. Young WB, Silberstein SD. Paroxysmal headache caused by colloid cyst of the third ventricle: case report and review of the literature. *Headache* 1997;37:15–20.
22. Mathiesen T, Grane P, Lindgren L, et al. Third ventricular colloid cysts: a consecutive 12-year series. *J Neurosurg* 1997;86:5–12.
23. Friedman DI. Pseudotumor cerebri. *Neurol Clin N Am* 2004;22:99–131.
24. Silberstein SD, Lipton RB, Goadsby PJ. Headache associated with non-vascular intracranial disease. In: *Headache in clinical practice.* London: Martin Dunitz, 2002:189–214.
25. Balcer LJ, Liu GT, Forman S, et al. Idiopathic intracranial hypertension: relation of age and obesity in children. *Neurology* 1999;52:870–872.
26. Scott IU, Siatkowsky RM, Eneyni M, et al. Idiopathic intracranial hypertension in children and adolescents. *Am J Ophthalmol* 1997;124:253–255.
27. Chiu AM, Chuenkongkaew WL, Cornblath WT, et al. Minocycline treatment and pseudotumor cerebri syndrome. *Am J Ophthalmol* 1998;126:116–121.
28. Keren T, Lahat E. Pseudotumor cerebri as a presenting symptom of acute sinusitis in a child. *Pediatr Neurol* 1998;19:153–154.
29. Kan L, Sood KS, Maytal J. Pseudotumor cerebri in Lyme disease: a case report and literature review. *Pediatr Neurol* 1998;18:439–441.
30. Wang SJ, Silberstein SD, Patterson S, et al. Idiopathic intracranial hypertension without papilledema: a case-control study in a headache center. *Neurology* 1998;51:245–249.
31. Jacome DE. Headaches, idiopathic intracranial hypertension, and pseudopapilledema. *Am J Med Sci* 1998;316:408–410.
32. Brodsky MC, Vaphiades M. Magnetic resonance imaging in pseudotumor cerebri. *Ophthalmology* 1998;105:1686–1693.
33. Kupersmith MJ, Garnell L, Turbin R, et al. Effects of weight loss on the course of idiopathic intracranial hypertension in women. *Neurology* 1998;50:1094–1098.
34. Corbett JJ. Headache due to idiopathic intracranial hypertension. In: Goadsby PJ, Silberstein SD, eds. *Headache.* Boston: Butterworth-Heinemann, 1997:279–283.
35. Friedman DI, Eller PE. Topiramate for treatment of idiopathic intracranial hypertension. *Headache* 2003;43:592.
36. Kelman SE, Heaps R, Wolf A, et al. Optic nerve decompression surgery improves visual function in patients with pseudotumor cerebri. *Neurosurgery* 1992;30:391–395.
37. Corbett JJ, Nerad JA, Tse DT, et al. Results of optic nerve sheath fenestration for pseudotumor cerebri: the lateral orbitotomy approach. *Arch Ophthalmol* 1988;106:1391.

38. Burgett RA, Purvin VA, Kawasaki A. Lumboperitoneal shunting for pseudotumor cerebri. *Neurology* 1997;49:734–739.
39. Higgins JN, Cousins C, Owler BK, et al. Idiopathic intracranial hypertension: 12 cases treated by venous sinus stenting. *J Neurol Neurosurg Psychiatry* 2003;74(12):1662–1666.
40. Mokri B. Low cerebrospinal fluid pressure syndromes. *Neurol Clin N Am* 2004;22:55–74.
41. Mokri B, Piepgras DG, Miller GM. Syndrome of orthostatic headaches and diffuse pachymeningeal gadolinium enhancement. *Mayo Clin Proc* 1997;72:400–413.
42. Ferrante E, Riva M, Gatti A, et al. Intracranial hypotension syndrome: neuroimaging in five spontaneous cases and etiopathogenetic correlations. *Clin Neurol Neurosurg* 1998;100:33–39.
43. Beck CE, Rizk NW, Kiger LT, et al. Intracranial hypotension presenting with severe encephalopathy: case report. *J Neurosurg* 1998;89:470–473.
44. Mokri B, Hunter SF, Atkinson JL, et al. Orthostatic headaches caused by CSF leak but with normal CSF pressures. *Neurology* 1998;51:786–790.
45. Atkinson JLD, Weinshenker BG, Miller GM, et al. Acquired Chiari I malformation secondary to spontaneous cerebrospinal fluid leakage and chronic intracranial hypotension syndrome in seven cases. *J Neurosurg* 1998;88:237–242.
46. Evans RW. Complications of lumbar puncture. *Neurol Clin* 1998;16:83–105.
47. Evans RW, Armon C, Frohman EM, et al. Assessment: prevention of post-lumbar puncture headaches: report of the therapeutics and technology assessment subcommittee of the American Academy of Neurology. *Neurology* 2000;55:909–914.
48. Turnbull DK, Shepherd DB. Post-dural puncture headache: pathogenesis, prevention, and treatment. *Br J Anaesth* 2003;91: 718–729.
49. Hilton-Jones D, Harrad RA, Gill MW, et al. Failure of postural maneuvers to prevent lumbar puncture headache. *J Neurol Neurosurg Psychiatry* 1982;45:743–746.
50. Cook PT, Davies MJ, Beavis RE. Bed rest and postlumbar puncture headache. The effectiveness of 24 hours' recumbency in reducing the incidence of postlumbar puncture headache. *Anaesthesia* 1989;44:389–391.
51. Spriggs DA, Burn DJ, French J, et al. Is bed rest useful after diagnostic lumbar puncture? *Postgrad Med J* 1992;68:518–583.
52. Vilming ST, Schrader H, Monstad I. Post-lumbar puncture headache: the significance of body posture. A controlled study of 300 patients. *Cephalalgia* 1988;8:75–78.
53. Dieterich M, Brandt T. Incidence of post lumbar puncture headache is independent of daily fluid intake. *Eur Arch Psychiatry Neurol Sci* 1988;237:194–195.
54. Fishman RA. *Cerebrospinal fluid in diseases of the nervous system,* 2nd ed. Philadelphia: WB Saunders, 1992.
55. Prager JM, Roychowdhury S, Gorey MT, et al. Spinal headaches after myelograms: comparison of needle types. *AJR* 1996;196: 1289–1292.
56. Jeanjean P, Montpellier D, Carnec J, et al. Post-spinal headache: a prospective, multicentre study in young adults. *Ann Fr Anesth Reanim* 1997;16:350–353.

57. Strupp M, Brandt T. Should one reinsert the stylet during lumbar puncture? *N Engl J Med* 1997;336:1190.

58. Engelhardt A, Oheim S, Neundörfer B. Post-lumbar puncture headache: experiences with Sprotte's atraumatic needle. *Cephalalgia* 1992;12:259.

59. Jager H, Krane M, Schimrigk K. [Lumbar puncture: the post-puncture syndrome. Prevention with an "atraumatic" puncture needle, clinical observations.] *Schweiz Med Wochenschr* 1993;123: 1985–1990.

60. Strupp M, Schueler O, Straube A, et al. "Atraumatic" Sprotte needle reduces the incidence of post-lumbar puncture headaches. *Neurology* 2001;57(12):2310–2312.

61. Choi A, Launto CE, Cunningham FE. Pharmacologic management of postdural puncture headache. *Ann Pharmacother* 1996;30:832–839.

62. Leibold RA, Yealy DM, Coppola M, et al. Post-dural-puncture headache: characteristics, management, and prevention. *Ann Emerg Med* 1993;22:1863–1870.

63. Camann WR, Murray RS, Mushlin PS, et al. Effects of oral caffeine on postdural puncture headache: a double-blind, placebo-controlled trial. *Anesth Analg* 1990;70:181–184.

64. Sechzer PH, Abel L. Post-spinal anesthesia headache treated with caffeine: evaluation with demand method. Part 1. *Curr Ther Res* 1978;24:307–312.

65. Feuerstein TJ, Zeides A. Theophylline relieves headache following lumbar puncture: placebo-controlled, double-blind pilot study. *Klin Wochenschr* 1986;64:216–218.

66. Tarkkila PJ, Miralles JA, Palomaki EA. The subjective complications and efficiency of the epidural blood patch in the treatment of postdural puncture headache. *Reg Anesth Pain Med* 1989;14:247–250.

67. Beards SCD, Jackson A, Griffiths AG, et al. Magnetic resonance imaging of extradural blood patches: appearances from 30 min to 18 h. *Br J Anaesth* 1993;71:182–188.

68. Olsen KS. Epidural blood patch in the treatment of post-lumbar puncture headache. *Pain* 1987;30:293–301.

69. Raskin NH. Lumbar puncture headache: a review. *Headache* 1990;30:197–200.

70. Tarkkila PJ, Miralles JA, Palomaki EA. The subjective complications and efficiency of the epidural blood patch in the treatment of postdural puncture headache. *Reg Anesth Pain Med* 1989;14:247–250.

71. Neuhauser H, Lempert T. Vertigo and dizziness related to migraine: a diagnostic challenge. *Cephalalgia* 2004;24:83–91.

72. Averbuch-Heller L, Daroff RB. Painful ophthalmoplegias, Tolosa-Hunt syndrome, and ophthalmoplegic migraine. In: Goadsby PJ, Silberstein SD, eds. *Headache.* Boston: Butterworth-Heinemann, 1997:285–297.

73. Goodwin J. Orbital pseudotumor and Tolosa-Hunt syndrome. In: Gilman S, ed. *MedLink neurology.* San Diego, MedLink Corp, 2004. Available at www.medlink.com.

74. Lewis J, Fourman S. Subacute angle-closure glaucoma as a cause of headache in the presence of a white eye. *Headache* 1998;38:684–686.

75. Daroff RB. Ocular causes of headache. *Headache* 1998;38:661.

76. Lee AG, Beaver HA, Brazis PW. Painful ophthalmologic disorders and eye pain for the neurologist. *Neurol Clin N Am* 2004;22:75–97.
77. Close LG, Aviv J. Headaches and disease of the nose and paranasal sinuses. *Semin Neurol* 1997;17:351–354.
78. Winstead W. Rhinosinusitis. *Prim Care* 2003;30(1):137–154.
79. Silberstein SD. Rhinosinus-related headache. In: Gilman S, ed. *MedLink neurology.* San Diego: MedLink Corp, 2004. Available at www.medlink.com.
80. Silberstein SD. Headaches due to nasal and paranasal sinus disease. *Neurol Clin N Am* 2004;22:1–19.
81. Clerico DM. Sinus headaches reconsidered: referred cephalalgia of rhinologic origin masquerading as refractory primary headaches. *Headache* 1995;35:185–192.
82. Israel HA. Temporomandibular disorders: what the neurologist needs to know. *Semin Neurol* 1997;17:355–366.
83. Stiles A, Graff-Radford SB. Head pain relating to oromandibular structures. In: Gilman S, ed. *MedLink neurology.* San Diego: MedLink Corp, 2004. Available at www.medlink.com.
84. Davidoff RA. Cranial neuralgias and atypical facial pain. In: Gilman S, ed. *MedLink neurology.* San Diego: MedLink Corp, 2004. Available at www.medlink.com.
85. Montalbetti L, Ferrandi D, Pergami P, et al. Elongated styloid process and Eagle's syndrome. *Cephalalgia* 1995;15:80–93.
86. Lance JW, Anthony W. Neck-tongue syndrome on sudden turning of the head. *J Neurol Neurosurg Psychiatry* 1980;43:97–101.
87. Lewis DW, Frank LM, Toor S. Familial neck-tongue syndrome. *Headache* 2003;43(2):132–134.
88. Pareja JA, Pareja J, Barriga FJ, et al. Nummular headache: a prospective series of 14 new classes. *Headache* 2004;44:611–614.
89. Lance JW. The red ear syndrome. *Neurology* 1996;47:617-620.
90. Evans RW, Lance JW. The red ear syndrome: an auriculoautonomic cephalalgia. *Headache* 2004; 44:835–836.
91. Drage LA, Rogers RS. Burning mouth syndrome. *Dermatol Clin* 2003;21:135–145.
92. Bird N, MacGregor EA, Wilkinson MI. Ice cream headache-site, duration, and relationship to migraine. *Headache* 1992;32:35–38.
92. Evans RW, Lance JW. The red ear syndrome: an auriculo-autonomic cephalgia. *Headache* 2004; 44:835–336.
93. Rapid responses. 1999-2004. bmj.com. to Hulihan J. Ice cream headache. *BMJ* 1997;314:1364.
94. Müngen B, Bulut S. Hot bath-related headache: four cases with headaches occurring after taking a hot bath. *Cephalalgia* 2003;23:846–849.
95. Pestronk A, Pestronk S. Goggle migraine. *N Engl J Med* 1983;308:226.

Other Secondary Headaches and Associated Disorders

Randolph W. Evans

This chapter covers other secondary headaches and associated disorders, including the following: cough, exertional, and sexual headaches; Chiari I malformation; infection and inflammation; metabolic disorders; sleep disorders; seizures; multiple sclerosis; and central pain syndrome (1,2).

COUGH, EXERTIONAL, AND SEXUAL HEADACHES

Introduction and Epidemiology

Headaches can be triggered by coughing, exertion, and sexual activity (3–5). The definitions of the International Headache Society (IHS) 2nd edition 2004 follow. The lifetime prevalence of benign cough headache, benign exertional headache, and headache associated with sexual activity is 1% for each (6). All three headache types occur most often in men. In 1996 Pascual et al. reported 72 benign and symptomatic cases of cough, exertional, and sexual headaches they had evaluated over a 15-year period (7). The findings are summarized in Table 15-1. The sexual headache reported is the explosive type. The one patient with a subarachnoid hemorrhage (SAH) had only a single headache; those with the benign type had multiple sexual headaches.

Cough Headache: Clinical Manifestations and Management

Primary (benign) cough headache is of sudden onset, lasting from 1 second to 30 minutes, brought on by and occurring only in association with coughing, straining, and/or Valsalva maneuver. Primary cough headache is usually bilateral and predominantly affects patients older than 40 years. In some cases, the onset may be after a respiratory infection with cough. The term *cough headache* is also used by many to include headache brought on by sneezing, weight lifting, bending, stooping, or straining with a bowel movement. Weight lifting can also cause an acute bilateral nuchal-occipital or nuchal-occipital-parietal headache that can persist as a residual ache for days or weeks, which may be due to stretching of cervical ligaments and tendons. Other secondary causes should be excluded as appropriate such as subarachnoid hemorrhage. Although primary cough headache is associated with an increase in intracranial pressure, the exact cause of the pain is not certain. Posterior cranial fossa overcrowding may be a contributing factor (8).

Primary cough headache may be diagnosed only after neuroimaging has excluded structural lesions such as posterior fossa tumor, Arnold-Chiari malformation (discussed later), platybasia, basilar impression, spontaneous intracranial hypotension, pneumocephalus, and subdural hematoma. Internal carotid stenosis

Table 15-1. Cough, exertional, and sexual headaches

Parameter	Cough headache		Exertional headache		Sexual headache	
	Benign	Symptomatic	Benign	Symptomatic	Benign	Symptomatic
Patients (n)	13	17	16	12	13	1
Age, range (years)	67 ± 11	39 ± 14	24 ± 11	42 ± 14	41 ± 9	60
	44–81	15–63	10–48	18–61	24–57	
Sex (% men)	77	59	88	43	85	100
Duration	Secs to 30 min	Secs to days	Min to 2 days	1 day to 1 month	1 min to 3 hours	10 days
Bilateral localization	92%	94%	56%	100%	77%	Yes
Quality	Sharp, stabbing, pulsating	Bursting	Pulsating, stabbing	Explosive,	Explosive + pulsating	Explosive + pulsating
Other manifestations	No	Posterior fossa signs	Nausea, photophobia	Nausea, vomiting, double vision, neck rigidity	None	Vomiting, neck rigidity
Diagnosis	Idiopathic	Chiari Type I malformation	Idiopathic	SAH, sinusitis, brain metastases	Idiopathic	SAH

From: Pascual J, Iglesias F, Oterino A, et al. Cough, exertional, and sexual headaches: an analysis of 72 benign and symptomatic cases. *Neurology* 1996;46:1520–1524, modified with permission.

and unruptured intracranial saccular aneurysms are questionable associations with unilateral cough headache. An MRI of the brain with contrast is the preferred imaging study to exclude secondary causes.

Benign cough headaches (and less often secondary cases) may respond to indomethacin 25 to 50 mg three times a day (9), lumbar puncture (10), methysergide (11), acetazolamide (500 to 2,000 mg per day in divided doses) (12), and perhaps topiramate (because of its weak carbonic anhydrase inhibition). Some patients may have an abrupt recovery after extraction of abscessed teeth.

Exertional Headache: Clinical Manifestations and Management

Primary (benign) exertional headache is brought on by and occurs only during or after physical exercise and lasts from 5 minutes to 48 hours. It is typically a throbbing bilateral headache and not attributed to another cause. Reported activities include running, rowing, tennis, and swimming. One particular activity may precipitate the headache in some individuals but not others. This headache type is prevented by avoiding excessive exertion, particularly in hot weather or at high altitudes. Exercise can be a trigger for a typical migraine for some migraineurs. Secondary causes to be excluded include SAH (Chapter 8), pheochromocytomas, cardiac ischemia, middle cerebral artery dissection (see Chapter 13), paranasal sinusitis, intracranial neoplasms, colloid cysts of the third ventricle, and hypoplasia of the aortic arch after successful coarctation repair. An MRI of the brain with MRA will assist in ruling out structural or vascular lesions.

In some cases, exertional headache may be prevented by a warm-up period. Some patients may choose to avoid the particular activity. Indomethacin (25 to 150 mg per day) may work as a preventive taken minutes to 1 hour before exertion. Prophylactic drugs used for migraine such as beta-blockers may be effective for some patients.

Sex Headaches: Clinical Manifestations and Management

The IHS 2nd edition criteria describe two types of primary headache associated with sexual activity (previously called benign sex headache or coital cephalalgia) in the absence of any intracranial disorder. A preorgasmic headache is a dull ache in the head and neck associated with awareness of neck and/or jaw muscle contraction, occurring during sexual activity, and increasing with sexual activity. An orgasmic headache is a sudden severe, explosive headache occurring at orgasm. Rarely, sexual activity can cause a CSF leak and result in a low-CSF-pressure-type headache (see Chapter 14).

In one study of patients with the primary orgasmic type, those who stop sexual activity with headache onset before orgasm had a duration of 5 minutes to 2 hours (13). Those who proceeded to orgasm had a severe headache for 3 minutes to 4 hours and a milder headache for 1 to 48 hours afterward. Forty percent of patients with the explosive type also have exertional headache (14). The headaches are usually bilateral but can be unilateral.

Occasionally, a dull headache can persist for up to a few weeks. A personal or family history of migraine is common in primary orgasmic headaches, which may be a migraine variant for some patients. Orgasmic headaches may occur more frequently when the person tries to have more than one orgasm after a brief interval.

Caution is necessary in diagnosing the first sex headache because sexual activity is the precipitant of up to 12% of ruptured saccular aneurysms and of up to 4% of patients with SAH resulting from bleeding arteriovenous malformations. Rarely, pheochromocytomas (Chapter 13) can present with paroxysmal hypertension precipitated by sexual activity. Extracephalic pain can be due to masturbation. Severe paroxysmal icepick-like pain has been described referred to the neck in a patient with compressive spondylitic cervical myelopathy and the groin and genitalia in another patient with a tethered cord (15). Other secondary causes include primary thunderclap headache, referred cardiac pain, nonhemorrhagic strokes, meningitis, encephalitis, hemorrhage into a cerebral tumor, glaucoma, myxedema, anemia, chronic obstructive pulmonary disease, sinusitis, hypoglycemia, Cushing's disease, and occlusion of the abdominal aorta. Medications that may cause sex headaches include phosphodiesterase-5 inhibitors (see later), amyl nitrate, amphetamine, marijuana, cocaine, amiodarone, birth control pills, and pseudoephedrine. Testing depending on the clinical context may include CT of the brain, lumbar puncture, MRI of the brain, and MRA.

The natural history of the benign explosive type of sexual headaches is variable. In one study of 26 patients, the headaches went away in 50% after 6 weeks to 6 months but recurred in 50% after remissions of up to 6 years (16). Headaches may be prevented in some patients by weight loss, an exercise program, a more passive role during intercourse, variation in posture, limitation of additional sexual activity on the same day, and medications (17). Indomethacin (25 to 50 mg), ergotamine tartrate, or a triptan given about 1 hour before sexual activity might be preventive (18). Propranolol (40 to 200 mg/day) and diltiazem (60 mg three times daily) (19) have been reported effective as a daily preventive if this headache type occurs frequently.

More Sex Headaches: Orgasm as a Treatment for Migraine

Although a pseudoheadache is often used as an excuse to avoid sex, those with migraine may want to have sex. Couch et al. reported on relief of migraine with sexual intercourse (20). Twenty-seven out of 57 women who reported having sexual intercourse during their migraine noted significant headache relief. Of these, 10 noted that orgasm produced complete remission of the migraine without recurrence, and 4 noted more than 50% improvement. The remainder noted temporary relief of approximately an hour or only modest relief.

Headache Due to Phosphodiesterase-5 Inhibitors (PDE-5)

PDE-5 inhibitors for erectile dysfunction (sildenafil, vardenafil, and tadalafil) cause headaches in about 15% of patients.

The risk of headache may be greater at higher doses of the medication. The headaches have not been classified in the studies. PDE-5 is the major enzyme responsible for the breakdown of cyclic guanosine monophosphate (cGMP). Thus PDE-5 inhibitors mimic one of the actions of nitric oxide: activation of soluble guanylate cyclase and increased cGMP formation.

Kruuse et al. triggered a migraine in 10 of 12 subjects with migraine without aura by administering sildenafil 100 mg (21). The median time to peak headache score was 4.5 hours after administration of sildenafil with a range of 2 to 9 hours. Usual headache medications (typically a triptan) had a good response in 9 of 10 subjects. Using transcranial doppler and SPECT, there was no initial dilatation of the middle cerebral artery. The authors propose that the triggering mechanism of the drug may reside within the perivascular sensory nerve terminals of the brain stem.

CHIARI TYPE I MALFORMATION AND HEADACHE

Epidemiology

Chiari type I malformation describes herniation of the cerebellar tonsils 5 mm or more below the level of the foramen magnum (22). Tonsillar descent less than 3 mm has no clinical significance, whereas descent of 3 to less than 5 mm is of indeterminate clinical significance. Although Chiari I malformation is usually congenital, reversible descent of the cerebellar tonsils below the foramen magnum (acquired Chiari I malformation) can occur due to lumbar puncture, overdraining CSF shunts, and spontaneous intracranial hypotension.

In one study, Chiari I was more common in women (3:2) and associated with syringomyelia in 40%, most commonly between the levels of C4 and C6 (23). All patients with tonsillar herniations greater than 12 mm and 70% of those with herniations of 5 to 10 mm were symptomatic. Information is unavailable about the prevalence of this disorder. With the advent of MRI, minimal tonsillar ectopia is frequently detected as an incidental finding.

Clinical Manifestations

Presentations include foramen magnum compression, central cord syndrome, cerebellar dysfunction, bulbar palsy, and paroxysmal intracranial hypertension (24). Syncope can occasionally occur with headache similar to basilar migraine or with Valsalva-like maneuvers or exercise.

In a study of 35 patients with Chiari I who subsequently underwent surgery (decompression of the foramen magnum, opening of the fourth ventricular outlet, and plugging of the obex), the frequency of clinical presentations in Chiari I were as follows: headache and neck pain, 73%; sensory dysesthesias/numbness, 56%; gait problems, 43%; upper-extremity weakness, 25%; cranial nerve dysfunction, 23%; blurred vision, 17%; and lower-extremity weakness, 15% (25). Significant improvement following surgery was described in 45% with syringomyelia and in 87% without syringomyelia.

Headaches have been reported in 15% to 75% of those with Chiari I. Stovner et al. described 20 patients with headaches out of 34 Chiari I patients seen with tonsillar herniation equal to or more than 5 mm. Many patients had several headache types. Fifty percent had short-lasting cough headache types (see earlier) of less than 5 minutes; 70% had headaches lasting 3 hours to several days; and 40% had continuous headaches. Associated symptoms present in some patients included intermittent dizziness, visual symptoms (visual field defects, oscilloscopia, diplopia, blurred vision, and skewed vision), and tinnitus. Long-lasting headaches were similar to cervicogenic headaches with occipital and neck pain, pain in the arm, and restriction of neck movement. Long-lasting headaches were unilateral in 50% and could shift sides. Those with long-lasting headaches averaged 6.25 attacks per month. The headaches, which were present in various locations—including below the eyes, eye(s), forehead, vertex, temple, and occiput—often were severe. The degree of tonsillar herniation was not correlated with the presence or absence of headaches or the presence of short-duration headaches. The headaches were improved in the five out of eight patients who had surgery.

Pascual et al. reported 26 patients with headaches out of 50 with Chiari I. Suboccipital-occipital headaches were present in 28%, with a duration that ranged from seconds to weeks and variable quality, including throbbing, dull, and lancinating pain (26). The pain was aggravated by Valsalva-like maneuvers in all the patients. This headache correlated with the degree of tonsillar herniation.

Thus a variety of headaches have been associated with Chiari I, including those that are similar to migraine with and without aura, are tension type, are cervicogenic, and result from high and low CSF pressure (27). Migraine and tension-type headaches can also occur unrelated to the Chiari I. If the tonsillar herniation is less than 5 mm, the physician should be wary of attributing the headache to Chiari I.

Biological Basis

Intermittent or persistent intracranial hypertension can be due to obstruction of CSF flow from the fourth ventricle to the cisterna magna or within the subarachnoid space at the level of the foramen magnum. The short-lasting cough headaches are due to a transient pressure dissociation between the intracranial and intraspinal compartments that causes further impaction of the cerebellar tonsils in the foramen magnum and produces pain by traction and pressure on pain-sensitive structures, such as the C1 and C2 nerve roots, cranial nerves, meninges, and vessels. The mechanism of recurrent, long-lasting headaches not induced by Valsalva-like maneuvers is not understood (28).

Pneumocephalus and Headaches (29)

Pneumocephalus or the presence of intracranial air may be located in the following locations: intraventricular, subdural, extradural, subarachnoid, and intracerebral. A pneumocele or areocele is well-circumscribed intracranial air. Sixty-five cc or more of air causes mass effect and is defined as tension pneumocephalus, which can result in cerebral herniation. Most cases of pneumocephalus are due to head trauma (over 70% of cases) or surgical procedures (such as intracranial procedures or nasal and sinus surgery with damage to the cribriform plate). Other causes include traumatic nasogastric and nasotracheal tube insertion, spinal and epidural anesthesia, lumbar puncture, tumors of the sinuses, bacterial meningitis, chronic otitis media, nasal continuous pressure-positive airway pressure, nasal oxygen cannula; colonic perforation in patients with a ventriculoperitoneal shunt, habitual performance of the Valsalva maneuver or coughing, recurrent sneezing, and barotrauma. A CT scan of the head can identify as little as 0.5 cc of intracranial air.

Symptoms of pneumocephalus include headache, visual disturbance, dizziness, seizures, confusion, and personality change. Sudden movement of the head may produce a "succussion splash" in 7% of cases.

HEADACHES DUE TO INFECTION AND INFLAMMATION

HIV and Headaches

A variety of headaches result from HIV infection (30). Primary headaches can also occur in those infected with HIV. Medication rebound should also be considered as a cause in those patients with chronic headaches or pain syndromes who frequently use pain medications.

HIV-Related Headaches

Two to 4 weeks after HIV-1 infection, up to 93% of patients develop an acute illness, often associated with headache, that lasts 1 to 2 weeks. Acute headaches with fever, meningeal signs, cranial nerve palsies, and CSF lymphocytic pleocytosis (20 to 300 cells/mm^3) can develop at any stage of the disease. In the late stages of the disease, the CSF may show no white blood cells because of lymphocyte depletion. Because CSF pleocytosis and elevated protein concentration can be seen in asymptomatic HIV-seropositive patients, this finding in a patient with headache does not exclude other etiologies. Up to 30% of HIV-seropositive people develop chronic headache and persistent pleocytosis.

Opportunistic infections and tumors can also cause headaches in HIV-1 disease. Meningitides include cryptococcal meningitis, tuberculous meningitis, syphilitic meningitis, and lymphomatous meningitis. Focal brain lesions that can cause headache include toxoplasmosis encephalitis, primary central nervous system lymphoma, progressive multifocal leukoencephalopathy, cryptococcomas, tuberculomas, and Candida abscess. Diffuse brain lesions that can cause headache include cytomegalovirus encephalitis, herpes simplex virus encephalitis, toxoplasmosis encephalitis, and HIV-associated dementia. Table 15-2 lists the frequency of headache with these various causes. Sinusitis, which is common in patients with AIDS, should also be considered as the cause of headaches.

A variety of medications taken by HIV-seropositive patients may be associated with headaches, including zidovudine, trimethoprim-sulfamethoxazole, fluoxetine, rifampin, ethambutol, methotrexate, and acyclovir. The protease inhibitors do not appear to cause or worsen headaches.

Table 15-2. Frequency of headache based on diagnosis in the HIV-infected individual

Diagnosis	Percentage with Headache
Cryptococcal meningitis	88
Neurosyphilis	88
Tuberculous meningitis	59
Toxoplasmosis encephalitis	55
Cytomegalovirus encephalitis	30
Progressive multifocal leukoencephalopathy	23
HIV-associated dementia	14

From: Ramadan NM, Khayr W. Headache associated with AIDS. In: Gilman S, ed. *MedLink neurology*. San Diego: MedLink Corp, 2004. Available at www.medlink.com, modified with permission.

Primary Headaches

Early in the AIDS epidemic in the United States, opportunistic infections such as cryptococcal meningitis were the most common cause of headaches. With better opportunistic and antiretroviral treatments, primary headaches have become more common. Stress and depression associated with HIV infection can certainly contribute to primary headaches.

In a prospective study of patients with headaches seen in a neuro-AIDS clinic performed by Mirsattari et al., primary headaches were present in 66% and secondary headaches occurred in 34% (31). Primary headaches have the following features: they are not uncommon in this population and are distinguished by the late age of onset, usual absence of family or personal history of headaches, and exacerbation following HIV infection; may present first in patients with severe immunosuppression; are unrelated to antiretroviral drug therapy; frequently do not respond to conventional treatments; and have a poor prognosis.

Diagnostic Evaluation

Diagnostic testing is often necessary to exclude secondary causes of headaches, especially in those patients with headache and a CD4+ cell count of less than 500 cells/mm^3 (also see Chapter 1). An MRI scan is preferable to a CT scan because of greater sensitivity in detecting lesions associated with HIV infection. If the findings of the scan do not explain the headache, a lumbar puncture is necessary, including routine CSF studies as well as bacterial, fungal, mycobacterial stains and cultures; sometimes viral studies and cytology; and cryptococcal antigen titers and venereal disease research laboratory (VDRL) titers. The CSF VDRL is nonreactive in 30% of cases of neurosyphilis. A nonreactive CSF-FTA-ABS or CSF-MHA-TP excludes neurosyphilis.

The diagnosis of tuberculous meningitis can be difficult. The sensitivity of acid-fast bacilli (AFB) stains is no more than 24%, and cultures may take 2 to 6 weeks for growth to occur. However, CSF polymerase chain reaction (PCR) for *Mycobacterium* tuberculosis has high sensitivity (variably reported as 32% to 100%) and specificity (about 8% false positives) for diagnosis.

In undiagnosed patients, HIV infection should be considered as the cause in patients with risk factors presenting with aseptic meningitis, cranial herpes zoster, facial pain associated with Bell's palsy, and new-onset or chronic progressive headaches. An enzyme-linked immunosorbent assay (ELISA) test, which is 99% specific and 98% sensitive when properly performed, is the initial test for HIV infection. Because false positives can occur, the diagnosis must be confirmed with more specific PCR or Western blot techniques. If the ELISA is negative, testing should be repeated in 6 months if there is sufficient concern because of the possible delay in the development of detectable serum antibodies.

Brain Abscess

Epidemiology

The annual incidence of brain abscess (32,33) is about 4 in 1 million. The most common age is the third decade of life. Abscesses due to paranasal sinus infection are most common between the ages of 10 and 30, whereas otogenic abscesses are most common in childhood and after 40 years of age. In children, the peak incidence is between 4 and 7 years of age, and 25% have cyanotic congenital heart disease.

Brain abscesses are usually the result of hematogenous spread of organisms from distant sites (e.g., bronchiectasis, lung abscess, and acute bacterial endocarditis) or spread from sinusitis (especially frontal, ethmoid, or sphenoid sinusitis), otitis, or mastoiditis through emissary veins. Less common causes include penetrating trauma, neurosurgical procedures, facial infections, and dental sepsis. In 20% to 30% of cases, no predisposing condition is identified. The microbiological profile, which includes a variety of aerobes and anaerobes, often reflects the origin of the infection. Multiple organisms may be present, especially when due to sinusitis or otitis. Infection in immunocompromised patients may be due to *Enterobacteriaceae, Pseudomonas aeruginosa,* and *Nocardia asteroides.* Brain abscesses in diabetics may be associated with *Cryptococcus neoformans, Candida, Mucor,* and *Aspergillus* species. Focal infections in AIDS are listed in the prior section.

Clinical Manifestations

Headaches, unilateral or bilateral, are present in about 75% of patients, and nausea and vomiting occur in about 50%. Fever is present in less than 50% of patients. Focal neurological signs are also present in less than 50%. About one third of patients present with seizures, which are usually generalized. Nuchal rigidity and papilledema are present in about 25% of cases.

Diagnostic Evaluation

CT and MRI scans are the key to diagnosis. CT scan classically shows a ring-enhancing lesion with a variable appearance, depending on the age and cause of the abscess. Early lesions may not show enhancement. Metastatic neoplasms may be difficult to distinguish from multiple brain abscesses. MRI is more sensitive than CT scans. T1-weighted images show hypodense areas with ring enhancement after gadolinium injection. T2-weighted images show a hyperdense central area surrounded by a capsule. Better imaging of the abscess allows more accurate estimates of its age and amenability to aspiration or drainage. Single photon emission computed tomography (SPECT) with thallium 201 is useful in distinguishing central nervous system lymphoma from toxoplasmosis. Lumbar puncture is contraindicated in the presence of a mass lesion because of the risk of herniation.

Meningitis and Encephalitis

Epidemiology

The annual incidence of meningitis and encephalitis (33,34) per 100,000 in the United States for various infections is as follows: bacterial meningitis, 5 to 10; viral meningitis, 10.9; and viral encephalitis, 7.4. Bacterial meningitis occurs more often in winter than during other seasons. Because of the *Hemophilus influenzae* type B vaccine, the median age of patients with meningitis due to *Hemophilus influenzae, Streptococcus pneumoniae, Neisseria meningitidis,* group B streptococcus, and *Listeria monocytogenes* has increased in the last 15 years from 15 months of age to 25 years. Pneumococcal meningitis is the most common cause of bacterial meningitis in the United States. Viral meningitis usually occurs during the summer and typically occurs in children and young adults. The most common organisms are enteroviruses (echo and coxsackie), mumps, and the arboviruses. Most cases of viral encephalitis occur in the summer and early fall. There are numerous causes of viral encephalitis, including mumps, arboviruses, enteroviruses, lymphocytic choriomeningitis, herpes simplex virus, Epstein-Barr virus, measles, influenza virus, varicella zoster, and mycoplasma. There have been increasing numbers of cases of West Nile virus encephalitis in the United States since the initial outbreak in New York City in 1999.

Clinical Manifestations

Bacterial meningitis in adults classically presents with fever, headache, meningismus, pain with eye movement, and altered mental status. The headache is usually generalized (but may be bifrontal), severe, and unremitting. Bacterial meningitis can present with a thunderclap headache. Young children and the elderly have headaches less often than young adults. Nausea, vomiting, photophobia, and myalgias are also common. Kernig's or Brudzinski's sign or both are present in about 50% of cases. Cranial nerve findings are found in less than 20% of cases. Subacute or chronic headache may be present in tuberculous or cryptococcal meningitis.

Viral meningitis typically presents with a severe, sudden-onset headache, fever, malaise, anorexia, pain with eye movement, phonophobia, photophobia, and nuchal rigidity. The features of encephalitis include headache, fever, alteration of consciousness, meningeal signs, focal neurological deficits, and seizures. Thunderclap headaches can also occur in viral encephalitis. About 20% of people infected with the West Nile virus develop a mild illness resembling the flu. Symptoms of mild illness or West Nile fever can include sudden onset of fever with headache, malaise, anorexia, nausea, vomiting, diarrhea, photophobia, neck pain and stiffness, myalgias, rash, and lymphadenopathy.

Diagnostic Evaluation

Patients with focal neurological findings, papilledema, or altered mental status should have a CT scan or MRI scan before a lumbar puncture. If there is a significant delay before the lumbar puncture or the patient is seriously ill, blood cultures should be taken and antibiotics started empirically when bacterial meningitis is suspected.

On lumbar puncture and CSF examination, the usual findings in bacterial meningitis are the following: an elevated opening pressure, increased white blood cells (WBCs) with neutrophilic predominance (1,000 to 5,000 cells/mm^3), increased protein level (100 to 500 mg/dl), and low glucose level (less than 40 mg/dl or a CSF-to-serum ratio of less than 0.3). Approximately 90% of patients will have more than 100 WBCs/mm^3; 65% to 70% will have more than 1,000 WBCs/mm^3.

Although the WBCs are predominantly neutrophils, initially 10% of patients may show mononuclear predominance, generally with cell counts of less than 1,000. CSF findings with a very high predictive value for bacterial meningitis include the following: glucose less than 34 mg/dl; CSF/serum glucose less than 0.23; WBCs more than 2,000/mm^3; and neutrophils more than 1,180/mm^3. Gram's stain of the CSF is positive in 60% to 90% of patients. Blood cultures may be positive in up to 50% of cases. Counterimmunoelectrophoresis (CIE) and latex agglutination tests of the CSF to test for bacterial antigens can be sensitive adjuncts, especially in partially treated meningitis.

On lumbar puncture and CSF examination, the usual findings in viral meningitis are the following: normal or slightly elevated opening CSF pressure; a mild pleocytosis (usually less than 1,000 cells/mm^3); protein either normal or slightly elevated; and glucose either normal or slightly decreased. Early in the course of the disease there may be neutrophil cell predominance, but this rapidly shifts to a lymphocytic pleocytosis.

On CSF examination, the usual findings in viral encephalitis include the following: a mild CSF pleocytosis (usually less than 200 cells/mm^3); protein concentration either normal or slightly elevated; and glucose level either normal or slightly decreased. The CSF typically shows a lymphocytic predominance, although a neutrophil predominance may be seen in the first 48 hours. MRI studies may show focal findings in focal encephalitides, such as herpes simplex or Eastern equine. Other useful studies include electroencephalogram, acute and convalescent sera, and CSF PCR. CSF PCR for herpes simplex virus encephalitis, with a sensitivity of 98% and a specificity of 94%, has supplanted the need for brain biopsy in these cases. The results may become negative once acyclovir has been started.

Drug-Induced Aseptic Meningitis

Numerous medications can cause an aseptic meningitis (35), including the following: nonsteroidal antiinflammatory drugs (ibuprofen, naproxen, diclofenac, sulindac, tolmetin, and ketoprofen); antibiotics (trimethoprim/sulfamethoxazole, sulfasalazine, cephalosporins, ciprofloxacin, isoniazide, ornidazole, and penicillin); intrathecal drugs and diagnostics (antineoplastics such as methotrexate and cytarabine, gentamicin, corticosteroids, spinal anesthesia, baclofen, repeated iophendylate for myelography, and radiolabeled albumin); intraventricular chemotherapy; intravenous immunoglobulin; vaccines (polio, measles, mumps, and rubella, and hepatitis B); and other drugs (e.g., allopurinol, carbamazepine, infliximab, muromonab CD-3, and ranitidine).

The clinical presentation is the same as that of viral meningitis. The CSF findings are similar to viral meningitis except for a neutrophil predominance in most cases. Aseptic meningitis due to intravenous immunoglobulin demonstrates eosinophils in the CSF. The prognosis in drug-induced aseptic meningitis is generally good.

Postmeningitis Headache

Following recovery from bacterial or viral meningitis, preexisting primary headaches can have an increased severity or new-onset headaches, including migraine, may begin within weeks after recovery (36).

Lyme Disease

Epidemiology

Lyme disease (37) is a multisystem infectious disease caused by the spirochete subspecies *Borrelia burdorferi sensu stricto* in North America. The disease is a zoonosis spread by hard-shelled Ixodes ticks with humans as the inadvertent host. Mature ticks usually attach to large mammals, such as bears or deer. Only 1% to 2% of humans with identified Ixodes tick bites become infected. About 17,000 cases are reported yearly in the United States to the Centers for Disease Control. Although cases have been reported from 47 states, most cases occur along the eastern seaboard from Maryland to Massachusetts, in the upper Midwest (primarily Wisconsin and Minnesota), and in northern California.

Clinical Manifestations

Up to 90% of infected people have a usually painless rash, erythema migrans, which starts as a red macule or papule and expands to form a large red ring with central clearing. During erythema migrans, headache is present in about 50% of patients.

About 15% of patients will develop nervous system involvement with all or part of the triad of lymphocytic meningitis, cranial neuritis, and painful radiculitis. Although any cranial nerve can be involved, cranial nerve VII is most common and can be bilateral. (Sarcoid and Guillain-Barré syndrome can also cause bilateral palsies.) Late or chronic neurological manifestations include a chronic encephalomyelitis (which is rare) and a mild peripheral neuropathy, which can be a symmetric distal polyneuropathy, more focal mononeuropathy multiplex, or a polyradiculopathy. A significant number of patients with chronic infection develop a mild encephalomyelitis with mild confusion and difficulty with memory and complex intellectual tasks. Headache occurs commonly with lymphocytic meningitis with or without cranial neuritis or painful radiculoneuritis or both and with encephalomyelitis.

Diagnostic Evaluation

Diagnostic testing is problematic for Lyme disease because of difficulties with the sensitivity and specificity of the tests. Patients with headache alone usually do not require testing. Serum antibody testing by ELISA, which can have both false positives and negatives, is the first step. Western blot tests confirm a positive ELISA or identify false positives. PCR, to detect bacterial DNA, has a sensitivity of about 60%. For neurological presentations, demonstration of intrathecal antibody production (the ratio of CSF to serum antibody) is very sensitive and specific.

Neurosarcoid

Sarcoidosis can affect any part of the central or peripheral nervous system. Neurosarcoid occurs in about 5% of cases. Sarcoid granulomas in the basal meninges, brain, and cranial nerves—the most common neurological manifestations—often cause headaches either directly or due to obstruction of CSF pathways and hydrocephalus.

Idiopathic Hypertrophic Pachymeningitis (38)

Idiopathic hypertrophic pachymeningitis is a rare idiopathic chronic inflammatory process that involves the dura mater diffusely or focally. The mean reported age is 50, with a range from 20 to 80 years with a male predominance. A severe headache is typically present at the onset that is variably associated with cranial nerve palsies and ataxia. Numerous other problems may be associated including hemiparesis, seizures, hydrocephalus, and memory loss. The MRI may show diffuse and/or nodular enhancement. The CSF shows variable elevation of protein and lymphocytosis. Corticosteroid treatment augmented as necessary with methotrexate or azathioprine improves most patients, although the benefit may be temporary and partial.

Other causes of thickened abnormally enhancing dura on gadolinium-enhanced MRI include the following: intracranial hypotension; infections (Lyme disease, syphilis, tuberculosis, fungal, cysticercosis, HTLV-1, malignant external necrotizing otitis due to *Pseudomonas*); systemic autoimmune/vasculitic disorders (Wegener's, rheumatoid arthritis, sarcoidosis, Behçet's, Sjögren's, temporal arteritis); malignancy (dural carcinomatosis, metastatic disease in adjacent skull bone, and lymphoma); and meningioma.

METABOLIC DISORDERS AND HEADACHE

Fever

Generalized headaches often occur with nonneurological disorders (39) such as pyelonephritis. The fever that results from the disorder in turn causes increased cerebral blood flow and headache.

Hypoxia

The IHS 2nd edition criteria for hypoxic headache include headache occurring within 24 hours after the acute onset of hypoxia with PaO_2 of less than 70 mm Hg or in chronically hypoxic patients with PaO_2 persistently at or below this level. Hypoxic headache can occur during exposure to reduced ambient oxygen or in patients with carbon monoxide exposure, pulmonary disease, anemia, cardiac failure, and sleep apnea. Hypoxia can also be a trigger for migraine and cluster headaches. Hypoxemia, especially when combined with an increased level of carbon dioxide, can produce headache due to dilation of arteries and arterioles.

Hypercapnia

Severe headaches can occur in some patients with hypercapnia caused by marked dilation of cerebral vasculature. Prolonged hypercapnia can be a secondary cause of pseudotumor cerebri.

Hypoglycemia

Missing a meal can be a trigger for migraineurs. Headache due to hypoglycemia can occur in diabetics, pancreatic islet cell tumors, hypopituitarism, adrenocortical insufficiency, hypothyroidism, and liver disease such as cirrhosis.

Carbon Monoxide Exposure

At levels of carboxyhemoglobin from 10% to 20% in acute carbon monoxide exposure, headache is present in 90% often accompanied by nausea and confusion. Seizures and coma develop at greater than 40% carboxyhemoglobin, and death can occur at greater than 60% carboxyhemoglobin. Acute carbon monoxide exposure is frequently followed by disabling neuropsychiatric symptoms. The headache is typically bilateral and/or continuous with an onset within 12 hours of exposure and resolution within 72 hours after elimination of carbon monoxide.

Hypothyroidism

Moreau et al. performed a prospective study of 102 adults with clinical and biological hypothyroidism (40). Thirty percent presented with headache 1 to 2 months after the first symptoms of hypothyroidism. The headache was slight, nonpulsatile, continuous, bilateral, and salicylate responsive and disappeared with thyroid hormone therapy.

Dialysis

Tension- or migraine-type headaches can be precipitated during dialysis. A new type of headache can also occur a few hours after dialysis, starting as a bifrontal aching and then a throbbing, sometimes with nausea and vomiting. In a study by Goksan et al., 48% of 63 chronic dialysis patients reported headaches during dialysis that were typically in a frontotemporal location with a throbbing quality, of moderate severity, and with a short duration of less than 4 hours (41).

High Altitude

Epidemiology

Acute mountain sickness (AMS) develops in about 25% of visitors to moderate altitudes (6,300 to 9,700 feet). Symptoms usually occur within the first 12 hours of arrival but may be delayed 24 hours or more. Those who are younger than 60 years of age, less physically fit, live at sea level, have a history of AMS, or have underlying lung problems are most likely to be affected (42). AMS leads to high-altitude cerebral edema (HACE) in perhaps 1.5% of cases. Alcohol use inhibits acute ventilatory adaptation to mild hypoxia at moderate altitude. High altitude can also be a trigger for migraines.

Clinical Manifestations

AMS, which usually occurs above 8,200 feet, is defined by the presence of a headache and at least one of the following symptoms: gastrointestinal symptoms (anorexia, nausea, or vomiting), fatigue or weakness, dizziness or lightheadedness, and difficulty sleeping (43). The headache is usually bilateral but may be unilateral. HACE, which is uncommon below 12,000 feet, is defined by the presence of a change in mental status and/or ataxia in a person with AMS or the presence of both mental status change and ataxia in a person without AMS. HACE, which can lead to coma and death, may be associated with abnormalities in limb tone, urinary incontinence, papilledema, cranial nerve palsies, and tremor.

High-altitude pulmonary edema, which can occur along with HACE, usually occurs above 9,840 feet. High-altitude retinal hemorrhage is common in people who go above 15,000 feet.

Biological Mechanisms

As the partial pressure of oxygen decreases with increasing altitude, ventilation increases, leading to respiratory alkalosis. Although hypocapnia alone results in cerebral vasoconstriction, hypoxia produces a net decline of cerebral vascular resistance and increased cerebral blood flow. Hypoxia can result in cerebral edema, which may be due to cerebral vasodilation and elevated cerebral capillary hydrostatic pressure. An increase in sympathetic activity follows, causing an increased heart rate, pulmonary vasoconstriction, and an initial increase and later decrease of cerebral blood flow (44).

Management

Altitude sickness may be prevented in those planning higher ascents by starting below 8,000 feet, resting the first day, and then ascending about 1,000 feet each day. Sleeping at a lower altitude at night may be helpful because hypoxia is worse with sleep. It is also important to keep well hydrated and avoid alcohol. Acetazolamide, at a dose of 250 mg twice a day starting 1 day before ascent (45) and continuing for 3 to 4 days, may prevent AMS and improve sleep. Dexamethasone 8 mg a day in divided doses may also reduce the incidence and symptoms of AMS. The combination of acetazolamide and dexamethasone is more effective than either alone. Aspirin may also prevent AMS. In one study, the incidence of headache was greatly reduced by giving aspirin 320 mg starting 1 hour before arrival at high altitude and then one every 4 hours for two doses (for a total of three doses) (46).

AMS may be treated symptomatically with rest, mild analgesics, alcohol avoidance, and adequate hydration. Depending on the severity of symptoms, it may be necessary not to go any higher, slow the rate of ascent, or descend. Acetazolamide may also help acute symptoms. In addition to descent, HACE may be treated with acetazolamide, dexamethasone, supplemental oxygen, and a portable hyperbaric bag.

AMS usually resolves after 16 to 72 hours at altitude. When descent is impossible and treatment is lacking, HACE and high-altitude pulmonary edema have a mortality rate of up to 50%.

Decompression Sickness

Decompression sickness (DCS), also referred to as the "bends" or caisson disease, usually affects divers and caisson workers but can occur in pilots during rapid ascent in a nonpressurized cabin. DCS, which can occur after diving to a depth of more than 25 feet, usually appears within a few minutes to a few hours after the end of a dive. Mild DCS (type I) is defined by pain usually in the joints (bends) and/or itching of the skin. Serious DCS (type II) is characterized by neurological problems. Involvement of the thoracic spinal cord, the most commonly affected area, leads to low back or pelvic pain and dysesthesias, which may be accompanied by sensory loss, weakness, and incontinence. Less often, the brain may be involved, resulting in various symptoms and signs, such as headache, confusion, lethargy, vertigo, speech disturbance, hemiparesis, visual impairment, and seizures, depending on the site of the insult (47).

Hyperventilation Syndrome

Introduction and Epidemiology

Hyperventilation syndrome (48), according to one consensus definition, is a "syndrome characterized by a variety of somatic symptoms induced by physiologically inappropriate hyperventilation and usually reproduced in whole or in part by voluntary hyperventilation" (49). Acute hyperventilation with obvious tachypnea accounts for about 1% of all cases of hyperventilation. The other 99% of cases are due to chronic hyperventilation in which there may be a modest increase in respiratory rate and/or tidal volume that may not even be apparent to the patient or a medical observer.

The hyperventilation syndrome occurs in about 6% to 11% of the general patient population. Most studies have reported hyperventilation syndrome occurring two to seven times more frequently in women than in men, with most patients ranging in age between 15 and 55 years. One large study reported that patients with acute hyperventilation syndrome ranged in age from 5 to 85 years and that this condition was particularly prevalent in women in their late teens (50). The prevalence of chronic hyperventilation is the highest in middle-aged women. In studies of patients with neurological symptoms of hyperventilation syndrome, the percentage of females ranged from 50% to 87%.

Hyperventilation syndrome is frequently associated with anxiety or stress, although some patients have no detectable psychiatric disorder and develop a habit of inappropriately increased ventilatory rate and/or depth. Common triggers of acute hyperventilation syndrome include anxiety, nausea and vomiting, and fever due to the common cold.

Clinical Manifestations

The manifestations of hyperventilation syndrome that include headaches are listed in Table 15-3. Patients with different symptoms may see different types of physicians. Primary care physicians may see an assortment of presentations. Cardiologists may see those with complaints of chest pain, palpitations, and shortness of breath. Neurologists frequently see patients describing dizziness, paresthesias, and pressure in the head. Ear, nose, and throat physicians may see those with dizziness.

Table 15-3. Symptoms and signs of the hyperventilation syndrome

General
> Fatiguability, exhaustion, weakness, sleep disturbance, nausea, sweating

Cardiovascular
> Chest pain, palpitations, tachycardia, Raynaud's phenomenon

Gastrointestinal
> Aerophagia, dry mouth, pressure in throat, dysphagia, globus hystericus, epigastric fullness or pain, belching, flatulence

Neurological
> Headache, pressure in the head, fullness in the head, head warmth
> Blurred vision, tunnel vision, momentary flashing lights, diplopia
> Dizziness, faintness, vertigo, giddiness, unsteadiness
> Tinnitus
> Numbness, tingling, coldness of face, extremities, trunk
> Muscle spasms, muscle stiffness, carpopedal spasm, generalized tetany, tremor
> Ataxia, weakness
> Syncope and seizures

Psychological
> Impairment of concentration and memory
> Feelings of unreality, disorientation, confused or dreamlike feeling, déjà vu
> Hallucinations
> Anxiety, apprehension, nervousness, tension, fits of crying, agoraphobia, neuroses, phobic, panic

Respiratory
> Shortness of breath, suffocating feeling, smothering spell, inability to get a good breath or breathe deeply enough, frequent sighing, yawning

The most common cause of distal symmetric paresthesias is hyperventilation syndrome. Although physicians generally recognize bilateral paresthesias of the face, hands, and feet as due to hyperventilation syndrome, many are unaware that hyperventilation can cause unilateral paresthesias. Unilateral paresthesias more often involve the left side. In a study of medical students, hyperventilation produced predominantly unilateral paresthesias in 16%, which involved the left side in more than 60% of control groups (51). Of those with hand numbness, often only the fourth and fifth fingers are involved. Unusual patterns of numbness reported include one side of the forehead, the shoulders, and one side of the abdomen.

Patients may report a variety of psychological complaints, commonly including anxiety, nervousness, unreality, disorientation, or they may describe feeling "spacey." Impairment of concentration and memory may be described as part of episodes or alternatively as symptoms of an underlying anxiety neurosis or depression. A patient's concern about the cause of the various symptoms of hyperventilation may result in feelings of impending death, fear, or panic, which may accentuate the hyperventilation. Patients with hyperventilation syndrome have a mean group profile very similar to patients with pseudoseizures: a neurotic pattern in which patients respond to psychological stress with somatic symptoms. Other complaints such as déjà vu or auditory and visual hallucinations are rare.

Biological Mechanisms

Acute hyperventilation produces a reduction in arterial PCO_2 resulting in alkalosis. Respiratory alkalosis produces the Bohr effect, a left shift of the oxygen dissociation curve with increased binding of oxygen to hemoglobin and reduced oxygen delivery to the tissues. The alkalosis also causes a reduction in plasma Ca^{2+} concentration. Hypophosphatemia may be due to intracellular shifts of phosphorus caused by altered glucose metabolism. In chronic hyperventilation, bicarbonate and potassium levels may be decreased because of increased renal excretion. Finally, stress can trigger a hyperadrenergic state that may cause hyperventilation through beta-adrenergic stimulation.

Central and peripheral mechanisms have been postulated for production of neurological symptoms during hyperventilation (52). Voluntary hyperventilation can reduce cerebral blood flow by 30% to 40%. Such symptoms and signs as headache, visual disturbance, dizziness, tinnitus, ataxia, syncope, and various psychological symptoms may be produced by diminished cerebral perfusion. Muscle spasms and tetany may be due to respiratory alkalosis and hypocalcemia. The finding that there is no relationship between the rate of fall of PCO_2 and the onset of dizziness and paresthesias suggests that symptoms may be due to hypophosphatemia. Hypophosphatemia can result in symptoms such as tiredness, dizziness, poor concentration, disorientation, and paresthesias. A hyperadrenergic state may result in tremor, tachycardia, anxiety, and sweating. Hypokalemia can cause muscle weakness and lethargy. The cause of bilateral and unilateral paresthesias is not certain. Evidence exists for both a central and peripheral mechanism, including a reduction in the concentration of extracellular Ca^{2+} and decreased cerebral perfusion.

Diagnostic Evaluation

The acute form of hyperventilation syndrome is easily recognized, even by the general public. However, the chronic form is less easily recognized, even by physicians, because the breathing rate is not reported as rapid or does not appear rapid and because the symptoms may appear to be atypical. For example, a respiration rate of 18 combined with an increased tidal volume of 750 mL per minute may lead to overbreathing that is not easily detectable. Because the chronic disorder is intermittent, spot arterial $PaCO_2$ or end tidal volume PCO_2 results can be normal.

The diagnosis depends on reproducing some or all of the symptoms with the hyperventilation provocation test and excluding other possible causes by either clinical reasoning or laboratory testing when indicated. The symptoms of panic attacks and hyperventilation syndrome overlap. In patients with prominent chest pain, cardiac disease should be considered.

The hyperventilation provocation test can be performed with either an increased ventilation rate of up to 60 per minute or simply deep breathing for 3 minutes. Dizziness, unsteadiness, and blurred vision commonly develop within 20 to 30 seconds, especially with the patient in the standing position; paresthesias start later. Chest pain is reported by 50% of patients after 3 minutes of hyperventilation and by all by 20 minutes. For clinical purposes, measurement of end tidal volume PCO_2 is unnecessary. In addition, there is no clear correlation between $PaCO_2$ and neurological signs. The hyperventilation provocation test should not be performed in patients with ischemic heart disease, cerebrovascular disease, pulmonary insufficiency, hyperviscosity states, significant anemia, sickle-cell disease, or uncontrolled hypertension.

Not infrequently, patients report only one or two symptoms, but on performing the hyperventilation provocation test, they report other symptoms appearing during their typical episodes that they did not remember to mention. For some patients with hyperventilation syndrome, symptoms cannot be reliably reproduced during the hyperventilation provocation test or even on consecutive tests. For others, antecedent anxiety and stress, not present during the test, may predispose to symptom formation, perhaps because of a hyperadrenergic state. Different patterns of hyperventilation with different respiratory rates, tidal volumes, and durations may induce different symptoms. In the individual case, if the hyperventilation provocation test fails to reproduce the symptoms but clinical suspicion persists, treatment such as breath holding, slow breathing, or breathing into a paper bag can certainly be suggested on a trial basis.

Management

Treatments for hyperventilation include patient reassurance and education; instructions to hold the breath, breathe more slowly, or breathe into a paper bag; breathing exercises and diaphragmatic retraining; biofeedback; hypnosis; psychological and psychiatric treatment; and such medications as beta-blockers, benzodiazepines, and antidepressants. Educational sessions, breathing techniques and retraining, and progressive relaxation may be helpful.

Most patients respond to reassurance, education (see patient information sheet in Chapter 18), and instructions to hold the breath, breathe more slowly, or breathe into a paper bag. If significant symptoms of stress, anxiety, or depression are present, use of appropriate medication and psychological or psychiatric referral may be helpful.

SLEEP AND HEADACHES

Headaches Occurring during Sleep

Secondary causes of nocturnal headaches (53,54) include drug withdrawal, temporal arteritis, sleep apnea, nocturnal hypertension-headache syndrome, oxygen desaturation, pheochromocytomas, primary and secondary neoplasms, communicating hydrocephalus, subdural hematomas, subacute angle-closure glaucoma, and vascular lesions (55). Migraine, cluster, hypnic, and chronic paroxysmal hemicrania are other primary headaches that can cause awakening from sleep. Hypnic headaches only occur during sleep (see Chapter 12). Migraine typically has associated symptoms and very uncommonly only occurs during sleep. Cluster headaches have autonomic symptoms and may occur during the day as well as during sleep. Chronic paroxysmal hemicrania occurs both during the day and at night, lasts for less than 30 minutes, and occurs 10 to 30 times a day.

Obstructive Sleep Apnea

Snoring and excessive daytime sleepiness are the most common symptoms of obstructive sleep apnea (OSA). Morning headaches are three times more common in those with OSA than in the general population (56) and may occur in 36% of those with OSA. However, Neau et al. found that headaches and morning headaches were not correlated with nocturnal respiratory or architectural sleep parameters or with excessive daytime sleepiness, but they were strongly correlated with mood disorders (57). More than two thirds of headaches improved with nasal continuous positive airway pressure treatment.

Sleep Bruxism

Bruxism (58) (grinding or clenching of teeth) during sleep occurs in up to 20% of the population as determined by visible tooth wear. Sleep bruxism is most common in children between the ages of 3 and 12 years and in adults between the ages of 19 and 45 years. Individuals are unaware of this behavior, which produces audible sounds in about 20% of episodes. Some patients report morning jaw discomfort and tension-type headaches that improve as the day goes on. Causes include dental factors (malocclusion and rough cusp ends), psychological and emotional factors, and systemic disorders (encephalopathies, hyperthyroidism, allergies, gastrointestinal disturbances, and nutritional deficiencies). Occlusal bite splints protect against damage. Medications that can be helpful at bedtime include propranolol, L-dopa, possibly bromocriptine, and, for acute exacerbations, diazepam. In severe, intractable cases, botulinum toxin injections may be beneficial.

Sleep Deprivation and Sleeping In

Lack of sleep can trigger migraine and tension-type headaches. In one study, 38.8% of medical and dental students reported headaches due to sleep deprivation (59). Some migraineurs find sleeping later than their usual time of awakening is a trigger.

Turtle Headache

Turtle headache is a bilateral headache that has been reported as occurring in the morning after awakening and going back to sleep with the covers over the head or retraction of the head under the blankets. Hypoxia is speculated as the cause (60).

Sleep to Relieve Migraine

Many migraineurs obtain relief from acute attacks by sleeping. In one study, 28% could terminate a migraine with sleep (61).

Parasomnias and Migraine

Somnambulism (sleepwalking) occurs in 28% of children with migraine and 5% of controls (62). Children with migraine also have a greater incidence of night terrors (71% vs. 11% in controls) and enuresis (41% vs. 16% in controls) (63).

Exploding Head Syndrome

Episodes of exploding head syndrome (64) awaken people from sleep with a sensation of a loud bang in the head, like an explosion. Ten percent of cases are associated with the perception of a flash of light. Five percent report a curious sensation as if they had stopped breathing and had to make a deliberate effort to breathe again. The episodes have a variable frequency and onset at any age, although the most common is middle aged and older. The episodes take place in healthy individuals during awakenings without evidence of epileptogenic discharges.

SEIZURES AND HEADACHES

Migraine and Seizures

The frequency of migraine in an epileptic population has been variably reported as 8.4% to 23%, and the reported frequency of epilepsy in a migraine population ranges from 1% to 17% (65). MELAS, arteriovenous malformations (Chapter 13), head trauma, and systemic lupus erythematosus can result in seizures and migraines or migrainelike headaches. Migraine with typical or prolonged aura, basilar migraine, and catamenial epilepsy can be triggers for seizures (66). Migraine can rarely cause a cerebral infarction that can cause seizures.

Benign occipital epilepsy, benign rolandic epilepsy, and temporal and occipital lobe epilepsy can cause seizures that mimic some features of migraine (67). A seizure is more likely if the aura lasts less than 5 minutes and is associated with alteration of consciousness, automatisms, and abnormal motor activity such as tonic-clonic movements. Migraine is more likely if the aura lasts more than 5 minutes and has positive (tingling, scintillations) and negative features (visual loss, numbness).

Ictal and Postictal Headaches

Hemicrania epileptica or synchronous ipsilateral ictal headache with migraine features is a cause of headaches resulting from a seizure. Most patients have both ictal headaches and some other seizure manifestations, although ictal headaches can be the only symptom. The seizure discharges, usually on the same side as the ipsilateral headache, begin and end simultaneously with the headache. The headaches usually last a few seconds to minutes. Unilateral or bilateral headaches can occur during a temporal lobe seizure (68).

Postictal headaches are common after partial complex and generalized tonic-clonic seizures, reported by 51% of subjects in one study (69). The headaches can resemble those of migraine or tension type.

In another prospective study, 34% of 341 patients with epilepsy experienced seizure-associated headache with a mean pain intensity of 6.1/10 and a duration of 12.8+/–15.7 (SD) hours (70). Seizures were always accompanied by headache in 60%. Headache occurred in 3% only preictally, in 27% periictally, and in 70% only postictally. In 55.7%, the headache could be classified as migraine and in 36.5% as tension type. The seizure-associated headache of migraineurs was identical to their migraine attacks. A history of migraine was a significant risk factor for seizure-associated headache.

In a study of headache in patients with temporal lobe epilepsy, the periictal headache was ipsilateral to the seizure onset in 90% of cases and usually conformed to the diagnostic criteria for migraine (71).

MULTIPLE SCLEROSIS AND HEADACHES

Acute Attacks and Headaches

Tension- and migrainelike headaches can occur with a first or subsequent attacks in 1.4% (72) to 7% (73) of cases. Some attacks with hemiparesis may raise the possibility of hemiplegic migraine.

Trigeminal Neuralgia and Multiple Sclerosis

A plaque at the point of entry of the trigeminal root, in the main sensory nucleus, or in the descending root of the trigeminal nerve can cause trigeminal neuralgia (74). Perhaps 1% of patients with multiple sclerosis have trigeminal neuralgia, and 2% of those with trigeminal neuralgia have multiple sclerosis. The pain becomes bilateral in about 14% of those with multiple sclerosis, compared with 4% of those without. New-onset trigeminal neuralgia under the age of 40 with normal facial sensation strongly suggests multiple sclerosis as the cause.

Migraine and Multiple Sclerosis

Migraine is twice as common in multiple sclerosis patients as in controls.

MIGRAINE AND TRANSIENT GLOBAL AMNESIA

Transient global amnesia (TGA) is characterized by the acute onset of anterograde amnesia or inability to incorporate new information with variable degrees of retrograde amnesia (75). Other aspects of cognition are only minimally involved. The patients are alert but appear confused and may get lost outside of familiar surroundings. During the attack, about 10% report a headache. Resolution is gradual with recovery occurring in two thirds within 2 hours to 12 hours and, in almost all, within 24 hours. Cases as short as 1 hour and as long as several days have been reported. Up to 18% of those with TGA will have at least one additional episode. Precipitating events, which are present in up to 84% of cases, include strenuous exercise, intense emotion, sexual intercourse, pain, swimming in cold water, taking a hot bath, cervical manipulation, coughing spells, and cerebral and cardiac arteriography. About 50% report Valsalva-like activities preceding TGA. Onset is usually after the age of 50 with a mean age of 60 years.

Patients with TGA have a significantly higher occurrence of migraine than normal and transient ischemic attack control subjects. TGA may also follow typical attacks of basilar migraine. Spreading depression could be a mechanism of TGA, which may be a heterogeneous disorder.

CENTRAL POSTSTROKE PAIN

Central lesions of the second-order trigeminal neurons, the quintothalamic tract, the ventrobasal nuclei of the thalamus, the parietal lobe, and even the cerebellum can cause diminished pain and burning sensations in the face and scalp. The ipsilateral extremities and trunk are usually also involved. Diminished pinprick and temperature sensation are usually present. Patients also report mechanical and thermal, especially cold, hyperalgesia. Central pain syndrome is a complication of 8% of strokes. The onset of the pain may be delayed for up to 6 months after the stroke. Multiple sclerosis can also cause central pain syndrome.

Treatment is often difficult. Medications that may be beneficial include tricyclic antidepressants (e.g., amitriptyline), antiepileptics (including lamotrigine, carbamazepine, oxcarbazepine, gabapentin, valproic acid, and topiramate), narcotics, clonidine, and neuroleptics (76).

TRIGEMINAL NEURALGIA

Trigeminal neuralgia has a 1.5 female to male ratio with ninety percent of cases beginning after the age of 40. There are about 15,000 new cases yearly in the United States. About 80% are due to vascular compression of the trigeminal nerve at the root entry zone most commonly by a branch of the superior cerebellar artery and about 5% of cases are due to tumors (epidermoid, acoustic neuroma, meningioma, and trigeminal neuroma).

The pain is a severe sharp, shooting, or electric shock-like sensation lasting seconds to 2 minutes usually in a unilateral maxillary and/or mandibular trigeminal distribution and uncommonly in the ophthalmic division. In about 90% of cases, trigger zones are present where nonpainful stimuli usually in the central part of the face around the nose and lips can trigger pain.

Stimuli can include talking, chewing, washing the face, brushing the teeth, shaving, facial movement, and cold air. After a paroxysm of pain, there is a refractory period lasting up to several minutes where stimulation of the trigger zone will not trigger pain. Facial grimacing or spasm may accompany the pain (tic douloureux). Between painful paroxysms, the patient is usually pain-free although dull aching may persist for a few minutes after long duration or multiple clustered attacks. Multiple attacks may occur for weeks or months. About 50% will have spontaneous remissions for at least 6 months. Physical examination is usually normal except for trigger zones although up to 25% of patients will have sensory loss.

Medications which may be effective alone and sometimes in combinations include the following with typical total dosage ranges per day: carbamazepine (400-800 mg); oxcarbazepine (900-1800 mg); baclofen (40-80 mg); phenytoin (300-500 mg); clonazepam (1.5-8 mg); divalproex sodium (500-1500 mg); topiramate (100-300 mg); lamotrigine (150-400 mg); gabapentin (900-2400 mg); and pimozide (4-12 mg). Low doses should be started and slowly increased. About 50% of patients fail medical treatment and may respond to one of the many surgical approaches available including extracranial peripheral denervation of trigeminal branches, radiofrequency thermocoagulation of the gasserian ganglion, glycerol trigeminal rhizotomy, percutaneous balloon compression of the gasserian ganglion, suboccipital retromastoid craniectomy for vascular decompression of the trigeminal nerve at the root entry zone, and gamma knife radiosurgery (77).

REFERENCES

1. Lance JW, Goadsby PJ. Other headaches without any structural abnormality. In: *Mechanism and management of headache,* 6th ed. Oxford: Butterworth-Heinemann, 1998:206–225.
2. Silberstein SD, Lipton RB, Goadsby PJ. Headache associated with non-vascular intracranial disease. In: *Headache in clinical practice.* London: Martin Dunitz, 2002:189–214.
3. Raskin NH. Short-lived head pains. *Neurol Clin* 1997;15:143–152.
4. Pascual J. Activity-related headache. In: Gilman S, ed. *MedLink neurology.* San Diego: MedLink Corp, 2004. Available at www.medlink.com.
5. Cutrer FM, Boes CJ. Cough, exertional, and sex headaches. *Neurol Clin N Am* 2004;22:133–149.
6. Rasmussen BK, Olesen J. Symptomatic and nonsymptomatic headaches in a general population. *Neurology* 1992;42:1225–1231.
7. Pascual J, Iglesias F, Oterino A, et al. Cough, exertional, and sexual headaches: an analysis of 72 benign and symptomatic cases. *Neurology* 1996;46:1520–1524.
8. Chen Y-Y, Lirng J-F, Fuh J-L, et al. Benign cough headache is associated with posterior cranial fossa overcrowding: a morphometric MRI study [abstract]. *Neurology* 2003;60:A157.
9. Mathew NT. Indomethacin-responsive headache syndromes. *Headache* 1981;21:147–150.
10. Raskin NH. The cough headache syndrome: treatment. *Neurology* 1995;47:1784.

11. Bahra A, Goadsby PJ. Cough headache responsive to methysergide. *Cephalalgia* 1998;18:495–496.
12. Wang S-J, Fuh J-L, Lu S-R. Benign cough headache is responsive to acetazolamide. *Neurology* 2000;55:149–150.
13. Lance JW. Headaches related to sexual activity. *J Neurol Neurosurg Psychiatry* 1976;39:1226–1230.
14. Silbert PL, Edis RH, Stewart-Wynne EG, et al. Benign vascular sexual headache and exertional headache: interrelationships and long term prognosis. *J Neurol Neurosurg Psychiatry* 1991;54:417–421.
15. Jacome DE. Masturbatory-orgasmic extracephalic pain. *Headache* 1998;38:138–141.
16. Ostergaard JR, Kraft M. Natural history of benign coital headache. *BMJ* 1992;305:1129.
17. Sami HR, Couch JR. Headache associated with sexual activity. In: Gilman S, ed. *MedLink neurology*. San Diego: MedLink Corp, 2004. Available at www.medlink.com.
18. Evans RW, Pascual J. Orgasmic headaches: clinical features, diagnosis, and management. *Headache* 2000;40(6),491–494.
19. Akpunona SE, Ahrens J. Sexual headaches: case report, review, and treatment with calcium blocker. *Headache* 1991;31:141–145.
20. Evans RW, Couch JR. Orgasm and migraine. *Headache* 2001; 41(5):512–514.
21. Kruuse C, Thomsen LL, Birk S, et al. Migraine can be induced by sildenafil without changes in middle cerebral artery diameter. *Brain* 2003;126(Pt 1):241–247.
22. Arnett BC. Tonsillar ectopia and headaches. *Neurol Clin N Am* 2004;22:229–236.
23. Elster AD, Chen MY. Chiari I malformations: clinical and radiologic reappraisal. *Radiology* 1992;183:347–353.
24. Milhorat TH, Chou MW, Trinidad EM, et al. Chiari I malformation redefined: clinical and radiographic findings for 364 symptomatic patients. *Neurosurgery* 1999;44:1005–1017.
25. Pillay PK, Awad IA, Little JR, et al. Symptomatic Chiari malformation in adults: a new classification based on magnetic resonance imaging with clinical and prognostic significance. *Neurosurgery* 1991;28:639–645.
26. Pascual J, Oterino A, Berciano J. Headache in type I Chiari malformation. *Neurology* 1992;42:1519–1521.
27. Khurana RK. Headache spectrum in Arnold-Chiari malformation. *Headache* 1991;31:151–155.
28. Ramadan NB. Unusual causes of headache. *Neurology* 1997; 48:1494–1499.
29. Jacome DE, Stamm MA. Malignant cough headache. *Headache* 2004;44:259–261.
30. Ramadan NM, Khayr W. Headache associated with AIDS. In: Gilman S, ed. *MedLink neurology*. San Diego: MedLink Corp, 2004. Available at www.medlink.com.
31. Mirsattari SM, Power C, Nath A. Primary headaches in HIV-infected patients. *Headache* 1999;39:3–10.
32. Greenlee JE. Brain abscess. In: Gilman S, ed. *MedLink neurology*. San Diego: MedLink Corp, 2004. Available at www.medlink.com.
33. Carlini ME, Harris RL. Central nervous system infections. In: Evans RW, ed. *Diagnostic testing in neurology*. Philadelphia: WB Saunders, 1999:405–417.

34. Silberstein SD, Dongmei L. Headache associated with meningitis, encephalitis, and brain abscess. In: Gilman S, ed. *MedLink neurology*. San Diego: MedLink Corp, 2004. Available at www.medlink.com.

35. Jain KK. Drug-induced aseptic meningitis. In: Gilman S, ed. *MedLink neurology*. San Diego: MedLink Corp, 2004. Available at www.medlink.com.

36. Neufeld MY, Treves TA, Chistik V, et al. Postmeningitis headache. *Headache* 1999;39:132–134.

37. Halperin JL. Lyme disease. In: Gilman S, ed. *Medlink neurology*. San Diego: MedLink Corp, 2004. Available at www.medlink.com.

38. Kupersmith MJ, Martin V, Heller G, et al. Idiopathic hypertropic pachymeningitis. *Neurology* 2004;62:686–694.

39. Nitu AN, Ramadan NM. Headache associated with metabolic disorders. In: Gilman S, ed. *MedLink neurology*. San Diego: MedLink Corp, 2004. Available at www.medlink.com.

40. Moreau T, Manceau E, Giroud-Baleydier F, et al. Headache in hypothyroidism. Prevalence and outcome under thyroid hormone therapy. *Cephalalgia* 1998;18(10):687–689.

41. Goksan B, Karaali-Savrun F, Ertan S, et al. Haemodialysis-related headache. *Cephalalgia* 2004;24(4):284–287.

42. Honigman B, Theis MK, Koziol-McLain J, et al. Acute mountain sickness in a general tourist population at moderate altitudes. *Ann Intern Med* 1993;118:587–592.

43. Sutton JR. High-altitude physiology and medicine. In: Evans RW, ed. *Neurology and trauma*. Philadelphia: WB Saunders, 1996.

44. Krasney JA. A neurogenic basis for acute altitude illness. *Med Sci Sports Exerc* 1994;26:195–208.

45. Basnyat B, Murdoch DR. High-altitude illness. *Lancet* 2003;7;361(9373):1967–1974.

46. Burtscher M, Likar R, Nachbauer W, et al. Aspirin for prophylaxis against headache at high altitudes: randomized, double blind, placebo controlled trial. *BMJ* 1998;316:1057–1058.

47. Greer HD, Massey EW. Neurological injury from undersea diving. In: Evans RW, ed. *Neurology and trauma*. Philadelphia: WB Saunders, 1996.

48. Evans RW. Hyperventilation syndrome. In: Gilman S, ed. *MedLink neurology*. San Diego: MedLink Corp, 2004. Available at www.medlink.com.

49. Lewis RA, Howell JBL. Definition of the hyperventilation syndrome. *Bull Eur Physiopathol Respir* 1986;22:201–204.

50. Hirokawa Y, Kondo T, Ohta Y, et al. Clinical characteristics and outcome of 508 patients with hyperventilation syndrome. *Nippon Kyobu Shikkan Gakkai Zasshi* 1995;33:940–946.

51. Evans RW. Neurologic aspects of hyperventilation syndrome. *Semin Neurol* 1995;15:115–125.

52. Beumer HM, Bruyn GW. Hyperventilation syndrome. In: Goetz CG, Tanner CM, Aminoff MJ, eds. *Handbook of clinical neurology,* vol. 19. Amsterdam: Elsevier Science, 1993:429–448.

53. Sahota PK, Dexter JD. Sleep and headache syndromes: a clinical review. *Headache* 1990;30:80–84.

54. Peres MFP. Sleep disorders associated with headaches. In: Gilman S, ed. *MedLink neurology*. San Diego: MedLink Corp, 2004. Available at www.medlink.com.

55. Gould JD, Silberstein SD. Unilateral hypnic headache: a case study. *Neurology* 1997;49:1749–1750.
56. Ulfberg J, Carter N, Talback M, et al. Headache, snoring, and sleep apnoea. *J Neurol* 1996;243:621–625.
57. Neau JP, Paquereau J, Bailbe M, et al. Relationship between sleep apnoea syndrome, snoring and headaches. *Cephalalgia* 2002;22(5):333–339.
58. Vaughn BV. Sleep bruxism. In: Gilman S, ed. *MedLink neurology*. San Diego: MedLink Corp, 2004. Available at www.medlink.com.
59. Blau JN. Sleep deprivation headache. *Cephalalgia* 1990;10: 157–160.
60. Gilbert GJ. Turtle headache. *JAMA* 1982;248:921.
61. Blau J. Resolution of migraine attacks: sleep and the recovery phase. *J Neurol Neurosurg Psychiatry* 1982;45:223–226.
62. Giroud M, Nivelon JL, Dumas R. [Somnambulism and migraine in children: a non-fortuitous association]. *Arch Fr Pediatr* 1987; 44:263–265.
63. Dexter JD. The relationship between disorders of arousal from sleep and migraine. *Headache* 1986;26:322.
64. Evans RW, Pearce JMS. Exploding head syndrome. *Headache* 2001;41(6):602–603.
65. Welch KMA, Lewis D. Migraine and epilepsy. *Neurol Clin* 1997;15:107–123.
66. Marks DA, Ehrenberg BL. Migraine-related seizures in adults with epilepsy with EEG correlation. *Neurology* 1993;43: 2476–2483.
67. Panayiotopoulos CP. Elementary visual hallucinations, blindness, and headache in idiopathic occipital epilepsy: differentiation from migraine. *J Neurol Neurosurg Psychiatry* 1999;66: 536–540.
68. Young GB, Blume WT. Painful epileptic seizures. *Brain* 1983; 106:537–554.
69. Schon F, Blau JN. Post-epileptic headache and migraine. *J Neurol Neurosurg Psychiatry* 1987;50:1148–1152.
70. Leniger T, Isbruch K, von Den Driesch S, et al. Seizure-associated headache in epilepsy. *Epilepsia* 2001;42(9):1176–1179.
71. Bernasconi A, Andermann F, Bernasconi N, et al. Lateralizing value of peri-ictal headache: a study of 100 patients with partial epilepsy. *Neurology* 2001;56(1):130–132.
72. Freedman MS, Gray TA. Vascular headache: a presenting symptom of multiple sclerosis. *Can J Neurol Sci* 1989;16:63–66.
73. Rolak LA, Brown S. Headaches and multiple sclerosis: a clinical study and review of the literature. *J Neurol* 1990;237:300–302.
74. Davidoff RA. Trigeminal neuralgia. In: Gilman S, ed. *MedLink neurology*. San Diego: MedLink Corp, 2004. Available at www.medlink.com.
75. Ardila A, Maher J, Hachinski VC. Transient global amnesia. In: Gilman S, ed. *MedLink neurology*. San Diego: MedLink Corp, 2004. Available at www.medlink.com.
76. Finnerup NB, Gottrup H, Jensen TS. Anticonvulsants in central pain. *Expert Opin Pharmacother* 2002;3(10):1411–1420.
77. Rozen TD. Trigeminal neuralgia and glossopharyngeal neuralgia. *Neurol Clin* 2004; 22:185–206.

What's My Headache?

Randolph W. Evans

Now it's time to play, "What's my headache?" the popular game enjoyed by millions of Americans yearly when they come to see their doctors. The focus is on diagnosis and management. A brief summary of a case based on patients I have seen is provided. Then you should decide on your diagnosis and management. What tests, if any, would you order, or can the diagnosis be made without testing? What treatment is appropriate? Final answer? You can then compare your answers with my diagnosis and management provided in the answers section at the end of the case presentations. The chapter (or chapters) dealing with the topic is also provided. The cases range from common to uncommon to rare causes and presentations of headaches.

Case Presentations

Case 1

A 31-year-old attorney complains of sinus headaches about three times monthly since her teens. She complains of a unilateral retroorbital pressure and throbbing of moderate to severe intensity associated with nausea, light and noise sensitivity, nasal stuffiness, and sometimes nasal drainage. The headache is worse with movement. Triggers include changes in the weather and her menses. She reports that her mother and two sisters also have sinus headaches. Over-the-counter sinus medications may dull the pain. The headaches last about 24 hours and may require bed rest. Medical history is otherwise negative except for a history of mitral valve prolapse, frequent anxiety, and panic attacks.

What is the diagnosis and what treatment is recommended?

Case 2

This 10-year-old boy was seen with a 1.5-year history of headaches that were all the same. He described a bifrontal pounding associated with a little nausea and with light and noise sensitivity. The headaches lasted about 1 hour and were helped by lying down and ibuprofen. The headaches usually occurred three or four times per month. During the prior 2 weeks, he had had five. The mother reported no increased stress or changes in schoolwork. There was a medical history of sinus symptoms and allergy treated with Bromfed. Family history is noncontributory. Neurological exam was normal.

What is the diagnosis? Would you order an imaging study? What treatment would you suggest?

Case 3

An 84-year-old woman was referred with a 2.5-week history of intermittent daily severe headaches described as a right retroorbital, hemicranial, and nuchal occipital pounding and pressure. She also reported pressure in the right posterior neck. Tylenol was of mild help. She thought she might have low-grade fever. She also complained of soreness of the right temporomandibular joint with eating. She denied any shoulder or pelvic girdle aching and had no recent weight loss. On examination, the right superficial temporal artery pulse was not present and the area was very tender.

What is the diagnosis? What studies are indicated? What is your treatment?

Case 4

This 31-year-old man complained of an 8-month history of daily severe headaches that often occurred in the afternoon. The headaches usually began bifrontally and then become a generalized throbbing with increased intensity with bending over or coughing. The headaches lasted several hours and could be associated with frequent nausea and occasional vomiting and photophobia. There was a history of occasional mild headaches. Neurological exam was normal.

What is the diagnosis? Would you recommend an imaging study? What treatment would you recommend?

Case 5

A 44-year-old woman is referred to the office with a 3-day history of a severe nuchal occipital and generalized throbbing ache associated with nausea and worse with movement. She had been seen in an emergency room the day before, where she was given a Stadol injection with only mild help. About 1 month earlier she had a similar but less severe headache that lasted 1 day. She otherwise had a history of occasional mild headaches. Neurological exam was normal.

What is your diagnosis? Would you recommend testing? Would you try giving a triptan?

Case 6

A 35-year-old woman complains of stress headaches. For the last few years, about one time a week, she develops a mild left-sided neck tightness that, after several hours, can spread to the left temporal area with moderate intensity. There is light and noise sensitivity and, sometimes, nausea. The headaches last about 8 hours and are minimally reduced by ibuprofen. She works full time and has three children. The headaches often occur in the late afternoon as she is rushing from work to picking up the children and preparing dinner.

What is your diagnosis? What treatment do you recommend?

Case 7

On the day before the consultation, this 47-year-old attorney had sex after a several-week abstinence. One minute before a second orgasm, he developed a bad, pounding nuchal occipital headache that increased in intensity with orgasm. The headache was bad for 1 hour and persisted as a mild nuchal-occipital ache when he was seen. He had no nausea, vomiting, or other symptoms. He had rare mild headaches in the past. Neurological exam was normal. The neck was supple.

What is your diagnosis? Would you recommend testing?

Case 8

This 33-year-old woman had a history of only occasional mild headaches. One year before presentation, she developed increasingly frequent headaches that were daily for the month before consultation. She described having daily mild to moderate bifrontal aching and throbbing headaches. About twice a week, the headache became a bifrontal and nuchal occipital pounding associated with nausea, light and noise sensitivity, and occasional vomiting. The mild to moderate headaches lasted about 2 hours if she took Excedrin Migraine. The severe headaches could last all day and she would go to bed. She was taking from two to six Excedrin Migraine tablets daily. In the year prior, she had seen an internist, a chiropractor, and another neurologist. A magnetic resonance imaging (MRI) scan of the brain was normal. No new medications were started. Neurological exam was normal.

What is your diagnosis? Would you recommend additional testing? How would you manage this patient?

Case 9

A 23-year-old woman in the middle of her menses presented with a 4-day history of a constant severe headache described as a generalized heaviness associated with noise sensitivity but no nausea, vomiting, light sensitivity, fever, or systemic symptoms. She reported occasional headaches in the past. She did have a history of two throbbing headaches on the top of her head followed by brief syncopal episodes at the ages of 8 and 18. With the last episode, testing, including an electroencephalogram and computed tomography (CT) scan, were reportedly negative. Family history was remarkable for two maternal aunts with migraine. Neurological exam was normal. Toradol 60 mg intramuscularly (IM) was given in the office. Within 30 minutes, the headache was reduced from an intensity rating of 10 to a level of 1.

What is your diagnosis? Would you recommend testing?

Case 10

This 18-year-old woman reported headaches every 2 weeks for the previous few years described as a bifrontal pressure relieved by ibuprofen. For the prior 2 years, every 3 or 4 months around her menses she had episodes of blurred vision in the right field of vision lasting 15 to 30 minutes without an associated headache or other symptoms. She presented with a 4-day history of an intermittent bitemporal and retroorbital pounding with noise sensitivity but no other symptoms. The headache was behind the right eye the day before the office visit and behind the left eye the next morning but had resolved by the afternoon office visit. The intensity was mild initially but became severe over a matter of a several hours. There was no history of similar headaches. She had no sinus or systemic symptoms. She had been on oral contraceptives for 4 months. Family history was noncontributory. Neurological exam was normal.

What is the diagnosis? Would you recommend testing?

Case 11

This 33-year-old man presented with a 6-year history of episodic headaches that occurred about every 1 to 2 years, often in the spring, and that recurred over an 8-week period. The current headaches were present for 10 days. He described a severe stabbing around the left eye and forehead associated with conjunctival injection, ipsilateral tearing of the eye, and clear drainage from the nares. The headaches lasted about 45 minutes, during which time he paced about and sometimes banged his head. He typically had two headaches per day, one in the afternoon and the other awakening him from sleep around 2 A.M.

What is your diagnosis? Would you recommend an imaging study? What treatment would you provide?

Case 12

This 35-year-old woman reported occasional mild headaches in the past. For the last few months, she has had a daily and fairly constant generalized nonthrobbing ache of moderate intensity without associated symptoms. She remembered the exact day of the onset but there were no precipitants such as respiratory infections or head trauma. Over-the-counter medications have been of little help and she stopped taking any medication. She drank occasional caffeinated beverages. She reports increased financial stress recently. Family history: 7-year-old daughter with chronic headaches. Neurological exam was normal.

What is your diagnosis? Would you recommend testing? What treatment would you suggest?

Case 13

This 27-year-old woman had occasional headaches in the past. She presented with a 3-month history of daily, intermittent nuchal occipital pressure-type headaches on the left more than the right that could occur any time of the day but did not awaken her from sleep. She reported being under increased stress. Her husband was being transferred out of state, her family was here, and she would prefer not moving. She has three small children. Exam showed left midsuperior nuchal line tenderness. Digital pressure produced pain similar to her headache. Neurological exam was otherwise normal.

What is the diagnosis? Would you recommend testing? What treatment would you recommend?

Case 14

This 26-year-old woman, 12 weeks pregnant, was admitted to the hospital by her obstetrician with a severe right nuchal-occipital and parietal pressure headache with nausea and vomiting present for 7 days. During the preceding 3 months, she had daily headaches. She had no fever or systemic symptoms. She was given intravenous (IV) morphine and phenergan, which did not help. She had a history of recurring generalized throbbing headaches with nausea, vomiting, and light and noise sensitivity lasting 3 to 4 days for the last 8 years. She saw a neurologist 4 months before admission and was diagnosed with migraine. Before this pregnancy, she was having headaches three times per month for the last 2 years. Neurological exam was normal.

What is the diagnosis? Would you recommend testing? What treatment would you recommend?

Case 15

A middle-aged man reports severe stabbing headaches shooting up from the palate lasting perhaps 30 seconds. The headaches are triggered by ice cream or yogurt. Although the headache is a 10, medical attention has never been sought. Neurological exam is normal.

What is the diagnosis? Would you recommend testing?

Case 16

This 24-year-old man came in with a 6-day history of a nuchal-occipital bad-aching headache associated with nausea and with sensitivity to light and noise. His concentration seemed off and he had intermittent blurred vision. One week earlier he had been in a motor vehicle accident in which he had bumped his forehead and briefly lost consciousness. That day he was seen in the emergency room and discharged on ibuprofen after a normal cervical spine series was obtained. Neurological exam is normal.

What is the diagnosis? Would you order an imaging study?

Case 17

This 30-year-old obese woman was seen with a 3-month history of rather constant, daily, generalized aching and throbbing headaches associated with intermittent brief graying out of vision. Neurological exam was normal except for bilateral papilledema.

What is the diagnosis? What tests would you recommend?

Case 18

This 11-year-old girl reported a history of four or five spells with the first at 7 years of age and the last 3 days before the consultation. The prior headache occurred 1 week previously. The episodes occurred while playing catch or running around except for the last one, which happened after she was dancing, laid down for a few minutes, and then got up. The episodes were described as an intense feeling of the right side of the head going to sleep or vibrating and lasting about 30 seconds. With all the episodes except the last, which was mild, she would fall down because of the pain. However, she did not believe there was any alteration in or loss of consciousness. Otherwise, her history was one of occasional mild headaches. There was no history of syncope, seizures, significant head trauma, or meningitis. Family history was negative for migraine and seizures. Neurological exam was normal.

What is the diagnosis? What tests would you recommend?

Case 19

This 35-year-old woman developed severe stabbing and throbbing pain in the left anterior neck and left side of the face, but not the head, lasting about 5 hours. For years she had experienced frequent right nuchal occipital pressure–type headaches associated with posterior neck tightness. She went to the emergency department, where the exam was normal and she was advised to see her doctor the next day. The next day her examination was normal.

What is the diagnosis? Would you recommend any testing?

Case 20

A 31-year-old woman has a 10-year history of mild headaches occurring about once a month. For the last 6 months, the headaches have increased in frequency and severity occurring 5 days per week and are described as a pressure around her eyes with nausea and light sensitivity typically of moderate intensity but severe once a week lasting many hours. There was no aura. There is no family history of migraine. Neurological exam was normal. A MRI scan of the brain was normal. She was started on topiramate 25 mg at bedtime to be increased by 25 mg per week to 100 mg per day.

When seen in follow-up 1 month later, the headaches were mild and had decreased to one or two per week. However, she reported having five episodes during the prior 3 weeks lasting 2 to 3 minutes and followed by a mild pressure headache behind her eyes lasting 30 to 45 minutes without medication. With three of the episodes, she felt like her entire body was too big and everything else was too small. With two of the episodes, she had a feeling her entire body was too small and everything else too big. During the episodes, however, everything actually looked normal and she was aware her abnormal feeling was not real. An EEG was normal.

On follow-up 5 weeks later, she reported eight episodes all lasting about 5 to 10 minutes. During four of the episodes she reported feeling too small and with two, too big. With two episodes, she would feel too big for about 5 minutes and then too small for about 5 minutes. All of the episodes were followed by a mild headache lasting about 1 hour.

What is the diagnosis?

Case 21

This 49-year-old woman was referred by her family physician for severe headaches. The patient reported an 11-day history of a right retroorbital and hemicranial throbbing headache that was worse with movement; she also experienced lightheadedness. She had nausea and vomiting for 2 days 4 days prior to the consultation. She had no fever, sinus symptoms, or systemic symptoms. She also complained of low-back soreness for 3 days. Her family physician gave her a cortisone shot for possible allergies, which did not help. A few days later she was given a Demerol injection, which also did not help. She then saw her allergist and was given Imitrex 50 mg orally and Medrol for 2 days without benefit. She was also prescribed Fiorinal #3 and Vicodin, which only dulled the headache, and Antivert, which did not help the dizziness. From her mid-20s until about 35 years of age, she had throbbing headaches on the top of her head associated with nausea and vomiting. Since then, she has had only occasional mild headaches. Neurological exam was normal. Her neck was supple.

What is your diagnosis? Would you recommend any testing? What treatment would you recommend?

Case 22

This 17-year-old young man presented with a 6-month history of bilateral throbbing headaches triggered by sneezing, coughing, weight lifting, or bowel movements lasting about 3 minutes.

About half of the time, a slight headache would persist for an additional 5 minutes. Before the visit, he was having about 10 headaches each week. He saw his family physician, who obtained a CT scan of the head with and without contrast, which was negative. He was placed on Inderal LA 60 mg daily without help. His father has cluster headaches. Neurological exam was normal.

What is your diagnosis? Would you recommend any additional evaluation or treatment?

Case 23

One evening I received a frantic telephone call from a friend who was in her Suburban en route to a pediatric emergency room. Her 9-year-old son was playing just a short time before at home when he accidentally bumped the back of his head on a table. There was no loss of consciousness. Within a couple of minutes, he developed a left frontal pain, nausea, vomiting, and sleepiness. There was no prior history of significant headaches or motion sickness. Family history was negative for migraine.

What would you tell the mother?

Case 24

This 45-year-old woman presented with a 4-day history of a right-sided throbbing headache with nausea and vomiting for 2 days. The day of the consultation, she complained of a right nuchal occipital and right frontal aching without nausea, fever, or systemic symptoms. There was a 15-year history of recurring headaches. The bad headaches had occurred about once weekly for the prior 6 months but were occasional for many years. She described a usually right-sided and occasionally left-sided throbbing associated with nausea and occasionally vomiting with light and noise sensitivity but no aura. The headaches usually lasted 1 day but could last up to 4. There were no triggers. Imitrex SC on one occasion did not help. Neurological exam was normal except for intensification of the headache with digital pressure over the right midsuperior nuchal line (over the greater occipital nerve).

What is your diagnosis? Would you recommend testing? What treatment would you suggest?

Case 25

A 54-year-old white woman was seen with a 10-year history of episodes of a burning sensation of the left ear. The episodes are preceded by nausea and a hot feeling for about 15 seconds and then the left ear becomes visibly red for an average of about 1 hour, with a range from about 30 minutes to 2 hours. About once every 2 years, she would have a flurry of episodes occurring over about a 1-month period during which she would average about five episodes with a range of one to six.

There was also an 18-year history of migraine without aura occurring about once a year. Neurological exam was normal.

What is the diagnosis?

Case 26

A 32-year-old woman has a 3-year history of headaches that are a bilateral occipital and retroorbital throbbing associated with nausea but no aura, vomiting, or light or noise sensitivity and lasting up to 2 days. Fiorinal #3 decreased but did not relieve the pain. The headaches occurred one or two times each week 1 year ago, but in the last year they have been infrequent, with the last occurring 4 months ago while she was taking amitriptyline and propranolol. She presented with a 4-day history of a severe bilateral occipital and retroorbital throbbing associated with light and noise sensitivity, nausea, but no aura or vomiting. She had not had any fever or systemic symptoms. Neurological exam was normal. She was admitted by her gynecologist and placed on parenteral narcotics without help.

What is the diagnosis? Would you recommend any testing? What treatment is indicated?

Case 27

This 61-year-old woman was seen with a 10-year history of a right mandibular sharp pain lasting seconds and extending from the chin to the TMJ area along the mandible. The pain was sometimes triggered by drinking water, talking, and chewing. There were no trigger zones to touch. She also had an intermittent right mandibular distribution dull ache at times. The pain would occur intermittently for a few months with up to 10 paroxysms daily and then go away for a few months but was almost daily for the prior year. She saw a dentist who gave her a partial bridge without help and then a second dentist who gave her a night guard without benefit. Neurological exam was normal.

What is the diagnosis? Would you recommend any testing? What treatment would you suggest?

Case 28

This 23-year-old woman was seen with a 5-day history of a severe bifrontal-temporal throbbing headache associated with nausea and photophobia, which was worse supine. She had no fever, sinus, or systemic symptoms. There was a history of occasional "sinus headaches" described as a hemicranial throbbing with nausea and light sensitivity occurring before her menses. She had been evaluated in the emergency department the night before the office visit. A CT scan of the brain and lumbar puncture and cerebrospinal fluid (CSF) evaluation were reported as normal. She was afebrile. Neurological exam was normal.

What is the diagnosis? Would you recommend any testing? What treatment would you suggest?

Case 29

A 69-year-old woman presented with a 6-month history of a recurring right retroorbital and occasionally nuchal-occipital piercing pain that could last up to 1 hour and often occurred at night. There was a history, going back a number of years, of posterior neck symptoms without upper-extremity complaints. Exam was normal except for marked right midsuperior nuchal line tenderness reproducing the headache.

What is the diagnosis? Would you recommend testing? What treatment would you recommend?

Case 30

This 60-year-old woman has about a 30-year history of episodes of vertigo with a spinning sensation and associated nausea occurring about twice per year and lasting about 1 day. The episodes either awaken her from sleep or are present upon awakening in the morning. There is no associated headache, pressure in the ears, tinnitus, or hearing loss. She recently saw an ENT physician and had a normal ENG and an audiogram showing mild bilateral high frequency sensorineural loss.

She has had a few severe headaches per year since about the age of 10 described as a unilateral throbbing with light and noise sensitivity but no aura or nausea that can last all day. She is not aware of any triggers. Acetaminophen dulls the headache but she has not tried any prescription drugs. There is a past medical history of ulcerative colitis for a few years and hypertension. Neurological exam is normal.

What is the diagnosis? What treatment would you recommend?

Case 31

This 38-year-old G2 P2 had a C-section 6 days previously for failure to progress. The epidural catheter was removed 1 day postpartum. She was breastfeeding. The day before I saw her, she developed a mild headache that within 30 minutes became a severe 10/10 generalized throbbing associated with nausea, light, and noise sensitivity and blurred vision. The headache was not better supine. She had no fever, back pain, or systemic complaints. This headache, the worst of her life, was still severe the next day when she was evaluated. There was a history of throbbing generalized headaches with nausea, vomiting, and light and noise sensitivity occurring several times per year but none since the first trimester. She was afebrile and had a supple neck. Neurological exam was normal.

What is your diagnosis? Would you recommend any testing? What treatment would you recommend?

Case 32

An 82-year-old man was seen with an 8-hour history of a mild dull right frontal headache that had been present since awakening. He had played golf that morning but did not feel quite right and shot a 92, about 10 strokes higher than his usual. (He had had a single-digit handicap when he was younger.) The headache was more intense when he bent over to pick up the ball or tee it up. There was no history of significant headaches. He was in good health except for hypertension controlled with medication. Neurological exam was normal.

What is your diagnosis? Would you recommend any testing? What treatment would you recommend?

Case 33

A 52-year-old overweight male police officer presented with a 2-month history of a dull intense bifrontal and retroorbital, rather constant headache that was worse with coughing or bending over. He had had occasional mild headaches in the past.

Neurological exam was normal except for the presence of papilledema. A MRI scan of the brain was normal.

What is your diagnosis? Would you recommend further testing? What treatment would you recommend?

Case 34

This 73-year-old woman presented with a 3-week history of a daily, mild to moderate, aching, generalized headache. She had experienced migraines for the last 15 years. There was a history of a mastectomy for breast carcinoma 3 years previously. Neurological exam was normal. A CT scan of the brain with and without contrast obtained by her primary care physician was normal.

What is your diagnosis? Would you recommend further testing? What treatment would you recommend?

Case 35

A 28-year-old woman is seen for evaluation of left-sided numbness. The patient developed a pounding bifrontal headache lasting about 5 hours. She went to sleep and the headache was gone the next morning. That afternoon she had the sudden onset of tingling of the left face and a numb and weak feeling on her left side. There was a history of occasional mild headaches. Neurological exam showed decreased sensation over the entire left face and left side of the body and decreased rapid alternating movements of the left side. A CT scan of the brain was normal.

What is your diagnosis? Would you recommend further testing?

Case 36

This 76-year-old woman underwent a left carotid endarterectomy for asymptomatic 95% internal carotid stenosis. There was no neurological deficit postoperatively. The next morning, she complained of a severe left frontotemporal-hemicranial aching headache without associated symptoms. Neurological exam was again normal.

What is your diagnosis? Would you recommend further testing?

Case 37

A previously healthy 42-year-old man was hospitalized with a 1-month history of right-sided headaches. Neurological exam was normal. A MRI scan of the brain revealed diffuse enhancement of the meninges.

What is your diagnosis? What further testing would you recommend?

The patient became progressively encephalopathic the day after admission and, by 2 weeks after admission, he was comatose. What is your diagnosis now?

Case 38

A 62-year-old man saw an orthopedist, complaining of a 4-month history of fairly constant neck pain, which he believed started after having his head propped at an angle for a long period of time. For the prior 2 months, he had had a constant dull ache behind the eyes, across the forehead, and sometimes on the top of the head. The neck pain, which frequently awakened him from sleep, was better with heat and ice and worse with bending the neck backward and to the left or right. Coughing or sneezing would cause a brief stabbing pain behind the left or right ear. His internist had tried him on naproxen with little help. On exam, the neck was nontender, with a decreased range of motion in all directions. Neurological exam was normal. A cervical spine series showed multilevel spondylosis. An erythrocyte sedimentation rate (ESR) was 1.

What is your diagnosis? What treatment would you recommend? Would you recommend any further testing?

The patient returned to see the orthopedist 2 weeks later with a 1-week history of complaints of intermittent slurred speech and difficulty eating, with problems coordinating his tongue and jaw. His wife was concerned that he might have had a stroke.

What would you recommend now?

Case 39

This 32-year-old woman was seen with an acute throbbing behind the left eye and across the forehead that was associated with nausea, vomiting, and light and noise sensitivity that had awakened her from sleep 9 hours earlier. This was the worst headache of her life and different from prior headaches. For 2 days previously she had had a mild constant bifrontal pressure headache. There was a history of left-sided throbbing headaches associated with nausea and noise sensitivity but no aura since 9 years of age. These headaches would begin 3 to 4 days before her menses started and last about 3 to 4 days. Imitrex 50 mg orally would help the headache, which would then recur. For the prior 5 years, she also had a left nuchal occipital parietal pressure headache about every other day that could last hours. She was taking 12 Tylenol per week and about 30 Fiorecet per month for the headaches. She had been on Prozac 20 mg daily for the prior year without reducing the headaches. Neurological exam was normal. She was afebrile.

What is your diagnosis? Would you recommend any testing? What treatment would you recommend?

Case 40

A 45-year-old woman presents with a 3 month history of a scalp pain. She describes a burning, stinging, itching, and sore pain of the mid posterior frontal and anterior parietal scalp in an elliptical distribution extending across both sides with a diameter of about 5 cm. The pain is present intermittently daily lasting hours at a time with an intensity of 5/10. At times, the area is sensitive when she brushes her hair. Ibuprofen may reduce the discomfort. She has seen two dermatologists who found normal skin examinations. There is no history of migraine or other headaches. Past medical history of hypertension. Neurological exam was normal with no abnormality of scalp sensation.

What is your diagnosis? Would you recommend any testing? What treatment would you recommend?

Case 41

The patient with the pilocytic astrocytoma diagnosed in pregnancy presented in case 14 had seen another neurologist 4 months before the diagnosis at 12 weeks gestation (i.e., 1 month before the pregnancy). Based on a history of typical nonprogressive headaches and a normal neurological exam, she was diagnosed with migraine. The patient requested a MRI scan of the brain, but the neurologist suggested she try treatment first.

Postpartum the first neurologist was sued for failure to diagnose. Plaintiff counsel argued that if the scan had been done as the patient requested, the neoplasm would have been diagnosed at an earlier stage increasing her chance of survival. In addition, she would have elected not to get pregnant at that time and her twins would not have been exposed to the myriad potential risks of a life-threatening illness during pregnancy.

What is the first neurologist's defense in this malpractice case?

Case 42

A 43-year-old woman was seen with a 5-month history of a noise in her head. On an almost nightly basis, as she was falling asleep, she would hear a loud noise like "electrical current running," lasting a second. Sometimes, her whole body would shake for a second afterward. Very occasionally, she would have an associated flash of light. Frequently, a second episode of the loud noise would occur shortly after the first. She could then fall asleep without any problem. The past medical history was positive only for hypertension controlled with medication. Neurological exam was normal. Diagnostic testing was not performed.

What is the diagnosis?

CASE STUDY ANSWERS

Case 1

Is she correct? Does she have sinus headaches? Stereotypical recurring headaches of moderate to severe intensity for many years are much more likely caused by migraine rather than sinus. Are the features of her headache consistent with migraine without aura? Absolutely. Her headaches meet the IHS migraine without aura criteria. The features of her headaches are found in the following percentages of migraines: unilateral, 60%; throbbing, 85%; moderate-severe, 80%; nausea, 80%; and light and noise sensitivity, 80%.

What about her complaints of nasal stuffiness and sometimes nasal drainage associated with her headaches? How could these symptoms be associated with migraine? Forty-five percent of migraineurs have at least one autonomic symptom (lacrimation, eye redness, ptosis, eyelid edema, nasal congestion, and rhinorrhea) during an attack. Of these, 45% have both nasal and ocular symptoms, 21% have only nasal symptoms, and 34% have only ocular symptoms. Migraine is commonly associated with autonomic symptoms because of parasympathetic activation of the sphenopalatine ganglion, which innervates the tear ducts and sinuses during an attack. Migraine is also misdiagnosed as sinus because the pain can occur in all distributions of the trigeminal nerve including the face.

What about her triggers? Eighty-five percent of migraineurs report triggers with a mean of 3. This patient's triggers are common. About 50% of women report menses as a trigger (14% have migraines only associated with their menses), and up to 50% of migraineurs report that a change of weather is a trigger.

Does her history of mitral valve prolapse, generalized anxiety, and panic attacks have any relationship to her migraine? Yes! There are many disorders with a greater than coincidental association, comorbidity, with migraine including stroke, epilepsy, systemic lupus erythematosis, Raynaud's syndrome, multiple sclerosis, and essential tremor. Psychiatric disorders comorbid with migraine include bipolar disease, major depression, generalized anxiety disorder, panic disorder, and simple and social phobia. Migraine may also be associated with hypertension, mitral valve prolapse, and patent foramen ovale.

The patient, however, insists she as well as her mother and two sisters all have sinus headaches. She said she was familiar with migraine, had friends with migraine, had seen television and print advertisements for migraine drugs, but she was certain of her sinus diagnosis. She is in good company with many migraineurs and even physicians in this misdiagnosis. Fifty percent of migraineurs do not know they have migraine. Forty-two percent of the undiagnosed self-diagnose themselves with sinus and 43% have received a diagnosis of sinus headache from a physician. Her family history was also unreliable. On further questioning, her mother and two sisters had long histories of stereotypical "sick" headaches often requiring bed rest. A denial of a family history of migraine is often inaccurate. Frequently, if one can obtain specific information about the headaches of first-degree relatives of migraineurs, one diagnoses migraine. In many instances, when parents, siblings, or children of migraineurs are present for the consultation, I inquire about their headaches and they discover for the first time they have migraine. (Chapter 2)

Case 2

This is a typical case of childhood migraine, which occurs in about 5% of boys. Migraines can be different in children from those in adults because the headaches have a shorter duration, often less than 2 hours, and are more often bilateral, frontal, and temporal (65% vs. 40% in adults) than unilateral. After discussion with his ear, nose, and throat (ENT) physician, who had started the Bromfed for atopic allergies, Bromfed was discontinued and he was started on Periactin 4 mg at bedtime. This is a treatment "two for" because Periactin is an antihistamine and an effective preventive migraine drug in children. (Other "two fors" are tricyclic antidepressants, for the treatment of migraine and depression; beta-blockers, for migraine and hypertension; and Depakote, for migraine and epilepsy.) After 2 weeks, the dose of Periactin was increased to 8 mg at bedtime. Within a few weeks, the frequency of the headaches decreased to two or three per month. (Chapter 10)

Case 3

A MRI scan of the brain was negative. The erythrocyte sedimentation rate (ESR) was 97 mm per hour. A superficial temporal artery (STA) biopsy was negative. The headache resolved within 24 hours of starting prednisone 60 mg daily. A repeat

ESR 2 weeks later was 55. The dose of prednisone was slowly tapered.

The diagnosis is temporal arteritis. Headaches are present in 60% to 90% of patients and jaw claudication is found in 38%. The false-negative rate of STA biopsy ranges from 5% to 44% in different series. Although other positive findings were present in this patient, the STA has a normal pulse and is nontender in about 50% of cases. The ESR has been reported as normal in 10% to 36% of cases. When abnormal, the ESR averages 70 to 80 and may be as high as 130 mm per hour. The C-reactive protein can also be very useful, providing additional sensitivity and specificity for the diagnosis, especially when the ESR is normal or only mildly elevated. (Chapter 12)

Case 4

This was the first headache patient I saw after completing my residency. Although the headaches are migrainelike, the daily occurrence does not fit for migraine. Medication rebound is a consideration, but he had stopped taking medications because nothing worked. A CT scan of the head demonstrated a colloid cyst of the third ventricle. He underwent craniotomy and transcollosal removal of the cyst. The headaches were gone post-operatively.

Colloid cysts of the third ventricle account for only 1% of primary intracranial mass lesions. Sudden death occurs in 5% of patients. Although you may never see a patient with a colloid cyst (some 40,000 patients later, I have seen only one other case), remember that the diagnosis of primary or benign headaches is one of exclusion. (Chapter 14)

Case 5

Statistically, this patient would probably have new-onset migraine even though migraines usually start before 40 years of age. She had a throbbing headache with nausea that was worse with activity. However, the criteria for migraine are based on a history of at least five attacks. This was her worst headache and warranted a "first or worst" evaluation. A CT scan of the brain was normal. Her neck was supple on exam. Have we now diagnosed migraine?

No! The probability of demonstrating subarachnoid hemorrhage (SAH) on CT scan is 74% on day 3. A lumbar puncture *must* be performed to exclude SAH. The lumbar puncture revealed xanthochromic CSF. A cerebral arteriogram demonstrated a 12-mm right middle cerebral artery aneurysm, which was successfully clipped. (Chapter 8)

Case 6

This is another case of migraine that is frequently misdiagnosed as stress or tension headaches by patients and physicians alike. Up to 75% of migraineurs report unilateral or bilateral posterior neck pain associated with the headache, which can be tightness, stiffness, or throbbing. The neck pain can occur during the migraine prodrome, attack itself, or postdrome, and it is typically relieved by migraine medication, such as a triptan. As noted, stress is reported as a migraine trigger by 50% of migraineurs. As she did not respond to over-the-counter medication, it is reasonable to try a triptan class medication, which has about an 80% chance of being effective. If she does not respond to one triptan, then she may respond to a different one. Her likelihood of having a rapid pain-free response will be greatly increased by taking the triptan when the headache is mild rather than waiting until the pain is moderate to severe. (Chapter 2)

Case 7
When a "first or worst" headache is associated with orgasm, SAH should be ruled out because sexual activity is the precipitant of up to 12% of ruptured saccular aneurysms and of 4% of bleeding arteriovenous malformations. To help remember the significance of this presentation, you may want to think of this as a "coming-but-going headache."

A CT scan of the head and lumbar puncture with CSF examination were normal. The headache resolved after 2 days. The patient then developed a severe post–lumbar puncture headache that was present for 3 days and resolved with a lumbar epidural blood patch. This is an example of the primary explosive type of sexual headache or primary orgasmic cephalalgia. The patient had a single recurrence of this type of headache and then experienced no further problems for the last 5 years. (Chapter 15)

Case 8
The headaches sound like a combination of tension and migraine type. However, with the frequent use of Excedrin Migraine (containing acetaminophen 250 mg, aspirin 250 mg, and caffeine 65 mg), medication rebound was the first consideration. (She was only drinking occasional caffeinated beverages.) She was advised to taper off the Excedrin Migraine and was started on nortriptyline 25 mg at bedtime. On an office visit 3 weeks later, she reported three headaches during the first week and then none for the next 2 weeks. She stopped nortriptyline on her own after 2 weeks due to constipation. She was seen again 2 months later. She had one migraine completely relieved by zolmitriptan 2.5 mg and six mild headaches for which she took no medication. When next seen 3 months later, she reported only three mild headaches.

In some cases, medication rebound headaches can dramatically and rapidly improve when the overused medication or beverages, foods, or medications containing caffeine are tapered off. (See the list of substances containing caffeine in Chapter 18.) Medication rebound headaches can be due to overuse of over-the-counter medications containing acetaminophen, aspirin, nonsteroidal antiinflammatory drugs, and caffeine as well as prescription drugs with these ingredients as well as others such as butalbital, narcotics, and benzodiazepines.

This patient's increased frequency of headaches coincided with her use of daily Excedrin Migraine, which she started taking after seeing a television commercial. She first thought she must have a brain tumor or aneurysm. She was very skeptical when advised to discontinue the Excedrin Migraine because she had never heard of medication rebound headaches. The medication warning label states, "Stop using this product and see a doctor if:

migraine headache pain worsens or continues for more than 48 hours." There is no warning about the potential for rebound headaches. Perhaps a more informative warning label on this and other over-the-counter medications used for headaches would be helpful for consumers.

Frequent use of symptomatic medications may also result in tolerance (the decreased effectiveness of the same dose of an analgesic, often leading to the use of higher doses to achieve the same degree of effectiveness); habituation; and dependence (respectively, the psychological and physical need repeatedly to use drugs). Habituation and dependence are a threat to the patient and a major aggravation for the physician. One example is patients who receive prescriptions from multiple physicians. Another example I have termed "Fiorinal fugax."

Over the years, the author has noticed that medication containing combinations of butalbital, aspirin, or acetaminophen, and caffeine with or without codeine (e.g., Fiorinal, Fioricet, Esgic, and Phrenilin) has an unusual propensity to flee or become lost in the manner of checks that are in the mail but never received. The patients with the disappearing medication are disproportionately women, although women suffer in greater numbers from headaches.

The following are some of the circumstances that have been reported: lost or stolen purses; medication falling out of the container either onto the ground or into the commode or sink; medication left at home when on trips or left out of town when returning home; home robberies in which only this medication is taken; dogs and cats who play with the medicine containers; and other family members, most commonly cousins, who borrow the medicine. Many of these disappearances are dutifully reported to the physician on Friday night or during the weekend when a new prescription is requested. Butalbital is especially unlucky for some women who have multiple purses stolen or lost in brief periods of time.

Interestingly, other drugs are rarely involved. How often do you receive calls from patients that their purse containing such drugs as Lipitor, Cozaar, Dilantin, and triptans was stolen or misplaced? Perhaps we should alert our patients to the risk of Fiorinal fugax when writing prescriptions (1). (Chapter 5)

Case 9

Although this was the first headache of this type for the patient, the headache seemed consistent with a migraine triggered by her menses. She had headache with syncope at 8 and 18 years of age that were probably of the migraine type. I advised the patient and her husband that this was probably a migraine but could not exclude other causes, such as SAH, meningitis, and sinusitis, without testing, such as a scan of the brain and possibly a lumbar puncture, which they declined. The headache returned that evening and was described as a right hemicranial and generalized pain with nausea and light sensitivity. A MRI scan of the brain demonstrated a hemorrhagic pituitary macroadenoma for which she underwent transphenoidal removal 1 month later.

Pituitary hemorrhage can result in pituitary apoplexy with headache and visual findings, be clinically silent, or, as this case demonstrates, present as a migrainelike headache without associated signs. Pituitary hemorrhage even in a macroadenoma can be overlooked and underimaged on a routine CT scan of the head for acute headache using 10-mm cuts. A MRI scan even without pituitary views routinely identifies the pathology. Sphenoid sinusitis, which can also cause a similar headache, is also well visualized on routine MRI scans of the brain but not necessarily on a routine CT scan of the head. (Chapter 14)

Case 10

There was a history of tension-type headaches every 2 weeks for a few years and perimenstrual migraine aura without headache for 2 years. She presented with a new type of headache for 4 days consistent with migraine, but there was no history of at least five similar attacks. A MRI scan of the brain was normal. The headache was gone the next day. The patient and mother declined a lumbar puncture. This was probably a first-time migraine headache of this type. It is possible that the oral contraceptive started 4 months previously was responsible for the new type of migraine.

Migraine often has different presentations in the same person. Seventy percent of patients with migraine with aura also have migraine without aura. Those with migraine aura without headache often have migraine headache with and without aura. Patients who usually have hemicranial migraines can also have occasional generalized headaches. Headaches can also be on one side or can move from one side to the other during an attack. The presence of associated symptoms, such as nausea, vomiting, and noise sensitivity, can vary from attack to attack. Those with typical migraine headaches without aura can develop transient migrainous accompaniments such as scintillating scotoma, numbness, dysarthria, and weakness for the first time after 45 years of age. (Chapter 12)

Case 11

This is a typical history of cluster headaches. The patient was started on verapamil sustained release 240 mg daily for prevention and a tapering course of prednisone. Use of 100% oxygen with a nonrebreathing mask for 15 minutes relieved the headaches. The headaches were gone within 2 weeks, at least until the next cluster attack. (Chapter 7)

Case 12

A MRI scan of the brain, a lumbar puncture and CSF examination, and blood studies were all normal. This presentation is consistent with new-onset daily persistent headache (2). Medication rebound, always a concern in patients with frequent headaches, was not a factor here. According to the IHS 2nd edition 2004 criteria, the criteria include a daily and unremitting headache from onset or from less than 3 days from onset with a duration of more than 3 months not attributed to another disorder. Testing is necessary to exclude mimics of new daily persistent headache with a normal neurological exam, especially when seen within the first 2 months, such as spontaneous intracranial hypotension, pseudotumor cerebri without papilledema, cerebral venous thrombosis, postmeningitis headache, chronic meningitis, brain tumors, leptomeningeal metastasis, temporal arteritis, chronic subdural hematoma, and sphenoid sinusitis. NDPH may be a presentation of another primary type such as migraine, tension, or benign thunderclap headache. An infectious trigger such as Epstein-Barr virus may be present in some cases. Symptomatic and preventive treatment for new daily persistent headache is the same as for chronic daily headache and chronic migraine. (Chapter 5)

Case 13

This patient also seemed to have new-onset daily persistent headaches with a muscle contraction component and left greater occipital neuralgia. The recent stress in her life could be the precipitant. I performed a left greater occipital nerve block and placed her on naproxyn. We discussed obtaining a scan of the brain, but she felt the headaches were due to stress and wanted to try treatment first. She called back 2 days later and the headaches were no better. She agreed to a MRI scan of the brain, which revealed a left cerebellar hemangioblastoma with mass effect. She underwent cerebellar hemispherectomy with a cure of the benign neoplasm that would have resulted in herniation and death in a short time without surgery. There was no family history or other lesions of the retina, spinal cord, kidneys, or pancreas to suggest Von Hippel-Lindau disease. Postoperatively, she had no neurological deficit. Two months later, she unhappily moved out of state but had no headaches.

Statistically, the odds were high that she had a benign headache type. However, there is about a 2% chance that a patient with chronic headaches and a normal neurological exam will have pathology such as a brain tumor. She was one of the 2%. When you obtain numerous normal scans on patients with headaches, it is easy to become frustrated and think you are wasting time and money. When you detect a case such as this, for a while you become paranoid about the possible presence of brain tumors in everyone you see with benign headaches.

In addition, it is easy to attribute all kinds of physical symptoms to stress. Although psychosomatic illness is common, everyone seems to have some stressors if you ask enough questions. The presence of stress is not diagnostic of a functional disorder, which is still a diagnosis of exclusion. (The use of the term *functional* is interesting. Although it seems to refer to a disorder of function, the term is used in neurology and psychiatry to indicate a nonorganic problem. This use dates to the 19th century. In his 1893 textbook of neurology, William Gowers divided neurological disorders into organic and functional disease. As another aside, he also described "Gowers's test," pulling on the pubic hair, for the detection of hysterical paraplegia. Disorders once believed to be functional, such as migraine, Tourette's syndrome, and dystonia, are now believed to have an organic basis.) (Chapters 1 and 14)

Case 14

This could be a case of transformed migraine or migraine status and new-onset daily persistent headaches. However, these are diagnoses of exclusion. A MRI scan of the brain demonstrated a pilocytic astrocytoma of the right cerebellar hemisphere with severe mass effect and hydrocephalus due to obstruction of the aqueduct of Sylvius. She was started on Decadron and underwent a ventriculoperitoneal shunt. Two days later, she underwent a craniotomy and resection of the neoplasm with clean margins. At 36 weeks, she underwent elective C-section with delivery of healthy twins. Two months postpartum, a follow-up MRI showed tumor recurrence. She had additional surgery and then radiotherapy. Six years later, she is doing well.

As in case 13, a normal neurological exam is not the same as the absence of pathology. Papilledema is present in only 40% of patients with brain tumors. Even in patients with mass effect such as these two, papilledema can be absent and the examination may be normal. Although neuroimaging should not be obtained without appropriate indications, when the indications are present, imaging should be performed. MRI scans during pregnancy have not been associated with any type of birth defects. (Chapters 11 and 14)

Case 15

This is a case of ice cream headache, also known as "brain freeze" or "slurpy headache." Ice cream headache (cold stimulus headache), first reported in 1850 as a hazard of eating ice cream, may be more common in migraineurs. This case description is my own, and I also have migraines with and without aura that are also of interest as I'll discuss later.

The point of the case is that pain is more easily tolerated when it is brief and the cause, especially when benign, is known. (Imagine working in the emergency room when a patient comes in and says, "Doc, I was eating some Haagen-Daz frozen yogurt and I got this terrible pain in my head.") Some patients may come to see you with an obvious migraine or even mild tension-type headaches. If you dismiss them without directly addressing their concerns about possible underlying pathology, they may still be quite anxious and may even obtain another opinion. It is important to find out if there is a hidden agenda or hidden concerns. They may think they have a brain tumor because their aunt had one, an aneurysm because their cousin had one, or sinus headaches because of all the television commercials they have seen. All you have to do is ask what they think may be causing the headache or if they have any other questions or concerns. I sometimes have a hard time convincing patients and/or their families that their headaches are actually of the migraine type and not due to something else. In some cases, they demand a scan of the brain even when they have a typical definite migraine history.

Why is it interesting that I have migraines? Evans, Lipton, and Silberstein performed a nationwide survey of neurologists and found a lifetime prevalence of migraine among male and female neurologists, respectively, of 47% and 63%. (3). Among headache specialists, the lifetime prevalence is about 75% . These numbers are sky high compared to the general population. Possible explanations include a personal history of migraine stimulating an interest in neurology (although 90% of respondents denied it) or an underestimation of migraine in the general population (although I doubt such a gross underestimation). Or perhaps neurology may be an attractive specialty for those with a rigid obsessional migraine personality. However, the available data argue against the presence of a migraine personality. Data on a neurologist personality are largely anecdotal. (Chapters 1 and 14)

Case 16

This presentation is consistent with a postconcussion syndrome. Because there is a 1% to 2% chance of a subdural or epidural hematoma, a CT scan of the brain without contrast was obtained with normal findings. The patient was initially placed on Tylenol #3 and Phenergan. The symptoms gradually resolved over a 3-week period. (Chapter 9)

Case 17

Pseudotumor cerebri, which occurs 90% of the time in obese women, was the most likely consideration. First, however, other causes need to be excluded, including tumor cerebri, cerebral venous thrombosis, and chronic meningitis. A MRI scan of the brain was normal. A lumbar puncture revealed an opening pressure of 36 cm, and the CSF analysis was normal. Examination by an ophthalmologist revealed enlarged blind spots. She was placed on oral Diamox 500 mg twice a day and advised to lose weight. Serial follow-up visits with the ophthalmologist and visual field testing are essential to detect the evidence of visual loss requiring more aggressive treatment, such as shunting or optic nerve sheath fenestration. A MRI scan of the brain is the preferred study rather than CT scan for the evaluation of this disorder because the MRI especially with MRV can detect the occasional case of cerebral venous thrombosis, which can be a fatal disease. (Chapters 13 and 14)

Case 18

A MRI of the brain was normal. An electroencephalogram was normal. After 3.5 years, she has had no further episodes. I do not know the cause of these episodes, which can be termed *short-lasting unilateral vibrating exertional headache* (SUV). Although the headaches were triggered by exertion, the features are different from benign exertional headaches, which are typically throbbing at the onset, bilateral, and last 5 minutes to 24 hours.

Occasionally, you may see a new type of headache that is unfamiliar to you. First, check with a neurologist (or another neurologist if you are one) and the literature to see if you can label the headache. Rarely, you might identify a new type of headache. In fact, many neurological disorders remain unrecognized, waiting for a first description by an astute physician. (Chapter 15)

Case 19

A MRI of the brain was normal. Magnetic resonance angiography (MRA) showed dissection of the upper left cervical internal carotid artery (ICA) but was otherwise normal. An arteriogram confirmed the left cervical ICA dissection but also demonstrated dissections of both distal vertebrals. She underwent extensive testing with no evidence of any underlying disorder as the cause of the spontaneous dissections. She was placed on Coumadin for more than 6 months, during which time serial MRA studies revealed resolution of the dissections.

Four years later, she developed right jaw pain. An arteriogram demonstrated a small short-segment dissection of the right ICA just superior to the carotid bulb. She was again placed on Coumadin.

Her initial presentation of anterior neck and facial pain raised concern about the possibility of an ICA dissection despite the absence of a Horner's syndrome or carotid bruit. Although the MRA demonstrated the ICA dissection, the vertebral dissection was only seen on the arteriogram. The occurrence of jaw pain 4 years later with this history raised concern about a recurrent dissection. Fortunately, she has never had any cerebral ischemic events from the dissections. The cause of her recurrent spontaneous dissections is unknown but may be due to cystic medial necrosis.

Head, face, orbital, or neck pain, usually ipsilateral to the site of the dissection, is the initial manifestation in about 80% of patients with extracranial ICA dissection. Focal cerebral ischemic symptoms occur in about 60% of patients and may follow the headache by up to 4 weeks or precede it. The presence of deficits is as follows: neurologically normal, 50%; mild deficits only, 21%; moderate to severe deficits, 25%; and death, 4%. An incomplete ipsilateral Horner's syndrome with ptosis and miosis but not anhidrosis is present in about 50% of cases due to damage of the sympathetic fibers. Either subjective or objective bruits or both are present in about 45% of patients. (Chapter 13)

Case 20

This is a case of "Alice in Wonderland" syndrome, a rare migraine aura in which patients experience distortion in body image characterized by enlargement, diminution, or distortion of part of or the whole body that they know is not real (4). The syndrome can occur at any age but is more common in children. The etiology may be migrainous ischemia of the nondominant posterior parietal lobule. The syndrome has also been reported after viral encephalitis (especially after Epstein-Barr virus) and as a seizure phenomenon.

Lippman first described the syndrome in 1952, which was named by Todd in 1955. The syndrome derives its name from the book *Alice's Adventures in Wonderland*, published in England in 1865 by Charles Lutwidge Dodgson (professor of mathematics at Oxford University) under the pseudonym of Lewis Carroll (the Latinization of Lutwidge Charles).

The neurological syndrome derives its name primarily from the opening scenes after Alice jumps down a rabbit hole and lands in a hallway where she finds a bottle that she drinks and causes her to shrink: "I must be shutting up like a telescope. And so it was indeed: She was now only 10 inches high." Later, she eats a piece of cake that makes her grow: "Curiouser and curiouser, cried Alice. Now I am opening out like the largest telescope that ever was! Goodbye feet! (For when she looked down at her feet they seemed to be almost out of sight they were getting so far off.)" (Chapter 10)

Case 21

The patient had a history of migraine without aura when she was younger. Status migrainosus, a possibility, is a diagnosis of exclusion. Other considerations included SAH, a subdural hematoma, neoplasm, and aseptic meningitis. Her complaint of low back pain raised concern of meningeal irritation due to SAH. I obtained a MRI of the brain with MRA on the day of the consultation because this study was available. A CT scan of the brain and, if negative, a lumbar puncture would have been appropriate alternative tests. (The probability that the CT scan would have shown evidence of SAH 11 days after the ictus is about 40%. The CSF would still be xanthochromic.) The MR studies showed a saccular aneurysm, which was confirmed on cerebral arteriography the next morning to be a 10-mm right supraclinoid internal carotid artery posterior wall aneurysm. The neck of the aneurysm was too wide for endovascular coil embolization. The next day, she underwent craniotomy. As the neurosurgeon approached the aneurysm, it ruptured, but the clip was placed successfully. She has no postoperative neurological deficit. (Chapter 8)

Case 22

Although this could be a case of benign weight lifter's headache, 50% of the headaches associated with Chiari I malformation are of this type. The CT scan, although normal, does not exclude Chiari malformation, which can be easily visualized on a routine MRI scan of the brain. (A CT scan with thin slices through the cervicomedullary region following injection of subarachnoid contrast, a myelogram, can detect this malformation.) The MRI of the brain was normal except for extension of the cerebellar tonsils through the foramen magnum to the level of the inferior surface of C2. MRI of the cervical and thoracic spine was otherwise negative with no evidence of syrinx. He underwent suboccipital craniectomy and C1 and C2 laminectomy followed by dural patch grafting. Postoperatively, the headaches were no longer present. (Chapter 15)

Case 23

I advised the mother this was probably a migraine triggered by the minor head injury ("footballer's migraine" originally described in adolescent boys with minor head injuries playing soccer but made world famous by Terrell Davis in the 1998 Super Bowl), although there was a small chance of a more serious problem (subdural or epidural hematoma). He was seen by a pediatric resident who found a normal neurological exam. The symptoms cleared completely within 2 hours. The resident did not recommend a scan of the brain. When I saw the mother and the boy a few weeks later, he was doing fine and had experienced no further headaches. If I had seen the child during the acute attack, I would have ordered a CT scan. (Chapters 9 and 10)

Case 24

This was a 15-year history of migraine without aura. The persistent aching headache present on the day of consultation was probably a muscle contraction type with occipital neuralgia triggered by the migraine. A right greater occipital nerve block completely relieved the headache within minutes. The patient was placed on amitriptyline 25 mg at bedtime, which reduced the frequency of the headaches to about twice monthly. Midrin at the onset decreased the headache. One year later, she was seen again with a similar history of a right-sided headache for 4 days with nausea and vomiting for the first 2 days. A greater occipital nerve block again promptly relieved the headache. (Chapters 1 and 9)

Case 25

This is an example of red ear syndrome, which was first described by Lance in 1995 who also proposes the term *auriculo-autonomic cephalalgia*. The disorder is characterized by episodic burning pain usually in one earlobe associated with flushing or reddening of the ear with a duration of less than 30 minutes to 3 hours in children and adults. In an individual, one ear or alternating ears or occasionally both ears can be involved in attacks that can occur rarely or up to 6 times a month. The redness can occur without pain. The syndrome can be primary, occur during migraine headaches, or be in association with upper cervical spine pathology. The cause is uncertain. (Chapter 14)

Case 26

On admission, the patient's temperature was 99.4°F. On the second hospital day, when I saw her initially, she had developed a fever of 101° with the same symptoms. Her neck was supple. Although the headache was very similar to her migraines, the light and noise sensitivity were new symptoms. Now with the development of fever, meningitis and SAH had to be excluded. A CT scan of the brain was normal. A lumbar puncture revealed an opening pressure of 24 cm and the following: glucose, 56; protein, 74; white blood cell count (WBC), 1,317, with 87% lymphocytes and 13% polymorphonuclear cells; and red blood cell count, 56. Gram stain, cryptococcal antigen, and meningitis latex screen were negative. She was placed on Rocephin, which was discontinued after 2 days with normal cultures and discharged with a milder headache. The headache resolved a few days following discharge.

The diagnosis was viral meningitis, probably due to an enterovirus. Diagnostic confusion can occur when viral meningitis causes a headache similar to migraine with low-grade fever or without fever. (Chapter 15)

Case 27

The diagnosis is trigeminal neuralgia. An MRI of the brain, obtained to exclude the occasional neoplasm, was normal. The patient was started on Tegretol XL 200 mg for 1 day, then one every 12 hours. The pain resolved within 1 day of starting Tegretol. (Chapter 15)

Case 28

What the patient described as "sinus headaches" was consistent with perimenstrual migraine. I wondered if this acute different type of headache was due to status migrainosus. However, a worse headache supine did not fit. An MRI scan of the brain revealed acute sphenoid sinusitis (complete opacification of the right and partial opacification of the left) that in retrospect was also present but not reported on the CT scan. She was seen that day by an ENT physician and was started on antibiotics and decongestants with resolution of the headache and sinusitis. In summary, a patient with a history of perimenstrual migraines, which she thought were sinus headaches, presented with a severe headache similar to migraine but due to acute sphenoid sinusitis.

Sphenoid sinusitis can mimic migraine, SAH, and meningitis. In patients presenting with "first or worst" headaches, sphenoid sinusitis should be specifically excluded. Nasal discharge is present in only about 30% of patients, and fever is present in more than 50%. Acute sphenoid sinusitis is an important diagnosis to make because complications include bacterial meningitis, cavernous sinus thrombosis, subdural abscess, cortical vein thrombosis, ophthalmoplegia, and pituitary insufficiency. Plain sinus X-rays may not detect sphenoid sinusitis in about 25% of cases. (Chapter 14)

Case 29

A new-onset headache in someone more than 50 years of age raises concern about such conditions as temporal arteritis and brain tumors. However, benign types of headaches can also occur. I suspected this headache was associated with neck muscle tightness and greater occipital neuralgia and performed a greater occipital nerve block with 3 ml of 1% lidocaine and placed her on Soma. The headache resolved. She returned 2 years later with an identical headache. I again performed an occipital nerve block and superior trapezius trigger point injection that decreased the headache. When the headache was still present 3 days later, she returned and the injections were repeated. The headache and neck discomfort resolved.

I saw another woman, 68 years old, with a similar headache that also resolved with an occipital nerve block. An ESR was 18. This patient returned a year later with a more intense hemicranial headache. The ESR was 40, a minimal elevation from the range of normal ([the woman's age + 10]/2 = 39) but significantly elevated from the year before. A superficial temporal artery biopsy was positive and the headache promptly resolved when she was started on prednisone. (Chapters 9 and 12)

Case 30

The history is consistent with migrainous vertigo (MV), which may occur at any age and has a female-to-male ratio variably reported as between 1.5 and 5 to 1 (5). Migraine typically begins earlier in life than MV, and, in some cases, MV may have an onset after patients have not had migraine headaches for years. MV is more common in patients with migraine without aura than in those with migraine with aura. The duration and frequency of attacks can vary between patients and in individuals over time. The duration of vertigo ranges from seconds to several hours up to several days with variable intervals between attacks of days, months, or years. Alternatively, attacks can occur in clusters for hours to days. The duration of vertiginous attacks are less than 5 minutes in 20% to 30%, 5 to 60 minutes in 10% to 30%, and hours or days in 20% to 50%.

Symptoms of vertigo may include rotational, positional, head motion intolerance, as well as other illusory self or object motion. Vertigo may precede the headache, begin with the headache, or occur late in the headache phase. Individuals can have attacks with and without headaches or some may never have an associated headache at all. Frequent episodes of MV may respond to the usual migraine preventative medications. For acute treatment, vestibular suppressants (e.g., meclizine, promethazine, and lorazepam) and perhaps triptans may be effective. (Chapter 14)

Case 31

The headaches occurring several times per year are consistent with migraine without aura. The acute headache, her worst ever, could be a migraine because migraines frequently are triggered by falling estrogen levels in the first week postpartum. When patients with migraine develop a new type of severe headache, this can certainly be migraine. Unfortunately, a history of migraine is not protective against other diseases that can cause severe headaches.

Complications of the epidural anesthetic should be considered. Although post–lumbar puncture-type headaches occur after about 20% of epidurals due to inadvertent puncture of the dura and although post–lumbar puncture headaches can be delayed for as long as 14 days, her headaches were not consistent with the diagnosis because they were not better supine. A lumbar epidural abscess causing meningitis and a headache is also a consideration, but she had a supple neck and no fever or back pain, which argue against that diagnosis. Pregnancy-induced hypertension can cause postpartum headaches, but her blood pressure was normal. Because up to 20% of aneurysmal ruptures occur during pregnancy or in the early postpartum period, SAH should also be ruled out. Cerebral venous thrombosis should also be considered because 90% of cases occur during the puerperium, most commonly in the second or third weeks postpartum.

An MRI of the brain, MRA, and MRV were normal. The lumbar puncture revealed a normal opening pressure and normal CSF. The headache resolved after two injections of Demerol and Phenergan 4 hours apart. The diagnosis is migraine. She was prescribed Vicodin if she were to have further migraines while pregnant. Triptans are relatively contraindicated while breastfeeding. (Chapter 11)

Case 32

This new headache in an elderly person warranted investigation even though the intensity was mild. A CT scan of the brain revealed a right frontal hemorrhagic infarction. I told the patient that he should get a "stroke handicap" for his round that morning.

Headaches commonly accompany stroke. In one study, headache occurred in 29% with bland infarcts, 57% with parenchymal hemorrhage, 36% with transient ischemic attacks, and 17%

with lacunar infarcts. The headache began before the event in 60% and at its onset in 25%. The headaches are equally likely to be abrupt or gradual in onset. The headache is usually unilateral and focal of mild to moderate severity, although up to 46% of patients may have an incapacitating headache. The headache may be throbbing or nonthrobbing and may rarely be stabbing. The headache is more often ipsilateral than contralateral to the side of the cerebral ischemia. Headache is more common in ischemia of the posterior than the anterior circulation, and it is more common in cortical than in subcortical events. The duration of the headache is longest in cardioembolic infarcts and thrombotic infarcts, of medium duration in lacunar infarction, and shortest in transient ischemic attacks. Associated symptoms in one study include nausea in 44%, vomiting in 23%, and light and noise sensitivity in 25%. Bending, straining, and jarring the head usually increase the intensity. (Chapter 13)

Case 33

Pseudotumor cerebri is a consideration but is less much less common in men than in women. Infectious causes of headache should be excluded. A lumbar puncture revealed an opening pressure of 35 cm. CSF analysis included a glucose of 30, protein of 65, and WBC of 350 (90% lymphocytes). CSF cryptococcal antigen was positive. The patient was HIV negative and otherwise healthy. A chest X-ray was negative. This patient was successfully treated with amphotericin B. Flucytosine is another treatment option.

Cryptococcal meningitis is rare in patients without AIDS. About 50% of these patients have an underlying association, such as lymphoma, diabetes mellitus, or chronic steroid therapy. Cryptococcal meningitis occurs in perhaps 5% of HIV-infected individuals. The CSF often shows minimal changes in AIDS patients, but in non-AIDS patients it typically shows a lymphocytic pleocytosis, low glucose, and elevated protein. CSF cryptococcal antigen is positive in 90% of patients without AIDS and in 90% to 100% of those with AIDS. Neuroimaging reveals nonspecific findings in about 30% of cases, including meningeal enhancement, hydrocephalus, cerebral edema, and mass lesions (cryptococcomas or cryptococcal abscesses). (Chapter 15)

Case 34

Because this is a new-onset daily headache in a patient more than 50 years of age, there should be a strong suspicion of a secondary headache type. A lumbar puncture was indicated to rule out infection or leptomeningeal metastasis as the cause of the headaches. An MRI scan of the brain could have been done before the lumbar puncture to further exclude the presence of neoplastic disease. A lumbar puncture revealed a normal opening pressure. The CSF evaluation showed the following: glucose, 15 mg/dl; protein, 60 mg/dl; and WBC 10. CSF cytology was positive for carcinoma. The patient was diagnosed with leptomeningeal metastasis and underwent whole-brain radiotherapy.

Breast cancer accounts for 39% of solid-tumor non–central nervous system primaries causing leptomeningeal metastasis. Headache, which is present in 33% to 62% of patients, is usually

not severe. A CT scan of the brain is usually normal in leptomeningeal metastasis, although meningeal enhancement with
contrast administration or hydrocephalus is sometimes present.
An MRI scan with contrast often demonstrates meningeal
enhancement. Initial CSF examination demonstrates elevated
WBCs in 51%, elevated protein in 73%, and hypoglycorrhachia
or decreased CSF glucose in 28%. CSF cytology is positive in
54% on the first lumbar puncture, is positive in an additional
30% after the second, and is positive in 1% more after the third.
Sending a relatively large volume of 5 to 10 ml of CSF for cytology may increase the yield. (Chapter 14)

Case 35

An MRI scan of the brain showed a small area of high signal
intensity in the left parietal periventricular area. A cerebral
arteriogram was normal. Blood work for vasculitis and an
echocardiogram were normal. CSF examination was normal.
Oligoclonal bands were absent. A visual evoked response study
showed a prolonged P wave latency on the right. Visual fields
demonstrated bilateral prechiasmal defects. The patient has
been subsequently followed for 13 years with relapsing/remit-
ting multiple sclerosis.

Although there was no history of migraine, the initial differential diagnosis included complicated migraine and the many other
causes of cerebrovascular disease. This case is an example of an
occasional acute strokelike presentation of multiple sclerosis.
Although headache can herald strokes, tension- and migrainelike headaches can occur with a first or subsequent attack of
multiple sclerosis in 1.4% to 7% of cases. (Chapters 13 and 15)

Case 36

A CT scan of the brain was normal. A benign ipsilateral frontotemporal intense headache may follow endarterectomy with a
latency of 36 to 72 hours. The headache may recur intermittently for up to 6 months. Headache can also develop postoperatively
because of intracerebral hemorrhage, which is a complication of
0.75% of operations. The hemorrhage occurs at a median of 3
days after surgery with a range of 0 to 18 days. Although the
latency of this patient's headache was shorter than the cases in
the literature, a benign postcarotid endarterectomy headache is
the best explanation. Although the cause is unknown, the
headache could be due to afferent impulses from the carotid
arterial wall or restoration of normal cerebral perfusion pressure. (Chapter 13)

Case 37

A lumbar puncture was performed revealing WBC 10, RBC
650, glucose 47, and protein 112. The opening pressure was not
measured. Cryptococcal antigen and venereal disease research
laboratory (VDRL) titers were negative. HIV was negative. A
meningeal biopsy showed acute and chronic inflammation. A
repeat lumbar puncture showed an opening pressure too low to
be recorded. The CSF showed 63 WBCs (61% lymphocytes), glucose 58, and protein 88. Starting the day after admission, the

patient became progressively encephalopathic. Two weeks after admission, he was comatose. Oculocephalics were intact. He withdrew all extremities to painful stimuli. Plantars were extensor bilaterally. A repeat MRI scan of the brain showed subdural accumulations of fluid, low cerebellar tonsils, and decreased fluid around the suprasellar cistern and the chiasmatic cisterns. An MRI scan of the cervical, thoracic, and lumbar spine showed no evidence of a CSF leak.

The patient underwent a lumbar epidural blood patch with injection of 50 ml of autologous blood. Within 1 day, the patient awoke and was confused. An MRI scan of the brain 3 days after the blood patch demonstrated some restoration of CSF in the chiasmatic and suprasellar cisterns and elevation of the brain stem. Two weeks later, he was alert and oriented. He had no recollection of the prior month. Neurological exam was otherwise normal except for a right-pupil-sparing third nerve palsy.

This is the first case reported of spontaneous intracranial hypotension (SIH) resulting in coma (6). An orthostatic headache, a headache when upright that is relieved when lying down, is the most common clinical feature. In some chronic cases, a daily headache is present without orthostatic exacerbation. In other cases, second half of the day headaches often with some orthostatic features may be present. Other types reported include exertional headaches without any orthostatic features, acute thunderclap onset, parodoxical orthostatic headaches (present in recumbency and relieved when upright), intermittent headaches due to intermittent leaks, and the acephalgic form or no headaches. Neck or interscapular pain may precede the onset of headache in some cases by days or weeks.

Other causes of thickened abnormally enhancing dura on gadolinium-enhanced MRI include the following: infections (Lyme disease, syphilis, tuberculosis, fungal, cysticercosis, HTLV-1, malignant external necrotizing otitis due to *Pseudomonas*); systemic autoimmune/vasculitic disorders (Wegener's, rheumatoid arthritis, sarcoidosis, Behçet's, Sjögren's, temporal arteritis); malignancy (dural carcinomatosis, metastatic disease in adjacent skull bone, and lymphoma); idiopathic hypertrophic pachymeningitis and meningioma. (Chapters 14 and 15)

Case 38

The patient went to physical therapy with a report of mild benefit. When I saw him on referral from the orthopedist, the neck was nontender with a decreased range of motion. The speech was slightly slurred and the tongue deviated to the right. An MRI scan of the brain revealed a skull base tumor on the right that was found to be a chordoma at the time of surgery.

This is a difficult presentation to diagnose without cranial nerve findings because skull base tumors can be associated with significant complaints of neck pain that may be more prominent than the headache. The tumor would have been detected with a cervical spine MRI. (Chapter 14)

Case 39

The patient had a history of migraine headaches without aura occurring around her menses for many years. She also reported a 5-year history of frequent left-sided headaches that could be of the tension type or related to medication rebound. The acute headache, the worst of her life, could have been a new type of migraine for her, but secondary causes could not be excluded without testing. I gave her a Demerol and Phenergan injection. An MRI scan of the brain with intracranial MRA was normal. A lumbar puncture produced clear CSF, which had normal constituents. She was then given an injection of Imitrex 6 mg subcutaneously that reduced the headache intensity from a 10/10 to a 2/10 within 20 minutes. I advised her to discontinue the Tylenol, Fiorecet, and Prozac and placed her on nortriptyline 25 mg at bedtime for headache prevention. When she was seen 2 weeks later, she had had no mild headaches and only one migraine. Thus she had episodic migraine, tension-type headaches with medication rebound, and the worst headache of her life due to a different presentation of migraine than previously. (Chapters 1, 5, and 8)

Case 40

An MRI of the brain was normal. Blood work was normal including the following: an erythocyte sedimentation rate was 12 mm/hour; rheumatoid factor 11 IU/ml; ANA screen negative; serum protein electrophoresis was normal; serum immunofixation showed no monoclonal immunoglobin; Sjögren's antibodies A and B negative; Vitamin B_{12} level 743 pg/mL; and TSH 1.5. The patient was placed on oral gabapentin 100 mg three times a day that she took as needed with a reduction in the level of pain to a 2/10.

This is an example of nummular headache (a coin-shaped cephalalgia) that is a rare, chronic, mild to moderate, pressure-like pain in a rounded or elliptical scalp area (most often the parietal region) of about 2 to 6 cm in diameter. The other cases reported are unilateral but this case is bilateral. Typically, the pain is continuous and persists for days to months with exacerbations described as lancinating pains lasting for several seconds or gradually increasing for 10 minutes to 2 hours. The affected area may show a combination of hypoesthesia and touch-evoked paresthesias. Spontaneous remissions may occur but the pain usually recurs. Diagnostic testing including MRI of the brain and blood work is normal. Although the cause is not known, the disorder is benign and may be due to a localized terminal branch neuralgia of the trigeminal nerve. (Chapter 14)

Case 41

When initially seen by the first neurologist, the patient had a long history of typical stable migraine with a normal neurological exam. There was no medical indication for neuroimaging. Indications to consider neuroimaging in migraineurs include the following: unusual, prolonged, or persistent aura; increasing frequency, severity, or change in clinical features; migraine status; first or worst migraine; migraine with a sudden onset and severe intensity ("crash migraine"); new onset over the age of 50 years; variants including basilar, confusional, hemiplegic, an aura without headache; late-life migraine accompaniments; and posttraumatic migraine. Therefore, this case is highly defendable: there was no neurological indication for neuroimaging.

Although migraine experts may agree, this does not mean a jury would come to the same conclusion. The plaintiff attorney with the help of a medical expert of his choosing might argue as follows. The patient wanted a scan and sensed that something was wrong but the doctor simply would not listen to her. Doctors are too busy to listen to us. They just want to rush us in and out to make money. Besides, the doctor may have been in cahoots with the insurance company to save money by not doing a scan. Additionally, isn't it obvious that patients with bad headaches should have a scan to check for a brain tumor or aneurysm? Then the poor twins, although seemingly healthy at birth, were exposed to all kinds of risk from the mother's treatment for the brain tumor. Perhaps they'll later have school problems. With the advice of the malpractice insurance carrier, the neurologist settled the case for $300,000 without going to trial.

Just because you do the medically correct thing does not protect you from malpractice suits. You can be struck by lightning in a case such as this in which a patient with migraine has an unrelated cerebral neoplasm. Unfortunately, this leads to the practice of defensive medicine and numerous normal scans of the brain are performed in patients with primary headache types who are concerned they have an underlying cause for their headache such as a brain tumor or aneurysm. It may be helpful to explain that secondary pathology is very unlikely and perhaps 2% of the general population has an incidental saccular aneurysm. In my practice, if a patient with headache without an indication still wants a scan after the explanation and either they or their insurance company are willing to pay for the scan, I order it. At least a normal scan may reassure an anxious patient and/or family members. (Chapter 1)

Case 42

This is a case of exploding head syndrome, a dramatic term coined by Pearce in 1988. Episodes of exploding head syndrome awaken people from sleep with a sensation of a loud bang in the head, like an explosion. Ten percent of cases are associated with the perception of a flash of light. Five percent report a curious sensation as if they had stopped breathing and have to make a deliberate effort to breathe again. The episodes have a variable frequency and onset at any age, although the most common is middle aged and older. The episodes take place in healthy individuals during awakenings without evidence of epileptogenic discharges. (Chapter 15)

CONCLUSION

I hope you enjoyed playing, "What's my headache?" The cases were selected to demonstrate the spectrum of primary and secondary headaches. If you are in primary care, most of your patients will have primary and benign headaches that can be easily diagnosed and successfully treated. However, you should be aware of the many secondary causes of headaches. If you are a neurologist, you can collect your own interesting series from the wide world of headaches.

REFERENCES

1. Evans RW. Fiorinal fugax. *Headache* 2000;40:328.
2. Evans RW. New onset daily persistent headache. *Curr Pain Headache Rep* 2003;7:303–307.
3. Evans RW, Lipton RB, Silberstein SD. The prevalence of migraine in neurologists. *Neurology* 2003:61:1271–1272.
4. Evans RW, Rolak LA. The Alice in Wonderland syndrome. *Headache* 2004; 44:624–625.
5. Neuhauser H, Lempert T. Vertigo and dizziness related to migraine: a diagnostic challenge. *Cephalalgia* 2004;24:83–91.
6. Evans RW, Mokri B. Spontaneous intracranial hypotension resulting in coma. *Headache* 2002;42:159–160.

The Headache Quiz

Randolph W. Evans

Review books based on questions and answers are becoming increasingly popular. Some of us learn better when it seems as though we are taking a test.

This chapter reviews many of the topics previously covered through questions and answers that are provided in outline form. If you do not like this style of questions, you can make up your own multiple-choice questions for extra credit. If you want to read more about the topic, refer back to the chapter that is cited.

1. What are the features of tension-type headaches? (Chapter 6)

Often bilateral, pressure or tight feeling
Prevalence, 90%; chronic type, 3%
Average age of onset between 25 and 30 years
Female-to-male ratio, 5:4
Seventy-five percent of those with chronic tension headaches are females
Prevalence in children through 11 years of age, 35%

2. How do you diagnose tension-type headaches? (Chapters 1 and 6)

Usually on clinical criteria
Early in course or if increased frequency, magnetic resonance imaging (MRI) or computed tomography (CT) scan
In those with chronic headaches and a normal neurological exam, yield on MRI or CT scan is about 2%
EEG not helpful

3. What is the epidemiology of migraine? (Chapter 2)

Prevalence, 18% for women and 6% for men
Prevalence for boys and girls before puberty, 4%
First migraine usually occurs before 40 years of age and 2% of the time after 50 years of age
Sixty percent of migraineurs do not know they have migraine—often called "sinus headache"

4. How do you diagnose migraine without aura? (Chapters 1 and 2)

IHS criteria
Simpler criteria for migraine without aura: presence of two out of four
    Unilateral site
    Throbbing quality
    Nausea
    Photophobia or phonophobia
Do not diagnose based on first attack
There should be no evidence of other causes

5. What are migraine triggers? (Chapters 1 and 2)

Present in 85%; median of three triggers/migraineur
Stress, 49%, or let-down headache
Certain foods, 45%
Alcoholic beverages, 52%
Menses for 48% of females
Missing a meal, 40%
Bright sunlight, 38%
Environmental factors: flickering lights, loud noise, high altitude, heat and humidity, smoky rooms, and strong odors
Lack of sleep or oversleeping
Medications such as NTG (nitroglycerin) or OCs (oral contraceptives)
Mild head trauma

6. What are the features of migraine? (Chapter 2)

Typically last 4 to 72 hours in adults without treatment and can last less than 2 hours in children
Unilateral in 60% and bilateral in 40%
Pulsating or throbbing in 50%
Nausea, 90%; vomiting, 30%; light and noise sensitivity, 80%
Migraine without aura, 80%

7. What are the features of migraine with aura? (Chapter 2)

Twenty percent of migraines are migraine with aura
Seventy percent of those with migraine with aura also have headaches without aura
Headache may be unilateral or contralateral to symptoms
Visual auras: photopsias (flashes of light), scotoma (partial loss of vision), teichopsia (fortification spectrum: scotoma that spreads outward with a scintillating edge of zigzag, flashing or occasionally colored)
Unilateral paresthesias and/or numbness often in ipsilateral hand, arm, and side of the face, especially involving the tongue and lips

8. What features of childhood migraine are different from those of adults? (Chapter 10)

Sixty-five percent bilateral (often bifrontal or bitemporal), 35% unilateral
Headache duration often less than 2 hours

9. What are some of the other types of migraines? (Chapters 10 and 13)

Typical aura without headache (acephalgic migraine)
Basilar-type
Retinal
Chronic: migraine headache occurring on 15 or more days per month for more than 3 months in the absence of medication overuse
Persistent aura without infarction: aura symptoms persisting for more than 1 week without radiographic evidence of infarction
Migrainous infarction: one or more aura symptoms associated with an ischemic brain lesion in an appropriate territory demonstrated by neuroimaging

10. What are the results of neuroimaging in migraine? (Chapter 1)

Yield on CT or MRI studies low: about 1%

White-matter abnormalities (foci of hyperintensity on both proton density and T2-weighted images in the deep and periventricular white matter due to either interstitial edema or perivascular demyelination) reported in 12% to 46% of migraineurs but also common in controls

11. What are the effects of the menses, menopause, and pregnancy on migraines? (Chapter 11)

Menses: strictly perimenstrual migraine in 7%, trigger for 48%

Menopause: two thirds improve

Pregnancy: improves or disappears, 60% (often during the second and third trimesters); no change, 20%; more frequent, 20%

12. What are the features of cluster headaches? (Chapter 7)

Percentage of all headache, 0.5%

Male-to-female ratio, 5:1

Unilateral severe stabbing pain usually in an orbital, retroorbital, or frontotemporal location

Usually accompanied by ipsilateral conjunctival injection, eyelid edema, tearing of the eye, and ipsilateral nasal congestion or clear drainage

Horner (miosis and ptosis) present in 30%

Attacks last 15 to 180 minutes and can occur one to eight times daily

Attacks often at the same time of day or night

Episodic: attacks for weeks to months

Twenty percent have chronic cluster with period exceeding 1 year without spontaneous remission or remissions for less than 2 weeks

Triggers: alcohol and NTG

Diagnosis usually by history

Secondary causes of clusterlike headaches: pituitary tumors, parasellar and upper cervical meningiomas, internal carotid artery and anterior communications artery aneurysms, and arteriovenous malformations

13. What are the features of greater occipital neuralgia? (Chapter 9)

Common and underdiagnosed

Aching, pressure, or throbbing nuchal-occipital and/or parietal, temporal, frontal, peri- or retroorbital distribution

Occasionally true neuralgia with shooting pain

Headache that can last minutes to hours to days

Headache that can occur after head and neck trauma or without trauma

Headache due to entrapment of nerve, myofascial trigger points, C2-3 facet joint, upper cervical spine, or posterior fossa pathology

14. What are the features of sinus headaches? (Chapter 14)

Acute frontal and maxillary sinusitis: frontal or maxillary pain with fever, yellowish green nasal drainage, and tenderness to palpation

Headache worse with shaking the head or bending head forward

Sphenoid or ethmoid sinusitis: pain may be behind and between the eyes and over the vertex. Can mimic migraine or meningitis

15. What are the features of trigeminal neuralgia? (Chapters 1 and 15)

Severe, sudden, intense, stabbing, or electrical burst of pain lasting less than 30 seconds

Unilateral pain, usually involving V2 or V3; less often, V1

Bilateral pain in about 3%

Trigger zones present

Talking, swallowing, chewing, brushing of teeth, or shaving may trigger

Can have multiple daily paroxysms

Typical onset after 40 years of age

Ratio of women to men, 1.6:1; incidence, 4.3:100,000

Three percent have multiple sclerosis, often with onset before 40 years of age

Eighty percent have vascular compression of the nerve at the root entry zone, usually by branch of superior cerebellar artery

Occasionally, tumors (schwannomas, meningiomas, lymphomas, lipomas, epidermoid, and metastatic and primaries of skull base) are cause

16. What are the features of medication rebound headaches? (Chapter 5)

Can occur in susceptible people taking over-the-counter or prescription medication for more than three doses daily for 3 or more days per week on a regular basis

Medications: ergotamine, butalbital, narcotics, alprazolam, lorazepam, acetaminophen, aspirin, triptans, and, less often, nonsteroidal antiinflammatory drugs (NSAIDs)

Caffeine (as little as 2 cups per day) can cause withdrawal headaches

17. What is the epidemiology of brain tumors? (Chapters 10 and 14)

About 18,000 primaries per year in the United States

Glioblastomas, 50%; astrocytomas, 10% (about 50% of these present with headache); meningiomas, 17%; pituitary adenomas, 4%; neurilemoma, 2%; ependymoma, 2%; and oligodendroglioma, 3%.

Over 100,000 new cases of metastatic brain tumors per year in the United States

    Eighty percent occur after diagnosis of primary

    Seventy percent have multiple cerebral metastases

Lung, 64%; breast, 14%; unknown, 8%; melanoma, 4%; colorectal, 3%, hypernephroma, 2%; other, 5%

Primaries in adults

Primaries in children

Most often from sarcomas and germ cell tumors

18. What are the features of headaches due to brain tumors? (Chapter 14)

Of those with brain tumors, 31% to 71% complain of headache

There is no specific brain tumor headache

Headache usually like tension type but occasionally like migraine

"Classic" brain tumor headache only in a minority

Headache can be unilateral or bilateral and in any location

Most headaches intermittent with moderate to severe intensity but can be mild and relieved by over-the-counter medications

Headache often associated with focal findings, seizures, confusion, prolonged nausea

19. What are the features of pseudotumor cerebri? (Chapter 14)

Ninety percent are women and 90% are obese

Mean age of onset, 30 years

Headache present in 94%

Headache usually generalized, severe, pulsatile, and daily

Other symptoms

Transient visual obscurations, 68%; pulsatile intracranial noises, 58%; photopsia, 54%; and retrobulbar pain, 44%

Signs

Papilledema in 95%

Sixth cranial nerve palsy in up to 20%

Enlarged blind spots and other field defects in 20%

Secondary causes

Venous sinus thrombosis, Addison's, hypoparathyroidism, steroid withdrawal, isotretinoin and vitamin A toxicity, anabolic steroids, and lupus

Evaluation

Normal MRI or CT scan. Empty sella or small ventricular system may be present

Normal CSF except for decreased protein concentration in some cases

On LP, opening pressure more than 20 cm in nonobese and more than 25 in obese

20. What are the features of post–lumbar puncture headache? (Chapter 14)

Usually starts within 24 hours and resolves within 7 days

Occurs in up to 40%

Decreased frequency with smaller Quincke needle and atraumatic needle such as Sprotte

Headache usually bilateral, better supine

Neck stiffness, low back pain, nausea, and occasionally blurred vision and tinnitus may be present

Rarely, meningitis or subdural hematoma can occur following lumbar puncture

21. What are the features of first or worst headaches? (Chapter 8)

Chief complaint of 1% of emergency room visits

Differential diagnosis

Subarachnoid hemorrhage, brain hemorrhage, pituitary apoplexy, acute subdural or epidural hematoma, acute severe hypertension, acute glaucoma, internal carotid dissection, acute ventricular obstruction, benign exertion or orgasmic headache, acute intoxications, acute noncephalic febrile illness, acute mountain sickness

More often subacute onset

Encephalitis, meningitis, sinusitis, periorbital cellulitis, cerebral vein thrombosis, optic neuritis, migraine, stroke, and cerebral vasculitis

Evaluation

CT or MRI scan first and if negative lumbar puncture unless acute meningitis suspected

22. What are the features of subarachnoid hemorrhage? (Chapter 8)

Eighty percent with nontraumatic SAH due to saccular aneurysm rupture that occurs in more than 30,000 people yearly in the United States with 18,000 deaths

General incidence of saccular aneurysms about 2%

Thirty-three percent of SAH during lifting, straining, or sex

Headache typically acute, severe, continuous, and generalized, often with nausea, vomiting, meningismus, focal neurological signs, and loss of consciousness

Eight percent have mild, gradually increasing headache

Headache may be unilateral

Neck or back pain may be present; 8% have no headache at onset

Stiff neck is absent in 36%

23. What are sentinel or warning leak headaches? (Chapter 8)

A sentinel or warning leak headache occurs up to 50% of time before major rupture

Headache usually lasts for several hours or days and can be associated with nausea, vomiting, and syncope

Neurological exam may be normal

Major SAH occurs in days or weeks after sentinel headache in up to 50%

Can easily be misdiagnosed as due to migraine, sinusitis, flu, hypertension, or cervical myositis

24. What does diagnostic testing reveal in subarachnoid hemorrhage? (Chapter 8)

CT scan without contrast

Day 0, 95%; day 3, 74%; 1 week, 50%; 2 weeks, 30%; 3 weeks, 0

Lumbar puncture should be performed if scan is negative

Xanthochromia due to breakdown of red blood cells with release of oxyhemoglobin and then bilirubin by third to fourth day

Xanthochromia present from 2 to 12 hours following bleed and 100% at 1 week, 100% at 2 weeks, 70% at 3 weeks, 40% at 4 weeks

Xanthochromia can be due to jaundice (total bilirubin 10 to 15)

CSF protein greater than 150 mg, dietary hypercarotenemia, malignant melanomatosis, and oral rifampin

Four-vessel cerebral angiogram necessary

Twenty percent have multiple aneurysms

Sixteen percent of initial angiograms may be false negative; should often be repeated after 2 weeks

MRA up to 88% sensitive in detecting aneurysms of or greater than 5 mm

25. What is a thunderclap headache? (Chapter 8)

A severe headache of sudden maximal onset with a normal CT or MRI scan and normal lumbar puncture

A very small percentage have an unruptured saccular aneurysm or cerebral vasospasm

Expansion, thrombosis, or intramural hemorrhage of aneurysm can cause headache without SAH

26. What types of headaches are associated with sex? (Chapter 15)

Various causes

Abstinence (according to some people)

Phosphodiesterase-5 inhibitors for erectile dysfunction in about 15%

Primary preorgasmic type

Twelve percent of subarachnoid hemorrhages

Primary orgasmic cephalalgia

Severe headache with an explosive onset; usually bilateral but can be unilateral

Occurs just before or at orgasm

Lifetime prevalence about 1%

Men more than women

More frequent with orgasms after the first during an encounter

A diagnosis of exclusion of other causes such as subarachnoid hemorrhage especially after the first headache

Other exertional headaches

Can occur with running, swimming, weight lifting

27. What are the features of headaches following mild head injury? (Chapter 9)

Headaches occur in 30% to 90% of those symptomatic after mild head injury

Headaches may occur more often and with longer duration with mild than with more severe trauma

Tension type often with greater occipital neuralgia in 85%

Cervicogenic: myofascial injury, cervical disc disease, cervical spondylosis, C2-3 facet joint injury (third occipital headache)

Footballer's migraine

Described in young soccer players after mild head injury

World famous as cause of Terrell Davis's 1998 Super Bowl migraine

Migraine with and without aura can be triggered de novo or an increased frequency of preexisting migraine can occur

Other causes
>   Supra- and infraorbital neuralgia, dysesthesias over scalp
>   lacerations, hematomas, cluster, carotid and vertebral
>   dissections

28. What are the features of subdural and epidural hematomas? (Chapter 9)

After mild head injury, the incidence for subdurals is about 1% ;
that for epidurals, less than 1%

Subdural hematomas
>   Nonspecific headache
>   Mild to severe, paroxysmal to constant
>   When unilateral, usually on same side as subdural

Epidural hematomas
>   Acute: lucid interval, then coma within 12 hours (talks,
>   then dies)
>   Chronic in up to 30%
>   >   May follow trivial head injury without loss of conscious-
>   >   ness in child or young adult
>   >   Persistent headache develops, often with nausea, vomit-
>   >   ing, and memory impairment, then focal findings

MRI more sensitive than CT scan, which can miss isodense
hematoma

CT scan usually preferred in acute setting

29. What are the features of headaches occurring in those past 50 years of age? (Chapter 12)

New-onset tension type rather common but migraine and cluster uncommon

Hypnic headaches
>   Onset usually past 45 years of age
>   Diffuse, throbbing pain but can be unilateral
>   Awakens patients from sleep same time every night, lasts
>   15 to 60 minutes

Secondary headaches
>   Mass lesions, temporal arteritis (TA), medication related,
>   trigeminal neuralgia, postherpetic neuralgia, systemic
>   disease (e.g., infections, acute hypertension, hypoxia or
>   hypercarbia, hypercalcemia, severe anemia, cervicogenic
>   headache, glaucoma, sinusitis, stroke)

30. What are the features of temporal arteritis and headaches? (Chapter 12)

Fifty percent of those with temporal arteritis (TA) have polymyalgia rheumatica (PMR)

15% with PMR have TA

Onset past 50 years of age, with mean age of onset 70 years

Prevalence in population past 50 years of age is 0.13%

Headaches present in 60% to 90%

Can be throbbing, sharp, dull, burning, or lancinating

Intermittent or continuous, more often severe than moderate or
mild

May have sensitivity of scalp and face (lying on pillow, combing
hair)

Fifty percent have tenderness of the superficial temporal arteries on exam

Location of headache is variable
> Only the temple, 25%; temple exclusively or inclusively, 54%; not the temple, 29%; generalized, 8%

Intermittent jaw claudication in 38%

31. How do you diagnose temporal arteritis? (Chapter 12)

American College of Rheumatology 1990 criteria
> Presence of three out of five gives sensitivity of 93.5% and specificity of 91%
>> Age of 50 years or more
>> New onset of localized headache
>> Temporal artery tenderness or decreased pulse
>> Erythrocyte sedimentation rate (ESR) at least 50
>> Positive histology

ESR
> Increases with age: upper limit of normal (divide man's age by 2; add 10 to woman's age and divide by 2)
> TA can be present with normal ESR in up to 36%
> When abnormal, average 70 to 80; can be 130

TA biopsy
> Demonstrates necrotizing arteritis
> False-negative rate, 5% to 44%
> Biopsy of contralateral artery increases yield up to 15%
> Pathology persists for at least 4 to 5 days after starting steroids

32. What drugs can trigger headaches? (Chapters 14 and 15)

Numerous drugs, some examples are provided

Cardiovascular: nitroglycerin, beta-blockers, calcium channel blockers, angiotensin-converting enzyme inhibitors, and methyldopa

Nonsteroidal antiinflammatory medications (NSAIDs), especially indomethacin
> NSAIDs, especially ibuprofen, can cause aseptic meningitis

Sex hormones: oral contraceptives, estrogen replacement therapy, tamoxifen

Amino acids: monosodium glutamate, aspartame (the sweetener)

Histamine receptor antagonists: cimetidine, ranitidine

Antibiotics: amphotericin, griseofulvin, tetracycline, sulfonamides

Phosphodiesterase inhibitors: dipyridamole, sildenafil

Serotonin antagonists: granisetron, odansetron

33. What headaches occur during sleep? (Chapter 15)

Secondary causes of nocturnal headaches: drug withdrawal, temporal arteritis, sleep apnea, oxygen desaturation, pheochromocytomas, primary and secondary neoplasms, communicating hydrocephalus, subdural hematomas, subacute angle-closure glaucoma, and vascular lesions

Primary headaches: migraine, cluster, hypnic, and chronic paroxysmal hemicrania

34. What is the association of headaches and multiple sclerosis? (Chapter 15)

Headaches can be associated with first or subsequent attacks in up to 7%, occasionally simulating migraine with aura

One percent of patients with multiple sclerosis have trigeminal neuralgia and 2% of those with trigeminal neuralgia have multiple sclerosis

Migraine is twice as common in multiple sclerosis patients as in controls

35. What is the lifetime prevalence of migraine among neurologists? (Chapter 16)

Much higher than in the general population

47% in male neurologists, 63% in female neurologists, about 75% in headache specialists

Patient Resources, Educational Materials, and Alternative Treatments

Randolph W. Evans

HEADACHE RESOURCES

American Council for Headache Education

The American Council for Headache Education (ACHE) is a nonprofit patient-health professional partnership dedicated to advancing the treatment and management of headache and to raising the public awareness of headache as a valid, biologically based illness.

ACHE's educational mission reaches out to health career policy makers, employers, opinion leaders, as well as to headache patients and their families. Its goals are to empower headache sufferers through education, and to support them by educating their families, employers, and the public in general. ACHE advocates individualized treatments, which combine the best of traditional medicine, alternative medicine, drug, and nondrug therapies. It does not advocate any specific approaches or medications. Through education in the causes and treatment of headache, sufferers can be empowered and equipped to seek effective therapies and knowledgeable health care providers who can aid them in achieving better quality of life.

19 Mantua Road
Mt. Royal, NJ 08061
Phone: 856-423-0258
Fax: 856-423-0082
Email: achehq@talley.com
Web site: http://www.achenet.org

Educational materials that are available include brochures, books, and a quarterly newsletter.

National Headache Foundation

The National Headache Foundation (NHF) disseminates free information on headache causes and treatments, funds research, and sponsors public and professional education seminars nationwide. In addition to functioning as a clearinghouse for information, NHF has audiotapes and videotapes, books, brochures, and other helpful materials available for purchase. A nationwide network of local support groups has been organized.

820 N. Orleans, Suite 217
Chicago, IL 60610-3132
Toll free: 888-NHF-5552
Fax: 773-525-7357

Web site: http://www.headaches.org
Email: info@headaches.org

Internet Web Sites

There are numerous additional internet Web sites with headache information. Here are a few with migraine information:

MAGNUM (Migraine Awareness Group: A National Understanding for Migraineurs): http://www.migraines.org
The Migraine Trust: http://www.migrainetrust.org
WebMDHealth: http://my.webmd.com/medical_information/
    condition_centers/migraines/default.htm
World Headache Alliance: http://www.w-h-a.org

CAFFEINE CONTENT OF SELECTED BEVERAGES, FOODS, AND OVER-THE-COUNTER AND PRESCRIPTION MEDICATIONS*

Daily use of caffeine in susceptible persons can cause frequent headaches, caffeine rebound headaches. People often recognize this headache as due to coffee. In fact, as few as two cups of coffee per day can be responsible. However, you may not be aware that caffeine is also present in a variety of other beverages, foods, and over-the-counter and prescription medications (see later). The headache typically is present in the morning and goes away after consuming caffeine. If you have this type of headache, slowly tapering off of caffeine can eliminate the headaches.

Coffee	
Brewed, 8 oz	135 mg
Instant, 8 oz	95 mg
Starbucks espresso, 1 oz	89 mg
Decaffeinated, 8 oz	5 mg
Soft drinks	
Coca-Cola, 12 oz	45 mg
Diet Coke, 12 oz	47 mg
Dr. Pepper, 12 oz	41 mg
Pepsi-Cola, 12 oz	37 mg
Sunkist Orange Soda, 12 oz	40 mg
Mountain Dew, 12 oz	55 mg
7-UP, 12 oz	0
Sprite, 12 oz	0
Tea	
Lipton tea, 8 oz	35–40 mg
Snapple iced tea, all varieties, 16 oz	48 mg
Celestial Seasonings herbal tea, all varieties, 8 oz	0

continued

*Source: The Center for Science in the Public Interest, product labels, and the *Physicians' Desk Reference*.

Lipton Natural Brew Iced Tea Mix, decaffeinated, 8 oz	<5mg

Chocolate

Hershey's Special Dark Chocolate Bar, 1.5 oz	31 mg
Hershey Bar, 10 mg.	10 mg
Hot chocolate, 8 oz	5 mg

Yogurt and Ice Cream

Ben & Jerry's No Fat Coffee Fudge Frozen Yogurt, 1 cup	85 mg
Starbucks Coffee Ice Cream, 1 cup	40–60 mg
Haagen-Dazs Coffee Fudge Ice Cream, 1 cup	30 mg
Dannon Coffee Yogurt, 8 oz	45 mg

Over-the-Counter Medications

NoDoz maximum strength, 1 tablet	200 mg
NoDoz regular strength, 1 tablet	100 mg
Excedrin Extra Strength, 2 tablets	130 mg
Exedrin Migraine, 2 tablets	130 mg
Anacin, 2 tablets	64 mg
Advil, Nuprin	0
Aleve	0

Prescription Medications

Fiorinal	40 mg
Esgic	40 mg
Cafergot	100 mg
Darvon Compound-65	32.4 mg

AN EXPLANATION OF HYPERVENTILATION SYNDROME[*]

Hyperventilation (overbreathing) attacks are the commonest cause of dizziness and often associated with headache. They can be overcome by recognizing the cause and following a few simple rules.

What are the symptoms?

A person may have any one or any number of the following symptoms:

Light-headedness, dizziness, faintness, giddiness
Tightness or pain in the chest
Shortness of breath or difficulty getting a good breath
Dry mouth
Faster heartbeat
Blurring of vision
Sweating
Trembling of hands and legs
Weakness ("jelly legs")
Pins and needles in hands, feet, and around the mouth
Headache

[*]From Lance JW, Goadsby PJ. *Mechanism and management of headache,* 6th ed. Oxford: Butterworth-Heinemann, 1998; modified, with permission.

Anxiety, fear, or panic
Sensation of being unable to breathe
Spasms of hands and feet
A feeling of having a heart attack, passing out, losing control, or
   being about to die

   When you overbreathe you may swallow air, causing:

Distension of the stomach
Burping
Passing gas

   What do we mean by overbreathing?

Deep, sighing breaths
Yawning often
Rapid shallow breathing
Deep breathing
There are two types of hyperventilation: acute, which affects 1%,
   and chronic, which affects 99% of patients
Acute hyperventilation is obvious when someone is breathing
   way too fast
Chronic hyperventilation is not obvious: You can breathe a little
   too fast and a little too deeply and cause hyperventilation, but
   neither you nor your doctor can tell just by looking at you dur-
   ing a spell

   When is this most likely to happen?

When you are tense, bored, or depressed
In crowds, at a party, or out shopping

   How does this cause symptoms?

Normally, nature takes care of the rate and depth of breathing.
   The carbon dioxide in your blood makes you breathe enough to
   eliminate it and get sufficient oxygen. If you override nature
   and breathe too much, you wash out too much carbon dioxide.
   This reduces the blood flow to your brain and makes you feel
   dizzy. It also reduces the available calcium in the blood, which
   can cause "pins and needles," numbness and tingling, and
   cause spasms of the hands and feet. Adrenaline increases in
   the bloodstream, causing a feeling of anxiety, sweating, and
   trembling, and makes the heart beat faster.
Contraction of muscles causes pain and tightness in the chest
   and headache.

   How can you stop it?

Look for the first signs of sighing or yawning
Do not:
      Open the windows.
      Run outside.
      Take deep breaths.
Instead:
Sit down.
Hold your breath and count to 10.
Breathe out slowly and say "relax" to yourself.
Then breathe in and out slowly every 6 seconds (10 breaths per
   minute).

If you wish, you may instead breathe into a lunch bag placed over your nose and mouth for a minute or so.

As soon as possible, forget about your breathing and let nature do it for you.

General principles

Take it easy. It is not a disaster if you forget someone's name, burn the dinner, or don't have time to mow the lawn. Talk more slowly. Walk more slowly. You have plenty of time.

Think positively. You can handle a problem as well as the next person.

Everyone else has problems, too. Spread out your workload through the day.

Give yourself enough time for each task. Remain calm.

Don't bottle up your feelings—discuss any worries or things that make you angry or upset.

Eat regular meals and don't hurry them. Limit caffeine in soft drinks, coffee, or tea.

Learn to recognize any tendency to overbreathe.

Learn to relax your muscles—no frowning or jaw clenching. Exercise regularly.

Take time out for social activities and holidays.

You can control your attacks completely by following these rules.

A HEADACHE DIARY

For patients with frequent headaches, a headache diary is very useful to document the frequency, possible triggers, and response to treatment. Headache diaries can range from just a piece of paper to a formal headache diary. On pages 386 and 387 is my headache diary which is printed on a 18 cm × 13 cm page with room to record 29 headaches.

A BRIEF DESCRIPTION OF ALTERNATIVE AND COMPLEMENTARY TREATMENTS USED FOR HEADACHES: ALTERNATIVE TREATMENTS FROM A TO Y

In the United States, 42% of the adult population used alternative therapy in 1997 (1). Thirteen percent used alternative treatments for headaches, including 42% who saw a medical doctor and used alternative therapy and 20% who saw a medical doctor and an alternative practitioner for headaches. According to a patient survey in the United States, alternative medicine users find these approaches to be more congruent with their own values, beliefs, and philosophical orientations toward health and life (2).

Despite advances, physicians and patients need all the help they can get in treating headaches. Consider the pharmacotherapy of migraine. Individual preventive medications have an efficacy of only about 60%, with a number of possible side effects. Triptans reduce or relieve migraine for 70% to 80%, depending on the route of administration, but what about the unaided 20% to 30%? In addition, chronic migraine and medication rebound are significant concerns.

Informed physicians can do their patients a service by providing unbiased information and suggesting and reading reference sources such as the books by Pikoff (3), Mauskop and Brill (4), and Jonas and Levin (5). As Jonas states, "Alternative medicine is here to stay. It is no longer an option to ignore it or treat it as something outside the normal processes of science and medicine" (6).

Although many alternative medicine treatments may have merit, others may be no better than expensive placebos. As Angell and Kassirer insist, "Alternative treatments should be subjected to scientific testing no less rigorous than that required for conventional treatments" (7). In a sense, there is no alternative medicine; there is only medicine that works and medicine that does not work.

Numerous alternative and complementary treatments are used for headaches (8). There are varying amounts of scientific evidence for effectiveness (9). A brief description of some of the treatments from A to Y follows.

Acupuncture

Acupuncture is a medical therapy developed in China more than 2,000 years ago. Hua Tuo, a 3rd-century A.D. Chinese surgeon, is credited with being the first to use acupuncture for headache. Acupuncture was introduced to physicians in the United States by William Osler in the late 19th century.

Very thin disposable needles of varying length are placed into the skin at specific points along meridians or channels. There are 12 main meridians that are believed to be connected to a specific organ system of the body. By needling acupoints of a particular meridian, a problem in a distant area of the body can be treated. Needles are usually kept in place for less than 30 minutes. Twirling or other motion of the needles is believed to enhance the effect. Acupuncture may be effective in reducing a variety of headaches (9), including migraine (10), tension (11), and posttraumatic.

In a large randomized prospective British study, up to 12 acupuncture treatments over 3 months were effective in reducing headache, improving quality of life, and reducing health care expenditures (12,13).

Aromatherapy

Practitioners believe that when essential oils from plants are inhaled or absorbed through the skin, they can alleviate headaches, including migraines and tension-type headaches (14). Aromatherapy may help reduce stress. Some people can have allergic reactions to the oils.

Biofeedback

Biofeedback is a Western approach to meditation (see later) with the goal of producing beneficial physiological changes. Monitoring equipment provides visual or audible signs of muscle and autonomic activity. The most common types of biofeedback are electromyography (surface electrodes are used to monitor muscle activity), thermal (measurement of skin temperature), electrodermal activity (measures changes in perspiration), finger pulse (measures pulse rate and the amount of blood in each pulse), and respiration feedback (measures the rate, volume, and rhythm of the patient's breathing).

EMG and thermal biofeedback are used for treatment of headaches. The therapist teaches relaxation techniques to use in conjunction with biofeeback. Biofeedback has been demonstrated to be effective in treating pediatric migraine (15) and tension headaches (16) and adult migraine and tension headaches (17,18), and it may be effective for chronic daily headache (19).

Chiropractic

Chiropractic (from the Greek for "done by hand") was founded in the 1890s in Davenport, Iowa, by D. D. Palmer. There are now some 50,000 chiropractors in the United States who saw 11% of the adult population in 1997. Misaligned vertebrae or subluxations are believed to interfere with the transmission of nerve impulses. "Straight" chiropractors focus almost exclusively on manual manipulation, whereas "mixers" use other treatments, such as nutritional counseling and exercise with manipulation. The hand is used to manipulate the spine with high-velocity, low-force recoiling thrusts or rotational thrusts with the hands or elbows. Some patients with headaches may benefit from chiropractic treatment (20). Studies have found benefit for cervicogenic headaches (21) but no benefit for treatment of episodic tension-type headache (22). Uncontrolled studies have reported benefit for migraine (23). One systemic review of randomized trials found that the data did not support any definite benefit for migraine, tension-type, or cervicogenic headaches (24).

Herbal Medicine

There are numerous herbs (plants or plant parts) with purported medicinal value. The use of herbal medicine has been documented as far back as the Neanderthals 60,000 years ago. More than one fourth of conventional pharmaceuticals come from herbs. There is insufficient evidence from randomized clinical trials that feverfew is effective in preventing migraines (25). A special butterbur root (Petasites hybridus) extract may be effective for migraine prevention using the Petadolex brand formulation at 25 mg twice a day (26).

Hypnosis

The induction of hypnotic states has existed at least since early recorded history. The Viennese physician Franz Mesmer popularized medical hypnosis in the late 1700s to treat imbalances of animal magnetism ("mesmerize"). Freud used hypnosis in conjunction with psychoanalysis in the early 1900s.

Hypnosis (from the Greek word for "sleep") is a state of focused attention or altered consciousness that makes the participant highly receptive to suggestion and allows a person to concentrate intently on a particular subject, memory, sensation, or problem. Patients can go to a hypnotherapist or learn self-hypnosis. Hypnosis can be effective in treating pediatric (27) and adult migraine (28).

Massage

Therapeutic touch can reduce headaches such as chronic tension type (29). The history of massage goes back 4,000 to 5,000 years. Hippocrates described massage as an effective treatment for sports and war injuries. There are numerous types of massage.

Swedish massage (devised by the 19th-century Swedish physician Per Henrik Ling) uses a system of long strokes, kneading, and friction techniques on superficial muscles and active and passive movements of joints. There are five types of strokes: effleurage (long, gliding stroke performed with the whole hand or thumb); petrissage (kneading and compression movements); friction (deep circular movements made with the thumb pads or fingertips); vibration (a fine, rapid, shaking movement); and tapotement (use of the hands to alternatively strike or tap the muscles).

Deep-muscle and connective-tissue massage uses deep finger pressure and slow strokes on contracted areas. Trigger-point therapy uses concentrated finger pressure on trigger points.

Shiatsu (Japanese for "finger pressure") and acupressure use finger pressure massage on special points along acupuncture meridians to unblock and balance qi, the body's hypothesized flow of energy.

Reflexology uses digital pressure on target points on the feet, which refer, or "reflex," to all areas of the body to help heal distant areas. Reflexology was started by an ENT physician, William Fitzgerald, in the early 20th century.

Rolfing, or structural integration, was devised by Ida Rolf, who had a doctorate in physiology, in the 1950s. The therapist uses fingertips, knuckles, elbows, and sometimes knees to knead muscle and tissue layers.

Meditation

Medicine and meditation have the same Latin root meaning "to cure" and "to measure" (in the sense of bringing the mind and body to its right inward measure). Most meditation techniques derive from Eastern religious practices and involve intense concentration on a breath, word, sound, prayer, or phrase while excluding all outside thoughts. Meditation can be practiced while sitting (Transcendental meditation); standing or lying down (e.g., qigong—the willful manipulation of the vital life force, or qi); or moving (tai chi chu'an—Buddhist mindfulness meditation). Meditation and other relaxation techniques may be effective in treating migraines, tension, and other headaches.

There are some Western approaches to meditation. The German physician Schultz developed autogenic training, which means "coming from the self." This is a simple exercise that combines verbal, visual, and sensory imagery to relax different parts of the body. In the late 1960s, the cardiologist Herbert Benson studied the beneficial physiological effects of meditation, which he termed the *relaxation response*. This response can be induced by a variety of techniques, including meditation, prayer, progressive muscle relaxation, hypnosis, and yoga.

Osteopathy

Andrew Taylor Still founded the first medical school for osteopathy (literally, "disease from the bones") in Missouri in 1874. Today medical school for osteopaths is similar to that for medical doctors with the addition of training in osteopathic medical manipulations or manual therapy, including soft-tissue technique, myofascial release, cranial osteopathy, lymphatic technique, thrust technique, muscle energy technique, counterstrain, and visceral techniques. Osteopaths can specialize in medical and surgical specialties or primary care.

Cranial osteopathy involves pressure and massage of the muscles and fascia surrounding the skull to take pressure off the nerves of the skull, improve blood flow, and improve the flow of cerebrospinal fluid within the head. Craniosacral therapy is also practiced by chiropractors.

Progressive Relaxation

Progressive relaxation, developed by Edmund Jacobsen in the 1920s, is a series of steps or exercises to relax the muscles that may be effective for tension- and migraine-type headaches (30,31). Relaxation techniques are often used in combination with biofeedback. An example of progressive relaxation exercises is provided in the next section.

Yoga

Yoga (from the Sanskrit word for "union") is an ancient Eastern philosophy and exercise of health and well-being that combines movements and simple poses with deep breathing and meditation to unite the soul with a universal spirit. A life energy, Prana, is believed to flow through and vitalize the body. Yoga may be beneficial for headaches, including migraines (32).

A SIMPLE MEDITATION EXERCISE*

This simple meditation exercise can be practiced by anyone.

1. Find a comfortable position—lying down or sitting either on the floor or in a straight-backed chair. If sitting, keep your back straight without being rigid and let your hands rest in your lap. If your feet don't reach the floor, place a stool or books beneath them so they rest on a firm surface.
2. Scan your body for tension from head to toe and relax your muscles. Unknit your eyebrows and unclench your jaw. Release your shoulders, arms, and belly. Let your spine lengthen, without becoming rigid, and your chin pull gently inward. Let your pelvis sink into the chair or ground.
3. Be aware of the sensation of your body touching the earth (or firm surface).
4. Close your eyes if you feel it's more comfortable.
5. Focus your mind on your breath as you inhale naturally. Breathe through your nose if you can. Feel the breath fill your chest and then your belly. Keep focused on the breath as you exhale, feeling it leave your belly and your chest. Alternatively, you can focus on the sensation of breath entering and leaving your nostrils.
6. Keep your eyes directed toward the end of your nose.
7. Keep your mind focused on your breath.

*From Mauskop A, Brill MA. *The headache alternative: a neurologist's guide to drug-free relief.* New York: Dell, 1997:276–277, with permission.

8. When thoughts cross your mind, gently note them, let them pass, and return to your breathing. Each time this happens, simply return to the breath.
9. Continue for 15 minutes. It's okay to check the clock every so often.
10. Sit quietly for a few minutes.

You can use the breath as a focus, or select a word. Any simple, positive word or name will suffice.

A PROGRESSIVE RELAXATION EXERCISE*

1. Get comfortable. Wear loose clothing, remove your shoes. Make sure you are neither too warm nor too cold. Find a quiet room where you won't be distracted for 15 minutes.
2. Sit in a comfortable chair or lie down on the ground on your back, using an exercise mat or soft carpet.
3. Take a few deep, easy breaths.
4. Tense all of the muscles in your body, from head to toe. Hold the tension for several seconds. Let your mind feel the sensation of this tension.
5. Holding on to the tension, inhale deeply and hold your breath for several seconds. Let your mind and body register the sensation of this tension.
6. Exhale slowly as you let the tension go by. Let your mind and body register the sensation of this relaxation.

Now work on individual muscle groups. As you tense the following muscles, try to keep the rest of your muscles as relaxed as possible. Repeat each of the following exercises three times.

1. Tighten your fists. Feel the tension radiating up your arms. Inhale deeply and hold the tension for several seconds. Exhale and let your hands relax.
2. Press your arms against the ground or chair. Inhale and hold the tension for several seconds, concentrating on the sensation. Exhale and let your arms relax.
3. Shrug your shoulders up to your eyes. Experience the tension in your neck and shoulders. Inhale and hold. Exhale and let your shoulders drop.
4. Frown and raise your eyebrows. Study the tightness in your face. Inhale and hold the tension. Exhale and release.
5. Press your eyelids closed as tightly as possible. Inhale and hold. Exhale and open your eyes gently.
6. Open your mouth as wide as possible. Inhale and hold. Exhale and release your jaw.
7. Clench your jaw, biting down with your teeth. Feel the tension spread across your skull. Inhale and hold. Exhale and release.
8. Inhale deeply into your belly, letting your chest expand. Hold the chest tension. Exhale and let your breath return to normal.
9. Tighten your abdominal muscles. Hold, then relax.

*From Mauskop A, Brill MA. *The headache alternative: a neurologist's guide to drug-free relief.* New York: Dell, 1997:264–265, with permission.

10. Arch your back, chest up and hips down. Inhale and hold. Exhale and release your back gently.
11. Tighten your hips and buttocks. Inhale and hold. Exhale and relax.
12. Tense your left leg, from thigh to heel. Inhale and hold. Exhale and relax.
13. Tense your right leg, from thigh to heel. Inhale and hold. Exhale and relax.
14. Curl your toes under. Inhale and hold. Exhale and relax.
15. Remaining still, scan your body. Experience the relaxation over your entire body. If you need to, return to areas of tension and repeat the exercise for that muscle group. Breathe naturally and deeply for several moments, experiencing the relaxed state. Gently and slowly stand up.

REFERENCES

1. Eisenberg DM, Davis RB, Ettner SL, et al. Trends in alternative medicine use in the United States, 1990-1997: results of a follow-up national survey. *JAMA* 1998;280:1569–1575.
2. Astin J. Why patients use alternative medicine: results of a national study. *JAMA* 1998;279:1548–1553.
3. Pikoff HB. Complementary headache therapy: a close look at the treatments and the evidence. Buffalo, NY: Data for Decisions, 2004.
4. Mauskop A, Brill MA. *The headache alternative: a neurologist's guide to drug-free relief.* New York: Dell, 1997.
5. Jonas WB, Levin JS. *Essentials of complementary and alternative medicine.* Philadelphia: Lippincott Williams & Wilkins, 1999.
6. Jonas WB. Alternative medicine: learning from the past, examining the present, advancing to the future. *JAMA* 1998;280: 1616–1618.
7. Angell M, Kassirer JP. Alternative medicine: the risks of untested and unregulated remedies. *N Engl J Med* 1998;339:839–841.
8. Henninger MI, Holroyd KA, Lipchik GI. Acupuncture and chiropractic treatments for headache. *Headache* 1999;39:357.
9. Melchart D, Linde K, Fischer P, et al. Acupuncture for recurrent headaches: a systematic review of randomized controlled trials. *Cephalalgia* 1999;19:779–786.
10. Baischer W. Acupuncture in migraine: long-term outcome and predicting factors. *Headache* 1995;35:472–474.
11. Vincent CA. The treatment of tension headache by acupuncture: a controlled single case design with time series analysis. *J Psychosom Res* 1990;34:553–561.
12. Wonderling D, Vickers AJ, Grieve R, et al. Cost effectiveness analysis of a randomised trial of acupuncture for chronic headache in primary care. *BMJ* 2004;328(7442):747. Epub 2004 Mar 15.
13. Vickers AJ, Rees RW, Zollman CE, et al. Acupuncture for chronic headache in primary care: large, pragmatic, randomised trial. *BMJ* 2004;328(7442):744. Epub 2004 Mar 15.
14. Schattner P, Randerson D. Tiger balm as a treatment of tension headache. *Aust Fam Physician* 1996;25:216–222.

15. Hermann C, Blanchard EB, Flor H. Biofeedback treatment for pediatric migraine: prediction of treatment outcome. *J Consult Clin Psychol* 1997;65:611–616.

16. Grazzi L, Leone M, Fediani F, et al.. A therapeutic alternative for tension headache in children: treatment and one-year follow-up results. *Biofeedback Self Regul* 1990;15:1–6.

17. Arena JG, Bruno GM, Hannah SL, et al. A comparison of frontal electromyographic biofeedback training, trapezius electromyographic biofeedback training, and progressive muscle relaxation therapy in the treatment of tension headache. *Headache* 1995; 35:411–419.

18. Grazzi L, Bussone G. Effect of biofeedback treatment on sympathetic function in common migraine and tension-type headache. *Cephalalgia* 1993;13:197–200.

19. Andrasik F. Behavioral treatment approaches to chronic headache. *Neurol Sci* 2003;24(Suppl 2):S80–S85.

20. Shekelle PG, Coulter I. Cervical spine manipulation: summary report of a systematic review of the literature and a multidisciplinary expert panel. *J Spinal Disord* 1997;10:223–228.

21. Nilsson N, Christensen HW, Hartvigsen J. The effect of spinal manipulation in the treatment of cervicogenic headache. *J Manipulative Physiol Ther* 1997;20:326–330.

22. Bove G, Nilsson N. Spinal manipulation in the treatment of episodic tension-type headache: a randomized controlled trial. *JAMA* 1998;280:1576–1579.

23. Chapman-Smith D. Chiropractic management of headache. *Chiropractic Rep* 1991;5:1–6.

24. Astin JA, Ernst E. The effectiveness of spinal manipulation for the treatment of headache disorders:a systematic review of randomized clinical trials. *Cephalalgia* 2002;22(8):617–623.

25. Pittler MH, Ernst E. Feverfew for preventing migraine. *Cochrane Database Syst Rev* 2004;(1):CD002286.

26. Diener HC, Rahlfs VW, Danesch U. The first placebo-controlled trial of a special butterbur root extract for the prevention of migraine: reanalysis of efficacy criteria. *Eur Neurol* 2004; 51(2):89–97.

27. Olness K, MacDonald JT, Uden DL. Comparison of self-hypnosis and propranolol in the treatment of juvenile classic migraine. *Pediatrics* 1987;79:593–597.

28. Reich BA. Non-invasive treatment of vascular and muscle contraction headache: a comparative longitudinal clinical study. *Headache* 1989;29:34–41.

29. Puustjarvi K, Airaksinen O, Pontinen PJ. The effects of massage in patients with chronic tension headache. *Acupunct Electrother Res* 1990;15:159–162.

30. Holroyd KA, Penzien DB. Pharmacological versus non-pharmacological prophylaxis of recurrent migraine headache: a metaanalytic review of clinical trials. *Pain* 1990;42:1–13.

31. Engel JM, Rapoff MA, Pressman AR. Long-term follow-up of relaxation training for pediatric headache disorders. *Headache* 1992;32:152–156.

32. Monro R, Ghosh AK, Kalish D. *Yoga research bibliography, scientific studies on yoga and meditation.* Cambridge, England: Yoga Biomedical Trust, 1989.

KEYS FOR HEADACHE DIARY

1. INTENSITY

   1 = Mild   2 = Moderate   3 = Severe

2. HEADACHE INTENSITY AFTER MEDICATION

   0 = None   1 = Mild   2 = Moderate   3 = Severe

3. EMOTIONAL STRESS TRIGGERS

1–Family or friends
2–Work
3–Social life
4–Financial difficulties
5–Relaxation after stress
6–Other

4. PHYSICAL TRIGGERS

  1–Fatigue
  2–Lack of sleep
  3–Oversleeping
  4–Bright/flashing lights
  5–Sun or glare
  6–Loud noise
  7–Strong smells
  8–Heat/high humidity
  9–Menstruation
10–Exercise or labor
11–High altitude
12–Travel
13–Vacation
14–Weekend
15–Other

5. FOOD AND DRINK TRIGGERS

1–Missing a meal
2–Chocolate
3–Cheese
4–Citrus fruit
5–MSG
6–Hot dogs or cured meat
7–Alcohol or beer
8–Wine
9–Other

HEADACHE DIARY

Patient's name_____ Date started_____

Date of Headache	Time Started	Time Stopped	1 Intensity	Medication Taken	2 Intensity after medication	3 Emotional stress triggers	4 Physical triggers	5 Food and drink triggers

Subject Index

Note: Page numbers followed by f indicate figures; those followed by t indicate tables.